PRENATAL ALCOHOL EXPOSURE

A Clinician's Guide

PRENATAL ALCOHOL EXPOSURE

A Clinician's Guide

by

Mansfield Mela, MBBS, M.Sc.Psych.

Director, Centre for Forensic Behavioral Science and Justice Studies
Professor, Department of Psychiatry, University of Saskatchewan
Diagnostic Research Lead, Canada FASD Research Network
Forensic Psychiatrist, Regional Psychiatric Centre
Saskatoon, Canada

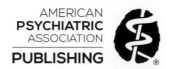

AMERICAN
PSYCHIATRIC
ASSOCIATION
PUBLISHING

If you wish to buy 50 or more copies of the same title, please go to www.appi.org/specialdiscounts for more information.

Copyright © 2021 American Psychiatric Association Publishing

ALL RIGHTS RESERVED

First Edition

Manufactured in the United States of America on acid-free paper
25   24   23   22   21   5   4   3   2   1

American Psychiatric Association Publishing
800 Maine Avenue SW, Suite 900
Washington, DC 20024-2812
www.appi.org

Library of Congress Cataloging-in-Publication Data
Names: Mela, Mansfield, author. | American Psychiatric Association Publishing, publisher.
Title: Prenatal alcohol exposure : a clinician's guide / by Mansfield Mela.
Description: First edition. | Washington, DC : American Psychiatric Association Publishing, [2021] | Includes bibliographical references and index.
Identifiers: LCCN 2020048844 (print) | LCCN 2020048845 (ebook) | ISBN 9781615372393 (paperback ; alk. paper) | ISBN 9781615373697 (ebook)
Subjects: MESH: Fetal Alcohol Spectrum Disorders—psychology | Prenatal Exposure Delayed Effects | Mental Disorders—diagnosis | Mental Disorders—therapy
Classification: LCC RG629.F45 (print) | LCC RG629.F45 (ebook) | NLM WQ 211 | DDC 618.3/26861—dc23
LC record available at https://lccn.loc.gov/2020048844
LC ebook record available at https://lccn.loc.gov/2020048845

British Library Cataloguing in Publication Data
A CIP record is available from the British Library.

Contents

PART I
History and Epidemiology

PART II
Etiology

PART III
Presentation

PART IV
Assessment and Diagnosis

PART V
Treatment

PART VI
Special Populations

PART VII
Systems of Care

Preface

This book provides clinically relevant information for mental health experts, but it goes beyond that to provide sufficient content to improve clinicians' level of comfort with information to which they have not hitherto been exposed. Clinicians in this context include professionals in the medical, mental, educational, vocational, legal and correctional, child welfare, and others in the health and social services sectors who encounter individuals with a hidden disability. The scope and course content of curricula needed to equip professionals are usually informed by the requisite skills and experience for optimum clinical care. Professionals require essential training to appropriately support patients who navigate the mental health system because of the consequences of prenatal alcohol exposure (PAE). Because curricula have only recently begun to incorporate this material, a text providing basic as well as advanced information is necessary. This book is significant because its content is useful for professional training across many mental health disciplines. It covers information missing from curricula about the long-term effects of PAE (fetal alcohol spectrum disorder ["FASD 101"]) and includes clinical information on the mental disorders relevant to FASD. Given the burgeoning research and knowledge in this area, the text also updates, synthesizes, and consolidates current information into one source. Even seasoned mental health professionals well versed in the research data can use this information to become better educated and informed on the intersecting mental health consequences of PAE.

Because a large number of individuals with neurobehavioral disorder associated with PAE/FASD also manifest overlapping features of mental disorders or have additional mental disorder diagnoses, advocating for a separate system that addresses their specific needs has lasting implications and benefits. Acknowledging the realities of life, educating and training mental health professionals to adapt their practices to recognize these needs is the next best thing. That is my hope for this text, with the future goal of stimulating innovation in the field.

The themes covered in this book outline a close and intricately complex relationship between PAE and mental disorder. The boundary between the two is open to various interpretations that potentially affect care and prognosis. The *interface* (discussed in several chapters of the book) refers to the overlapping and enmeshed relationship between the recognized effects of PAE and the additional mental health problems that can manifest.

Introduction

Terminology

Over the five decades that the complications of prenatal alcohol exposure (PAE) have been recognized in the scientific literature, terms used to describe these entities have changed. It is helpful for the reader to understand the acronyms referred to in this textbook. FASD is universally accepted as standing for fetal alcohol spectrum disorder, the recognized term used in this text to encompass the representative diagnostic forms—fetal alcohol syndrome [FAS], fetal alcohol effects (FAE), partial FAS (pFAS), alcohol-related neurodevelopmental disorder (ARND), and alcohol and related birth defects (ARBD)—of conditions caused by PAE. FASD was elevated to a diagnostic term in 2016 by the Canadian Diagnostic Guidelines (Cook et al. 2016); these guidelines have been adopted in a number of international jurisdictions. Neurobehavioral disorder associated with PAE (ND-PAE) is the official mental disorder in DSM-5 (American Psychiatric Association 2013). Most studies prior to 2013 (when ND-PAE was introduced in the literature) used FASD in reference to patients with PAE who were diagnosed medically. In this text, using the term FASD and its diagnostic forms applies to evidence, research findings, and discussions derived from subjects differentiated as having FASD before the option of ND-PAE was available. Hence, using FASD sequesters research and clinical and policy outcomes to the pre–ND-PAE period.

By now, mental health clinicians and professionals have become acquainted with the term *neurobehavioral disorder associated with PAE*. In its strict usage, ND-PAE refers to the 2013 criteria found in Section III of DSM-5 ("Conditions for Further Study"). This term can be easily confused with *neurodevelopmental* disorder associated with PAE, which has raised a number of criticisms, responses, and reactions. Research articles, conference presentations, policy briefs, and clinical case series have used these terms interchangeably. Available to clinicians and researchers, DSM-5 allows conditions associated with PAE to be clinically diagnosed under the formal rubric of other neurodevelopmental disorders (other specified and unspecified categories).

ND-PAE/FASD is used frequently in the text to recognize the bridging of FASD at the interface of PAE and its mental disorder sequelae. The inconsistencies of the terms will likely remain unresolved, given the different perspectives adopted for the physical, cognitive, and mental expressions of PAE. For instance, Mukherjee (2016) observed and commented on this inconsistency: "Recently, the term neurodevelopmental disorder associated with prenatal alcohol exposure (NDPAE) has also been used to describe FASD; this may become the agreed term alongside FAS in the future, but it has yet to be fully implemented" (p. 4).

Clinical Management

With terminologies understood and put aside, this text targets and provides clinicians with information relevant to managing disorders associated with PAE. Whatever the outcome of PAE, it is dependent on the interaction between the exposure and several contributory factors. The diagnostic consequences of PAE and the mental disorders emanating from minor or major contributions of PAE are interrelated. Quite literally, the flow of the expression of PAE intermingles with risk factors of mental disorder to produce a plethora of consequences. Understanding the pathophysiology is key to interpreting the outcomes, which in turn informs the relevant prevention and intervention strategies. Although current available evidence continues to present PAE and the development of mental disorder in a sequential, linear manner, weaved throughout this text is the proposition that the effects of PAE vary according to the differential impacts of other biopsychosocial factors. When PAE is significant, it could be a precursor to, risk factor of, or unrelated to the mental disorder, and this correlation can vary throughout the person's lifetime. This clinical guide should be understood as being as current as the available evidence on gene-environment interaction allows.

It is my hope that mental health professionals reading this text will take an interest in, and study, the significance of PAE and in turn develop a better understanding of the clinical and therapeutic perspectives of their patients.

To emphasize this clinical and practical goal, clinical scenarios are frequently used. Fashioned from composite clinical features, these vignettes are meant to stimulate a logical question: What else could it be? Given the reported high rates of misdiagnosing PAE and its mental disorder sequelae, post-vignette discussions expound on clinical patterns of differential diagnoses. Clinicians and diagnosticians are encouraged to recognize the warning signs (red flags) associated with PAE. Additionally, these vignettes may help catalyze appropriate interventions and to encourage clinicians to ask the question: What difference does our new knowledge about PAE make for clinical management? To this end, suggestions for evidence-based and practice-based supports are included (modifications), and future research is encouraged. By providing examples of challenging cases, clinicians are offered a reality-based understanding and suggestions for treatment at a standard of care that ensures acceptable quality of life for patients in the context of PAE.

Virtually all organs of the body are adversely affected by the teratogenic effect of PAE. FAS was the first diagnostic entity ascribed to PAE, and it comprised the full features of physical and neurodevelopmental abnormalities. Terms used to describe the full or partial manifestations of these effects have changed to accommodate classification systems and changes in and advancement of the knowledge of disorders associated with PAE. Nonclinical reasons for adjusting classification systems include meeting critical thresholds for the criteria required to qualify for insurance and thus satisfy guaranteed billing purposes. Better and more reliable estimates of the rates of individuals affected by PAE and its consequences (FASD) are now available, and innovative therapies are being appropriately used to intervene in individual cases. Completed research has revealed varying and unusually high rates of FASD in some specific populations (e.g., preschool, school, youth, offenders, low socioeconomic communities) and systems (e.g., child welfare, foster care, mental and addiction services). Incremental changes are expected to guide future policy and system planning.

Interaction of Alcohol and Other Substances in the Prenatal Environment

Progressive research has also revealed that alcohol alone is very rarely the only psychoactive substance to which an affected fetus is exposed during gestation. Increasingly high rates of co-occurring substance use (e.g., nicotine, cannabis, opiates, stimulants, solvents) in nonpregnant individuals correlate with findings of multiple substances consumed by pregnant women. Isolating the effect of one such substance from the multitude, or delineating a highly specific pattern unique only to alcohol exposure, continues to preoccupy clinical researchers, especially because those findings are highly clinically relevant to mental health practice. In addition, separating the effects of the different environmental factors affecting the developing fetus and understanding the contribution of combined biological and nonbiological risk factors in the final fetal outcome are areas that require ongoing study. Along with many other substances, the fetus is exposed to many non-psychoactive substances and environments during pregnancy. Factors associated with the prenatal environment, such as medications (traditional and complementary/alternative), nutrition, lifestyle factors, levels of stress, exposure to violence and vulnerabilities, raise the important question as to how one best studies the mechanism of the outcome from exposures. The estimated magnitude of the effect of one substance or environment and the interrelated contribution of each (singly or jointly) to the outcome remain active areas of research. Advances in epigenetics, in understanding the developmental origins of health and abnormalities and early childhood adversities, and in animal models of stress-diathesis offer helpful insights into the pathogenesis and longitudinal effects of exposure to alcohol and other substances on the fetus.

Correlation of PAE With Mental Disorder

Overrepresentation of mental disorders in individuals exposed to alcohol prenatally and diagnosed with the most predominant consequence of PAE (FASD) was recognized in early longitudinal and cohort studies. The strength of the association and the inclusion of a researchable diagnostic term in DSM-5 highly suggested that FASD and mental disorder may be on a spectrum. The consequences of PAE and mental disorders reflect complementary neurocognitive deficits, theories of developmental origins, and current intervention strategies. The writing of this text was motivated by the desire to understand the exact nature of the relationship, classification, and etiological underpinnings of mental disorder and PAE. A large proportion of patients in the mental health system, identified or not, has been affected by the adverse consequences of PAE. By using several vignettes and providing practical responses to identification, classification, and algorithmic intervention, this book helps readers (especially clinicians) acquire a more FASD-informed knowledge to galvanize their active case findings and provide effective interventions. Interventions are competent if they include appropriate and informed support, but the current state of knowledge of mental disorder classification (atheoretical etiology) is insufficient in addressing all the questions arising from the association between FASD and mental disorder.

Symptomatology and Diagnosis

Existing classification systems identify multiple variations of the potential symptomatology associated with PAE. Various diagnostic labels have been applied to differentiate levels of gestational alcohol exposure, severity of neurocognitive deficits, and the presence or absence of growth or dysmorphic facial features. Attempts to improve reliability, validity, and acceptability of FASD diagnoses have led several researchers to study pathognomonic patterns in populations with FASD. Findings to date have suggested that facial dysmorphic features present the most pathognomonic corollary of PAE. That unique profile may serve as a biomarker of PAE. Additionally, many have pursued neurocognitive profiling, anticipating that it could provide greater ease of identification and classification. The outcomes have yet to be successful; "diffuse neurocognitive damage" is the best explanatory term used to refer to FASD thus far. No specific and pathognomonic clinical presentations are seen consistently in all individuals affected by the consequences of PAE.

Assessment and Diagnosis

The best efforts at valid diagnosis currently involve the comprehensive functional assessment of neurocognitive deficits, medical examination, and the collection of clinically relevant interview data. Conducted using the different expertise of the members of a multidisciplinary team, the assessment seeks to identify common pathological deficits associated with PAE. Diagnostic efforts also recognize the multiple factors contributing to the deficits during the lifespan and involving neurodevelopmental domains. The social, biological, historical, and psychological perspectives presented through these assessment methods form the basis for identifying patients' relevant deficits and strengths, which in turn informs treatment recommendations made to support those patients, their families, and their communities.

The settings for these comprehensive assessments are varied: they may include rural and urban centers, schools, medical clinics, correctional environments, and employment centers. The number of specialty clinics has increased over time, and collaborations within those clinics have provided a ready source of research. Given that there has been only approximately four decades of research activities in the field, such collaborations yield immediate benefits and have significant long-term advantages. It is expected that with DSM-based recognition and advancement in biologically based nosology, mental health professionals will pay closer attention to ND-PAE/FASD. Advanced and current research findings in electrophysiological and neuroimaging studies should soon assume clinical importance and anticipated utility. Electrophysiological and functional and structural imaging continue to illuminate areas that clinical tests cannot. For instance, eye-tracking studies have been used to differentiate individuals with FASD from those with other disorders such as ADHD. By detecting microstructural abnormalities of white matter and neural pathways, diffusion tensor imaging is revolutionizing our knowledge of the abnormalities in connectedness associated with alcohol teratogenesis.

An exhaustive assessment typically uses two forms of investigations: psychological and laboratory. Data are combined with the comprehensive clinical interview to corroborate the diagnosis and identify potential comorbid conditions. Psychological assessments are essential to confirm that the observed deficits meet the threshold of "significant impairment" from PAE-induced neurodevelopmental damage. Several cognitive functional domains —adaptive skills, executive function, intelligence, memory, attention, language, communication, and affect—are clinically assessed and compared with the norm. Significant deviations from the mean are accepted as the threshold for diagnosis using current diagnostic schemes. Assessment results also remain relevant and essential in treatment planning. Given the multiple co-occurring disorders that may be present (e.g., genetic, hormonal, cardiovascular, musculoskeletal, renal), laboratory investigations assist in recognizing wider consequences of the effects of PAE.

Treatment Interventions

Physical and neurodevelopmental assessments inform the treatment recommendations of expert clinicians and multidisciplinary teams. Various interventions are considered effective. Some interventions target specific deficits, whereas others focus on the person affected or the person's circle of care. Still others involve pharmacological treatment or combine pharmacological and nonpharmacological approaches. Psychological treatments, such as family intervention, social skills training, friendship, and safety training, promote improvements in functioning but in a nonspecific way. Targeted interventions using technological approaches (e.g., GoFAR [focus and plan, act, and reflect], MILE [Math Interactive Learning Experience]) ameliorate educational, affective, and cognitive deficits and support functioning (see Chapter 14, "Psychological Treatment"). Computer-based interventions are evolving and provide more evidence for effectiveness in children and youth. Pharmacological approaches utilize knowledge of neurotransmitter abnormalities associated with various ligands—norepinephrine, dopamine, and serotonin—to improve the balance of the feedback mechanisms. Combination therapy appears most successful when social supports such as housing, finances, employment, and mentoring are combined with supervision and structure.

The place for innovative clinical services related to PAE and its outcomes in the general health system remains unclear. Specific FASD teams assume the roles of assessment and intervention with all ages and accept referrals based on the confirmed history of PAE. Most of these teams assess children and adolescents and are insufficient when specific issues arise that require the expertise of other mental health specialists (e.g., anxiety, mood, conduct, and substance use disorders). Relevant specialist teams have been formed in areas with an overrepresentation of FASD, such as pediatrics, family medicine, psychiatry, geriatrics, and forensic psychiatry. Depending on the health care system, professionals with expertise in addictions and developmental disability disorders also embrace individuals diagnosed with ND-PAE/FASD as their clientele. These specialist teams provide a reasonable clinical pathway for patients with ND-PAE/FASD. Unfortunately, individuals who do not conform to the expectations of those services are excluded. Surprisingly, many patients fall within this category; they exist in a "no-man's land." The argument can be made that because of failures in several systems, a separate and all-encompassing special stream of services dedicated to understanding the all-encompassing, lifelong challenges of the ND-PAE/FASD patient population should be considered and developed.

References

American Psychiatric Association: Diagnostic and Statistical Manual of Mental Disorders, 5th Edition. Arlington, VA, American Psychiatric Association, 2013

Cook JL, Green CR, Lilley CM, et al: Fetal alcohol spectrum disorder: a guideline for diagnosis across the lifespan. CMAJ 188(3):191–197, 2016

Mukherjee R: The relationship between ADHD and FASD. Thrombus 8:4–7, 2016

Acknowledgments

The subject of prenatal alcohol exposure and its relationship to long-term mental disorder and criminal consequences has seemed to occupy the past 15 years of my clinical and academic life. What I did not know and have come to realize is that authoring a book is not the endeavor of one person, but it is the task of many people. This was definitely the case with this book. Help came from unexpected places. I was struck by how I met the people who helped me immensely. I am bound to forget a few, so I offer my apologies in advance. My dear wife, Halima, who captained the ship of my household during my very real and physical absence, deserves red roses on a daily basis. She has a great imagination and the ability to make that gift come alive. My three active boys (Yaddak, Faidai, and Fonon) were most accommodating, especially during final examinations of high school, to allow me to disappear so "Dad can write his book." They were patient with my idiosyncrasies during that time, always asking "Are you done with your book?" My siblings and in-laws were front and center carrying the torchlight of support. During a 3-week absence from the country, while my brother and his wife and children attended the inauguration of the new members of parliament in Nigeria, I was fortunate to have the use of their residence. My nephew, my brother's namesake, Ivan, constantly asked to pray and persistently asked about the progress of the writing. These encouraging prompts were not insignificant in providing motivation for "this first-time lone writing." All of you were in the long-distance race with me and never stopped. My brother from another mum, Pastor Ralph Peters, was like Aaron holding up the hands of Moses. Thank you.

I took two writing retreats that were made possible by the generous offer from Pastor Dallas and Leah Beutler of their residence while they were on a 4-month sabbatical in Thailand. Indeed, their home was quiet for the project. However, on second thought, I should have gone to Thailand for the writing project. The memories of their house will not leave me for a while. They live near a forestry park and suggested walking in the park could reinvigorate my writing ability when I felt fatigued, but that year was one of the Saskatchewan prairie's deep winters, so I dared not venture out even once. Unexpected friends also took a strong interest, and your support was really oil for the engine.

As a person entering a new experience with elements of anxiety, I knew from day one that, as in the Bible story, I needed a few people to "hold up Moses' hands." Literally, this was necessary to overcome fatigue, thought blocks, distraction, and diminished motivation. For the group of men and women who responded to my call to pray, you were indeed prayer warriors and superb at it because I felt the answers. As the saying goes, "Your reward is in heaven." Senior colleagues, friends, and brethren really held up "the hands of Moses": Jason Stinson, Marvin Wodja, Lanre Okunola, Segun Oyedokun, Gene Marcoux, Jordan Bako, Busola Olabimtan, Joanna Bogunjoko, Ben Samuel, Brent Cooper, Akin Peluola, Lydia Maikenti, Hauwa Bwala, Enid Pierce, Naomi Mela, Ron Sprentz, Lou Leventhal, Aunty Shatu Garba, Hussaini Musa, Tony Best, Kevin Aubrey, Helen Bako, Busola Adelugba, Jide Adelugba, Bola Obayan, and all their families. To so many, too many to list, I remain grateful.

The exercise of writing this book came with some interesting surprises. I had heard of the few medicolegal gurus of our time, one of whom was in New Zealand. We were on a panel together, and I immediately felt drawn to him. Professor Brookbanks is well known in the field and has written about various aspects of the interaction between FASD and the law. I asked him to provide me with the guidance and supervision I felt I needed. He did not falter, was prompt in review, and supportive, and I owe him a great deal for making me a better writer. Professor Gutheil, Professor Luther, and Ms. Pam Buttinger, along with Professor Brookbanks, are the real reason you are able to follow the writing and understand it. Left to my own writing skills, the material would have been convoluted, redundant, and harder to read, with awkward sentences. They helped me to imagine "the naïve reader holding my hand as I took him or her through the text." You can only imagine what these reviewers went through before the final product. Thank you for volunteering and actively engaging in this process. You are an integral part of the writing and deserve a lot of credit. Thanks also to Andrea DesRoches who undertook additional revisions.

CanFASD, a collaborative interdisciplinary research network, helped me to inculcate the attitude of striving for excellence and current evidence. The University of Saskatchewan, by allowing me to take the sabbatical and approving the project, clearly helped me move from desire to actuality. My able research coordinator Tara Anderson and the staff of the FASD network were excellent in supporting several projects, and the FASD diagnostic team in Cold Lake deserves a special mention. I changed my schedule several times, and as "my closest FASD family," they accommodated my needs.

My patients, their families, and caregivers deserve a special thank you. Learning is more challenging once you have been doing the same thing for a while. In writing, I have had to relearn and to revisit many scenarios, made possible only because of the experience of learning from my patients. My hope is that many more patients will be helped by those who read and apply the content of this book.

Finally, I was motivated periodically by an internal awareness that I needed to do my part, as though I had a purpose bigger than myself. Knowing that my abilities are a gracious gift and that my achievements come because the all-powerful God decides to step in and rescue me and then help me, I am grateful for the answers to prayers and the effect this book will have on those who read it and on those who directly or indirectly benefit from its content. As you can imagine, the creative, innovative, and artistic abilities, as endowed and sustained by Him, all the benefits and the best to come out of and be associated with the content of this book is returned unreservedly to the source of all wisdom, love, and real meaning, to God Himself be the glory. TGBTG!

Mansfield Mela, MBBS, M.Sc.Psych.

PART I

History and Epidemiology

CHAPTER 1

History of Fetal Alcohol Spectrum Disorder and Mental Disorders

WHAT TO KNOW

The deleterious effect of alcohol on the unborn child was known before there was a clinical description.

Historically, the first mental health symptoms to be associated with PAE were suicide and epilepsy.

The effects of PAE were included in psychiatric nosology at only two points during a 60-year time span.

A long-standing issue remains: understanding the distinction between contributors to FASD and contributors to mental disorders.

The Biblical account (Judges 13:7) of the warning given to Samson's mother not to drink wine has been suggested as the earliest historical documentation of the awareness of the deleterious effect of PAE. The role of PAE in specific mental disorder manifestations is, nonetheless, attributed to Aristotle's *Problemata*. In that thesis, Aristotle referred to women who drank alcohol, even when not associated with pregnancy, as "foolish, drunken, or haire-brain women" (Brown et al. 2019; Burton 1845). Aristotle asserted that they gave birth to languid and morose offspring. Specific mental health effects of alcohol use during pregnancy were discovered and reported during the increased consumption of gin in the eighteenth century. During this "gin epidemic," as it was then called, the College of Physicians in London documented and presented evidence about the consequences of PAE, which was blamed for producing "weak, feeble and distempered" children (Royal College of Physicians of London 1726, p. 253). Joint responsibility was placed on both male and female drinking because the nature of the report adopted a public health perspective. Thus, early writings focused globally on male and female alcohol use, highlighting the distribution of drinking by social class and identifying specific consequences of prenatal alcohol consumption (Lemoine 2012).

The initial mention of the features of mental disorders associated with PAE coincided with the suspicion that alcohol was a teratogen. Alcohol used in pregnancy interfered with fetal development and was associated with malformations. This idea of teratogenicity had previously and briefly been considered by physicians in the nineteenth century but was soon abandoned in favor of the concept of hereditary syphilis (herodosyphilis); it was common to ascribe the characteristic facial dysmorphology identified at birth to the sexually transmitted disease rather than to PAE (Sullivan 2011). Of note, syphilis regularly co-occurred with alcohol use, but it was given causal primacy over PAE. In the nineteenth century, the mechanism of dysmorphology associated with syphilis was ascribed to maternal or parental alcohol use. Although male alcoholism was the most dominant parental alcohol use at the time, its effect was still shrouded in doubt. As early as 1899, William Sullivan, a prison physician, noted that parental alcohol use was detrimental to offspring. He recommended incarcerating pregnant women with alcoholism as a treatment to reduce this negative outcome. Relevant among the reported outcomes in offspring of mothers with alcoholism at that time were suicide, epilepsy, and early mortality. These outcomes constituted the best description of the mental health effects of PAE at the time.

In 1967, Paul Lemoine, a French pediatrician who studied and clinically described the first cases of FAS, identified psychological disorders, microcephaly, intellectual deficits, and maladaptive behavior persisting into adulthood as surprising manifestations. These symptoms occurred whether or not offspring had syndromal physical features. It was established around that time that FASD occurred more often in populations characterized by poverty, social exclusion, and colonial legacies. Description of the clinical phenotype did not enter into any diagnostic system until much later. The phenotype was based on the description of eight children who were heavily exposed to alcohol prenatally. In 1973, two physicians (Kenneth Jones and Charles Smith) detailed the clinical features of these children, and this provided a significant impetus for the recognition of the diagnostic outcomes of PAE (Lemoine 2012).

Although the diagnostic schemes for FASD and mental disorders were independently developed, the two interestingly intersected (Lange et al. 2017). It took almost three decades of classification of psychiatric disorders using DSM, from 1952 to 1980, before the psychiatric aspect of PAE was included in the third edition (DSM-III) (American Psychiatric Association 1952, 1968, 1980). From that point on, the goal of DSM was to reproduce observational and atheoretical diagnoses. Therefore, including a diagnosis relating to consequences of PAE, the premise of which was almost entirely etiological in its framework, signaled a departure from the theoretical format of previous editions. It is unclear how the acceptance of this lone diagnosis and recognition came about in spite of the etiological connotations (Mela 2006). In 1978, the all-encompassing and amorphous category of fetal alcohol effects (FAE) was introduced in the FASD literature. Whether the term FAE influenced the DSM mention is not clear; the two fields (FASD and mental disorders) did not commonly relate their findings to each other. Indeed, FASD and the consequences of PAE were easily attributable based on medical reasoning, but they usually remained diametrically separate from a mental health standpoint, where a psychodynamic psychological frame of reference dominated (Astley and Clarren 2000). The DSM category lasted only 7 years, and PAE appeared as an etiological factor in DSM-III and was removed from the classification of mental disorders (DSM-III-R American Psychiatric Association 1987). Two more versions of DSM (DSM-IV and DSM-IV-TR; American Psychiatric Association 1994, 2000) did not consider or include FASD or the consequences of PAE. During the decade in which DSM was reviewed and upgraded twice (1990–2000), very little changed in the classification of FASD as a medical diagnosis. It was after DSM-IV that the Institute of Medicine proposed its criteria in 1996 (Stratton et al. 1996). Limitations to various existing classifications of FASD led to a new system, the 4-digit code, which is similar to the DSM classification in many respects.

Proposed as a more objective measurement of the components of FASD diagnosis, the four-digit code reflected the diverse continuum of the combinations of four key diagnostic features. To diagnose FASD, the scheme ranked growth deficiency, facial dysmorphia, CNS damage/dysfunction, and alcohol exposure in different categories. Using a varying combination of the ranking of these features, this scheme yielded 256 possible diagnostic codes. These were reclassified into 22 categories (A–V), which were further subdivided into nine unique diagnostic outcome categories (Astley 2004). The four-digit code, especially the 2004 version, ushered in more rigorous assessment measures such as normed growth charts and the ranking of facial characteristics, which were then computed as z-scores. Ethnic representation of facial features, postnatal risk factors, and facial measurement using computer software

TABLE 1–1.   Important historical events related to PAE

YEAR	IMPORTANT EVENT
1973	First clinical description of unique features of fetal alcohol syndrome
1978	Introduction of unspecific term fetal alcohol effect
1996	Publication of Institute of Medicine diagnostic criteria
	Publication of landmark study on outcomes of PAE
1999	Publication of four-digit diagnostic code and lip-philtrum guide
2005	Publication of various diagnostic guidelines (e.g., Hoyme criteria)
2013	Identification of mental disorder
2016	Description as whole-body disorder

(facial photographic analysis) were additional features of the multicategory four-digit code. One of the FASD categories, neurobehavioral disorder, grouped those features of mental disorder associated with definite significant PAE (Astley 2004). By comparison, the existing DSM-IV classification had 383 categories. Table 1–1 gives some of the historical events and landmarks associated with the understanding of the effect of PAE.

Almost immediately following the four-digit code system, two distinct yet related methods of diagnosis were introduced to the field of FASD: the Canadian Diagnostic Guidelines (CDG) for FASD and the Hoyme criteria (Hoyme et al. 2005), both released and published in 2005. The CDG used a consensus process and harmonized features of the four-digit code and Institute of Medicine criteria (Chudley et al. 2005; Cook et al. 2016). A major recommendation promoted multidisciplinary team assessments as the gold standard to which clinicians should strive. Closely related to mental health, neurocognitive deficits in the following neurodevelopmental domains are required for diagnosis: hard and soft neurological signs, sensorimotor signs, brain structure, cognition, communication, academic achievement, memory, executive functioning, attention, and adaptive behavior. These deficits, including affect regulation, added in the 2016 revision, reflect CNS abnormalities. The diagnostic threshold is a minimum of three domains with standard scores two standard deviations below the mean of the normed scores (Chudley et al. 2005; Cook et al. 2016). The Hoyme criteria contained the fewest references to features of mental disorder, focusing on the structural criteria of CNS impairment over cognitive and behavioral deficits (Hoyme et al. 2005).

After two more updated versions of DSM (DSM-IV and DSM-IV-TR) from the time the mention of FASD was excised, DSM-5 (American Psychiatric Association 2013) adopted FASD in various forms. In the section

"Neurodevelopmental Disorders," under "Other Neurodevelopmental Disorders" prenatal alcohol use is identified as a causal factor so that codes 315.8 and 315.9 are available for clinicians to identify patients with PAE and intellectual deficits. PAE is recognized as a risk factor or predisposing to motor coordination disorder and ADHD. A future research-based condition in DSM-5 Section III, "Neurobehavioral Disorder Associated With Prenatal Alcohol Exposure," bears the closest resemblance to FASD (American Psychiatric Association 2013). Self-regulation, neurocognition, and adaptive function are referred to as superdomains; they correlate with the existing neurodevelopmental domains of the revised CDG. The superdomains were indeed instrumental in determining the domains in the revised and updated CDG, which also includes affect regulation as a new specific domain to be assessed. The criteria for affect regulation are based on the presence of a lifelong diagnosis of anxiety and mood disorders according to DSM-5 criteria, meaning they are of a pervasive quality. The intersection of the 10 domains of the CDG and the superdomains of the DSM-5 research criteria (self-regulation, neurocognition and adaptive function) arose from several research findings. Current basic science and clinical evidence suggest that the impairment in affect regulation induced by PAE is through the deficit of the hypothalamic-pituitary-adrenal (HPA) axis feedback mechanism (Temple et al. 2019; Weinberg et al. 2008). This same deficit is also found in anxiety and mood disorders.

Science of FASD and Mental Disorder

The sections of DSM-5 list various criteria for identifying mental disorders. These disorders are diverse, but each may contain features that can easily be identified among the neurocognitive deficits of PAE. Instead of listing all of the associations PAE has with all DSM-5 diagnoses, a few will be highlighted to set the stage for understanding the intricately complex etiology and pathogenesis shared by both. These overlaps have historical trajectories that can shape future research and clinical endeavors.

In a final report to the Centers for Disease Control and Prevention, Streissguth and colleagues in 1996 reported a high rate of mental disorder diagnosis among patients diagnosed with FASD. In that seminal work, they recruited 473 FASD-diagnosed individuals and completed a life history interview with 415 (Streissguth et al. 1996). After about 25 years, 16% of the cohort met the criteria for developmental disability (called mental retardation in DSM-IV; an individual's IQ score ≤70). The study population was divided according to diagnosis of either FAS or FAE. The mean IQ score for the FAS group was 72 (IQ range 29–120). The mean score was 92 (IQ range 42–142) for individuals diagnosed with FAE. Additional mental diagnoses were overrepresented in the study sample, with 94% of the sample having a mental disorder, 60% with ADHD and a high rate of clinical depression. The study also reported that 43% of the sample had threatened suicide and 23% had attempted suicide (Streissguth et al. 1996). Over the years since this study was published, replication studies have found similarly high rates of mental disorders (Clarke and Gibbard 2003). Studies of mental disorder in children and adolescents with FASD reported rates of conduct disorder, anxiety, or features of attachment disorder higher than those in the general population (O'Connor 2014).

The overrepresentation of alcohol and substance use disorders in the FASD-affected population has been an interesting area of research. In one sample, 30% of adults who had been diagnosed with FASD under the age of 12 were found to have alcohol use disorder (Streissguth et al. 1996). In another sample, adult males and females diagnosed with FASD were noted to have substance use disorders at a rate of 53% and 70%, respectively (Lange et al. 2017). These figures set the stage for inquiry about the relationship between mental disorder, substance use disorder, and FASD. Over the past two decades, intense research efforts have sought to understand the mechanism of and distinguish the role played by each disorder in the various outcomes of the phenotypes. Studies show that in adults diagnosed with FASD for whom lower IQ (or intellectual disability) was controlled, a variety of mental disorders (mood, psychotic, and personality disorders) were diagnosable and at notably high rates (Famy et al. 1998).

Clinical investigators studying the different factors related to FASD and caring for patients with FASD and diagnosable mental disorders report the difficulties of teasing apart the weight and importance of those factors. Because of the historical inability to align theories about etiology, pathophysiology, treatment, and prognosis, the interface between FASD and mental disorders has raised many questions. These issues are being addressed, albeit slowly. The history of FASD and its relationship with mental disorders is characterized by the differing multiple attributions associated with a person having comorbid conditions. These attributions have broad implications, which include misclassification and consequently inappropriate support and treatment.

Clinical Vignette

A patient presents with prominent features of mental disorder. Symptoms of neurodevelopmental maladaptive abnormalities are prominent. Perhaps the patient has also been diagnosed with substance use disorder, and following a major accident, the patient also experiences neuropsychiatric sequelae of head trauma. The latter manifest as significant deficits in behavior control. The likelihood of a poor therapeutic alliance—and worse outcome than in the absence of these intervening characteristics—is high. The patient will typically be given the label "noncompliant." In the past, and in keeping with the clinician's expertise and knowledge of the various known and unknown risks and contributors, a number of differential diagnoses were possible. Etiology is considered relatively important in the obvious traumatic brain injury. The focus on phenomenology overshadows the search for causes of the presentation. Therefore, PAE and its consequences will essentially be concealed from the clinical inquiry, and the preferred diagnosis will not include PAE as a major contributor. Thus, the clinician is likely to invoke different diagnosable mental disorders even if criteria are not completely fulfilled.

In more recent times, and especially among clinicians working in centers adopting FASD-informed approaches, clinicians may respond quite differently. Sensitized by knowledge of brain damage from PAE, those clinicians attend to such clinical presentations differently. With the introduction of ND-PAE, broader differential diagnoses can be imagined. A patient who presents with the clinical history described in this vignette will rarely receive a single DSM mental diagnosis (e.g., personality change due to another medical condition, substance use disorder). Neurodevelopmental disorder will now feature prominently in the list of differential diagnoses. This provides an explanatory model and offers support linked with the patient's disability. The patient's unexplained "noncompliance" now is embedded in a framework that allows for therapeutic support. Recognizing symptoms as attributable to ND-PAE also acknowledges the chronic nature of the deficits. These patients are then spared the daunting expectation that they can exert control over their challenging behavior. Intervention at this stage involves a lifelong model of support rather than an immediate treatment expected to resolve the behaviors.

Training mental health and addiction workers to recognize and employ differential approaches to accommodate the neurocognitive deficits of PAE is a requisite component of system transformation. Because FASD with other comorbid mental disorders is generally the rule rather than the exception, it is valuable to teach workers to recognize the presence of FASD alongside other challenges rather than exclude the option of FASD when other challenges are prevalent. Comorbid findings originally derived from work by Anne Streissguth of Seattle, Washington, have been replicated (O'Connor et al. 2002; Weyrauch et al. 2017). More than 400 subjects diagnosed with FASD were followed up for more than two decades. Multiple and varied mental disorders were identified in these subjects over time. The disorders more commonly reported were anxiety, mood, personality, and substance use disorders. The replication samples of the findings cut across settings and were from different countries. The results have produced research directed at exploring the interface of the commonality and coexistence of mental disorders in individuals exposed to alcohol prenatally. Care for people affected by this interface fell to mental health professionals. Unfortunately, the professionals surveyed were noted to have minimal awareness of the diagnosis or the outcomes of PAE (Tough et al. 2003). Recently, however, surveyed mental health professionals were shown to be better at recognizing the deficits of PAE in their clinical cases (Brown and Harr 2018). Their responses also revealed that they were more knowledgeable about PAE than those professionals surveyed a decade earlier and were evaluated as better placed to diagnose and treat the complex issue of comorbidity. Mental health professionals are often the gatekeepers and triage links for patients with mental health struggles; early and appropriate recognition of the consequences of PAE is crucial to improve outcomes and prevent misdiagnosis. Accurate identification leads to appropriate support, on which the future of individuals with PAE is dependent.

Returning to the clinical vignette, the potential list of risk factors that contribute to the clinical picture includes some or all of the following: PAE, potential genetic inheritance of alcohol and substance use disorders from parents, consequences of psychosocial trauma, head injury, societal adversity, and the use of alcohol and substances by the affected person. The list is expanded because etiology is actively considered in conceptualizing the case. The framework for managing this patient depends on the type of service the patient encounters first and the availability of relevant clinical specialties.

In alcohol and substance use services, a patient with the presentation described in the vignette is traditionally expected to maintain a period of sobriety before accessing support services. If that is possible, the next phase of intervention requires the patient to demonstrate some ability to engage cognitive faculties. This is because traditional treatment approaches now expect the patient to reason out motivations for change using cause and effect thinking abilities. This cause and effect process is well known to be absent or significantly impaired in people with FASD, and thus engagement in this type of treatment is negatively impacted. Most of the neurocognitive deficits may not be obvious to the unsuspecting clinician.

Expectations that the patient commit to treatment and act accordingly also interfere with treatment. Commitment to change will likely be determined by actions such as attending individual and community group therapy appointments on time and actively participating in residential group program activities, including completion of homework tasks. Instructions given during residential treatment that are meant to keep all patients safe are usually presented verbally, including the expectation to strictly adhere to house rules about living. Patients in residential rehabilitation treatment are required to sign treatment agreements. This means zero tolerance of the use of alcohol and substances during therapy. Nonadherence or breaches of these agreements typically result in the person being suspended or expelled from the program. Although behaviorally motivating to some patients, this treatment plan does not take into account the hidden cognitive issues arising from PAE, and it will ultimately be unsuccessful without appropriate modifications that respect an individual's specific deficits. Attrition and incomplete program participation are well established as significant risk factors for negative outcomes (Grant et al. 2014; Substance Abuse and Mental Health Services Administration 2014). In a study among women attending addiction services, individuals with a history of PAE or diagnosed with FASD were less likely to attend and complete inpatient and outpatient addiction treatment (Grant et al. 2013). By adopting an FASD lens when planning treatment, potentially obstructive expectations can be avoided or modified as required for effective learning to occur.

Red Flags: What Else Could It Be?

Attributions of symptoms to align with diagnostic criteria can be highly subjective and often depend on the clinician's level of knowledge about specific diagnoses. When little attention was paid to the findings of neurocognitive deficits, clinicians interpreted treatment-interfering behaviors as deliberate and under the patient's control. Clinicians more likely to apply this approach to behavioral abnormalities tried to explain why the patient did not avoid obvious misjudgments. Differing attributions are also dependent on the clinician's social and moral perception of causation. The different perspectives applied to the constellation of features existing in one individual engender a plethora of attributions. Clinicians need to understand their personal biases and how these biases affect how they view and interact with patients.

However, over time, information about PAE and knowledge about the effect of deficits associated with FASD have been incorporated into the clinical toolkit of professionals who care for patients in mental and addiction services. The documentation and trajectory of treatment can look different depending on when that knowledge was acquired. A clinician lacking an understanding of PAE and its consequences may attribute intentionality, responsibility, blame, symptom management, and self-control to a patient. Also influencing such attributions are a clinician's competence and perspective. These skills originate in and are reinforced through training and paradigms associated with features that form clinical patterns. Clinicians with knowledge about the biological components of the neurodevelopmental disorder are better informed about the effects of the deficits and less likely to attribute unreasonable responsibility to the patient assessed with neurocognitive deficits than clinicians without knowledge of the relationship between FASD and mental disorders.

To make any definite treatment modification, a comprehensive assessment of deficits and strengths is essential and should be requested for individuals with PAE. The assessment process should thoroughly examine past failures in treatment and identify critical success factors. Addressing these factors is best done by incorporating successful existing evidence-based interventions for individuals with neurocognitive deficits.

Modifications to Care: What Difference Does It Make?

An obvious follow-up to identifying red flags is to determine how to apply the knowledge to effect a substantial improvement in outcome. The value of the knowledge lies in understanding how the manifesting features and biological dimensions of the disorder coalesce. Clinicians are armed with advance information that enables them to adjust their intervention approaches to patients who have significant cognitive deficits and addictions. Recognition of the biological domain of FASD not only fundamentally changes the way treatment is approached but also releases patients from the frustration associated with "just not trying hard enough" (Miresco and Kirmayer 2006). Clinicians who are better equipped and informed about alternative approaches have the potential to provide much-needed relief to patients and families who may experience feelings of guilt and shame associated with the consequences of PAE. The modification of interventions takes into account the biological basis of FASD, applies appropriate psychological strategies, and ensures a vital supportive response to the patient. These fundamental benefits reflect an evolution of treatment in the history of mental disorders and FASD. The neurocognitive deficits of PAE that contribute to failed treatment and noncompliance can now be isolated and given the attention they deserve. Consequently, patients can be appropriately supported.

Specific approaches may involve modified communication to ensure comprehension. Because patients' suggestibility contributes to poor judgment, efforts are directed at reducing the influence of negative peers during treatment. Thus, the chances of better engagement, reduced rates of attrition, and improved outcomes are increased. Informed clinicians will be aware of obstacles to treatment. For instance, patients may be easily swayed to leave the treatment center to indulge in alcohol or drugs. Prompted by the suggestions of a cognitively competent patient, impaired patients are likely to go along. Because they signed a treatment agreement not to violate the house rule of abstaining from alcohol and drugs, suspension is one approach to dealing with such "blatant" breaches. Identifying the neurocognitive deficit of executive function that contributed to these patients' poor judgment and suggestibility, clinicians can modify the approach. Protection from other, more sophisticated treatment group members and increased supervision and structure during residential treatment optimize chances of success. A stepwise response to patients' failures could include strategies such as restricting access to friends likely to negatively influence them, written lists of expectations, and limiting outings; however, it should be noted that consequences should be linked to each defaulting act both in terms of immediacy and relevance. To maintain therapeutic alliance, consistent emphasis on an individual's strengths (identified during comprehensive assessment) is the best known ingredient of success. Clinicians should embrace the proven elements of success—hope, resilience, and flexibility—as they modify their approach to cognitively impaired patients.

History and Future of Research

FASD research has changed, prompted by events in the social and health sectors. Policy and services have been impacted. Abstinence from alcohol is now recommended, and all health professionals are encouraged to routinely inquire about alcohol use during pregnancy and in women considering pregnancy. It is not a coincidence that as the U.S. Surgeon General advised women to limit their alcohol use during pregnancy in 1981, the number of academic articles on the consequences of PAE started to explode. The research interest of multiple institutions (e.g., Canada FASD Research Network, Centers for Disease Control and Prevention, National Institutes of Health, World Health Organization) has helped propel the field forward. The use of innovative technology, such as interactive computer games, neuroimaging, and artificial intelligence in screening and diagnosis, advances our understanding of the disorder and how to prevent and intervene.

Conclusion

The recognition of the harm caused by PAE began with accepting that alcohol was a teratogen. Once clinicians recognized that PAE is associated with a number of negative outcomes, the question that remained was how to modify treatment approaches to support the person affected. Now, diagnostic classifications and treatment modalities are in place to meet the needs of patients grappling with the consequences of PAE. Going forward, combined basic and clinical research hold the promise of a better future for many individuals with PAE.

CLINICAL PRACTICAL APPLICATIONS

- Clinicians should learn about the diagnostic classification of PAE and how this benefits the majority of their patients.

- PAE-related diagnoses provide explanatory models that can inform current treatment of patients with PAE.

- In making attributions of symptoms, knowledge of the relationship between PAE and mental disorder, and the weight ascribed to each, can enhance the clinical approach.

References

American Psychiatric Association: Diagnostic and Statistical Manual: Mental Disorders. Washington, DC, American Psychiatric Association, 1952

American Psychiatric Association: Diagnostic and Statistical Manual: Mental Disorders, 2nd Edition. Washington, DC, American Psychiatric Association, 1968

American Psychiatric Association: Diagnostic and Statistical Manual of Mental Disorders, 3rd Edition. Washington, DC, American Psychiatric Association, 1980

American Psychiatric Association: Diagnostic and Statistical Manual of Mental Disorders, 3rd Edition, Revised. Washington, DC, American Psychiatric Association, 1987

American Psychiatric Association: Diagnostic and Statistical Manual of Mental Disorders, 4th Edition. Washington, DC, American Psychiatric Association, 1994

American Psychiatric Association: Diagnostic and Statistical Manual of Mental Disorders, 4th Edition, Text Revision. Washington, DC, American Psychiatric Association, 2000

American Psychiatric Association: Diagnostic and Statistical Manual of Mental Disorders, 5th Edition. Arlington, VA, American Psychiatric Association, 2013

Astley SJ: Diagnostic Guide for Fetal Alcohol Spectrum Disorders: The 4-Digit Diagnostic Code, 3rd Edition. Seattle, WA, University of Washington Publication Services, 2004. Available at: http://depts.washington.edu/fasdpn/pdfs/guide04.pdf. Accessed September 26, 2020.

Astley SJ, Clarren SK: Diagnosing the full spectrum of fetal alcohol-exposed individuals: introducing the 4-digit diagnostic code. Alcohol Alcohol 35(4):400–410, 2000

Brown J, Harr D: Perceptions of fetal alcohol spectrum disorder (FASD) at a mental health outpatient treatment provider in Minnesota. Int J Environ Res Public Health 16(1):E16, 2018

Brown JM, Bland R, Jonsson E, Greenshaw AJ: A brief history of awareness of the link between alcohol and fetal alcohol spectrum disorder. Can J Psychiatry 64(3):164–168, 2019

Burton R: The Anatomy of Melancholy. London, Thomas Tegg, 1845

Chudley AE, Conry J, Cook JL, et al: Fetal alcohol spectrum disorder: Canadian guidelines for diagnosis. CMAJ 172(5 suppl):S1–S21, 2005

Clarke ME, Gibbard WB: Overview of fetal alcohol spectrum disorders for mental health professionals. Can Child Adolesc Psychiatr Rev 12(3):57–63, 2003

Cook JL, Green CR, Lilley CM, et al: Fetal alcohol spectrum disorder: a guideline for diagnosis across the lifespan. CMAJ 188(3):191–197, 2016

Famy C, Streissguth AP, Unis AS: Mental illness in adults with fetal alcohol syndrome or fetal alcohol effects. Am J Psychiatry 155(4):552–554, 1998

Golden J: Commentary: observing the effects of alcohol abuse and pregnancy in the late 19th century. Int J Epidemiol 40(2):292–293, 2011

Grant TM, Brown NN, Graham CJ, et al: Screening in treatment programs for fetal alcohol spectrum disorders that could affect therapeutic progress. Int J Alcohol Drug Res 2(3):37–49, 2013

Grant TM, Brown NN, Graham JC, Ernst CC: Substance abuse treatment out comes in women with fetal alcohol spectrum disorder. Int J Alcohol Drug Res 3(1):43–49, 2014

Hoyme HE, May PA, Kalberg WO, et al: A practical clinical approach to diagnosis of fetal alcohol spectrum disorders: clarification of the 1996 Institute of Medicine criteria. Pediatrics 115:39–47, 2005

Lange S, Probst C, Gmel G, et al: Global prevalence of fetal alcohol spectrum disorder among children and youth: a systematic review and meta-analysis. JAMA Pediatr 171(10):948–956, 2017

Lemoine P: The history of alcohol fetopathies: 1997. J Popul Ther Clin Pharmacol 19(2):e224–e226, 2012

Mela M: Accommodating the fetal alcohol spectrum disorders in the Diagnostic and Statistical Manual of Mental Disorders (DSM V). J FAS Int 4:1–10, 2006

Miresco MJ, Kirmayer LJ: The persistence of mind-brain dualism in psychiatric reasoning about clinical scenarios. Am J Psychiatry 163(5):913–918, 2006

O'Connor MJ: Mental health outcomes associated with prenatal alcohol exposure: genetic and environmental factors. Curr Dev Disord Rep 1:181–188, 2014

O'Connor MJ, Shah B, Whaley S, et al: Psychiatric illness in a clinical sample of children with prenatal alcohol exposure. Am J Drug Alcohol Abuse 28(4):743–754, 2002

Royal College of Physicians of London: Annals. London, Royal College of Physicians, 1726, p 253

Sprague HB, McGinn S: The apical chest lead as the chief aid in the diagnosis of coronary occlusion. N Engl J Med 218(13):555–560, 1938

Stratton K, Howe C, Battaglia FC (eds): Fetal Alcohol Syndrome: Diagnosis, Epidemiology, Prevention, and Treatment. Washington, DC, National Academies Press, 1996

Streissguth AP, Barr HM, Kogan J, Bookstein FL: Understanding the Occurrence of Secondary Disabilities in Clients with Fetal Alcohol Syndrome (FAS) and Fetal Alcohol Effects (FAE), Final Report to the Centers for Disease Control and Prevention (CDC) (Tech Rep No 96-06). Seattle, University of Washington, Fetal Alcohol and Drug Unit, 1996

Substance Abuse and Mental Health Services Administration: Addressing Fetal Alcohol Spectrum Disorders (FASD) (Treatment Improvement Protocol [TIP] Series 58, HHS Publ No SMA 13-4803). Rockville, MD, Substance Abuse and Mental Health Services Administration, 2014.

Sullivan WC: A note on the influence of maternal inebriety on the offspring: 1899. Int J Epidemiol 40(2):278–282, 2011

Temple VK, Cook JL, Unsworth K, et al: Mental health and affect regulation impairment in fetal alcohol spectrum disorder (FASD): results from the Canadian national FASD database. Alcohol Alcohol 54(5):545–550, 2019

Tough SC, Clarke M, Hicks M: Knowledge and attitudes of Canadian psychiatrists regarding fetal alcohol spectrum disorders. Can Child Adolesc Psychiatry Rev 12(3):64–71, 2003

Weinberg J, Sliwowska JH, Lan N, Hellemans KGC: Prenatal alcohol exposure: foetal programming, the hypothalamic-pituitary-adrenal axis and sex differences in outcome. J Neuroendocrinol 20(4):470–488, 2008

Weyrauch D, Schwartz M, Hart B, et al: Comorbid mental disorders in fetal alcohol spectrum disorders: a systematic review. J Dev Behav Pediatr 38(4):283–291 2017

CHAPTER 2

Epidemiology

WHAT TO KNOW

Initial rates of prevalence of mental disorder among those with PAE indicated that more than four out of five individuals with PAE had a mental disorder diagnosis.

In the mental health system, more than a quarter of mental health patients will report PAE and are diagnosable with ND-PAE/FASD.

Epidemiology pinpoints access and support issues relevant to the clinical picture of those with ND-PAE/FASD that are also relevant in the addiction and mental health systems.

Risk factors associated with ND-PAE/FASD include living in a colonized country, intergenerational trauma, domestic violence, and health inequalities (more common in specific populations).

Understanding the predictors and moderators of expressed mental disorders among individuals with PAE may inform policy decisions. Among these moderators are efforts at prevention. Diagnosed mental disorders or neurocognitive deficits related to PAE exist on a comorbid continuum or spectrum. Mental health professionals can contribute to estimating prevalence rates by recognizing the affected patients in their practice. Patients

vary in their presentation to different health and social services. The implication is that the rates of patients with PAE found later to have mental disorders differ from those of patients with mental disorders found later to
have PAE. PAE occurs among many who are diagnosed with mental disorders and who are involved in the mental health system. Knowledge among
mental health clinicians of its frequency and sequelae in patients diagnosed
with mental disorders is increasing, and therefore detection and appropriate support for these patients will likely increase also.

Relevance of Mental Disorder in ND-PAE/FASD Service Provision

Studies conducted to determine the distribution of ND-PAE/FASD have
generally followed up subjects initially selected because of PAE in whom
rates of mental disorders were calculated (Astley 2010; Famy et al. 1998;
Mela et al. 2013). The rates of FASD found in the general population in
case ascertainment studies (2%–5%) are one-fourth to one-tenth of the
current rates of mental disorder (20%) in the general population (Kessler
et al. 2003; Steel et al. 2014; Weyrauch et al. 2017). Identifying individuals
in the mental health system who were exposed to alcohol prenatally is now
increasingly of interest to researchers. Rates of PAE and diagnosed sequelae
among mentally ill patients indicate the frequency of co-occurring disorders. Current findings show that 75%–95% of people initially diagnosed
with FASD will experience an additional mental disorder diagnosis, usually
multiple diagnoses (Chasnoff et al. 2015). Among patients in the mental
health system, at least one-quarter of those in the samples studied are diagnosable with ND-PAE/FASD (O'Connor and Paley 2009; O'Connor et al.
2006). Given reduced detection, misdiagnosis, and system barriers, the latter figure clearly underestimates the actual frequency. Accurately calculated
rates of the two disorders coexisting should inform clinical management,
policies for service development, and prevention programs (Anderson et al.
2017; Burd et al. 2007).

Over the years, FASD clinicians and specialists understood and responded to the overrepresentation of mental disorders among individuals
with PAE. They studied the rates and implications, adjusted their diagnostic schemes, and initiated therapeutic interventions. These interventions
are directed at the shared neurocognitive deficits as well as features unique
to each disorder, as they can also manifest differently (Pei et al. 2011). Researchers have not established the most efficacious interventions for patients with both disorders (Popova et al. 2013). As practice-based evidence
is generated from the results of these interventions, evidence from epide-

miology provides a complementary approach. Improving availability and access to the appropriate support services is an approach dependent on information generated through epidemiological studies (Rangmar et al. 2015). Findings from studying patients found at the interface of PAE and its mental disorder outcomes highlight the need for the development of specialty care (Mukherjee et al. 2019). Given the complexity associated with the health care management of these patients, specific epidemiological studies of the interface also hold the potential for simplifying preventive, diagnostic, treatment, and rehabilitative services. These approaches are needed across the lifespan, and they require multidisciplinary involvement and engagement of policymakers.

Mental Disorder Rates Among Patients With PAE and ND-PAE/FASD

Virtually all epidemiological studies detect and report significantly higher rates of mental disorders among individuals with PAE and its outcomes (Roozen et al. 2016). For instance, when 415 patients diagnosed with FASD were reassessed after two decades, 94% reported having an additional mental diagnosis (Streissguth et al. 1996). These findings were replicated in several retrospective and prospective studies (Clark et al. 2004; Streissguth et al. 2004). When clinical assessment used standardized instruments rather than self-report, prevalence rates of diagnosed mental disorders fell to between 50% and 75% (Weyrauch et al. 2017). In children and adolescents in whom most of the initial FASD diagnosis findings were identified, the instruments used to determine mental disorders included the Composite Diagnostic Scale (CDS), Computerized Diagnostic Interview Schedule for Children, Composite International Diagnostic Interview (CIDI), and Mini International Neuropsychiatric Interview (MINI) (O'Connor et al. 2002). Table 2–1 depicts the findings of lifelong higher prevalence of issues and disorders associated with PAE.

Large numbers of patients diagnosed with FASD were subsequently assessed for other mental disorders recognized in DSM. In a study with over 1,400 patients, Astley (2010) identified 82% with mental disorders. ADHD, the most representative diagnosis, was noted in almost 54% of the sample (Astley 2010). Another cohort study examined the odds of having a diagnosed mental disorder in the offspring of mothers who consumed alcohol heavily during pregnancy (Barr et al. 2006). Among 1,529 pregnant women, 500 offspring exposed to heavy alcohol use were assessed using the Structured Clinical Interviews for DSM-IV (SCIDs), including both the SCID for Axis I and Axis II personality disorders (First et al. 1997a, 1997b). At the

TABLE 2–1. Lifelong perspective of epidemiologically prevalent issues and disorders associated with PAE

Preconception	Alcohol dependence and social inequalities
Prenatal environment	Maternal depression, mental disorder, and domestic violence
Childhood	Sleep and mood disorders, externalizing, internalizing behavior, ADHD, oppositional defiant disorder, reactive attachment disorder
Adolescence	ADHD and conduct, mood, and substance use disorders
Adulthood	Personality and mood disorders, alcohol abuse, social anxiety
Elderly/Older adult	Early-onset neurocognitive disorders

mean age of 25.7 years, Barr et al. (2006) reported that one or more episodes of binge drinking were associated with double the odds of psychiatric disorders. The odds were stable after controlling for confounders in the diagnoses of Axis I substance dependence or abuse disorders and Axis II passive-aggressive and antisocial personality disorders or traits. From an epidemiological perspective, PAE constitutes a risk factor for specific psychiatric disorders and traits in early adulthood (Barr et al. 2006).

Similarly, Famy et al. (1998) examined the rates of mental disorders among individuals with FASD (excluding intellectual disability). Adults in these types of studies were usually those diagnosed with FASD during the developmental period. In adults with FASD (mean age 28.8; range 19–51 years), whose IQ was >70 (mean IQ 86.6; range 73–110) assessed using a standardized instrument (SCID) to diagnose mental disorders and personality disorders, comorbid mental disorders were diagnosed among 92% of the sample. The rates of alcohol and drug use disorder (60%), major depressive disorder (44%), psychosis (40%), and avoidant personality disorder (48%) were the highest noted (Famy et al. 1998).

In a case-control nationally based registry study, Rangmar et al. (2015) compared 79 patients with FAS (mean age 32 years) with 3,160 subjects matched by age, gender, and place of birth in Sweden. Compared with the non-FAS group, psychiatric disorders and the likelihood of receiving a psychotropic drug was two- to sixfold higher in those with FAS. Researchers also identified other disadvantages and vulnerabilities for participants with FAS, including being on disability insurance, receiving special education, and being unemployed, and 81% had been involved with the child welfare system (Rangmar et al. 2015).

Weyrauch et al. (2017) recently conducted a systematic review of 26 different studies that met criteria for reporting one of 15 DSM diagnoses. The sample included more than 5,000 participants, with a mean age of 10 years. The authors found an overrepresentation of mental disorders in individuals with PAE. ADHD was the most represented disorder, at 10 times the general population rates. Other mental disorders included anxiety, depression, PTSD, oppositional defiant disorder (ODD), and learning and intellectual disorders, with prevalence rates ranging from 10% to 45% (Weyrauch et al. 2017). This epidemiological finding has a number of service and policy implications. Notably, the overrepresented disorders are the same disorders that patients commonly present to mental health services. Identifying those patients allows for appropriate support and intervention and prevents adverse outcomes. These negative consequences occur commonly in individuals receiving inappropriate care and who have a history of misdiagnosis due to PAE. In any event, mental health providers should be well informed and actively seek out patients whose complex presentations fit the comorbid conditions associated with PAE.

Popova and colleagues (2017) performed a meta-analysis of epidemiological studies up until 2016 and compared the pooled rates of mental disorders among subjects with PAE with those rates in the general population. ODD, conduct disorder, and antisocial personality disorder were frequently represented (Popova et al. 2017). The most prevalent disorder was ADHD. The prevalence rates of the 15 disorders studied ranged from 2-fold to 15-fold higher in the PAE group than in the general population, representing a significant burden on the pediatric mental health care system. The authors requested a cautionary interpretation of these results because of the inherent challenges of studying comorbidity in a population without specific diagnostic criteria and pathognomonic features to distinguish ND-PAE from other neurodevelopmental disorders. The samples were mostly referred cases, which may introduce selection bias. The lesson, however, is that the consequences of PAE should be considered in individuals who act up and are commonly disruptive.

Clinical Vignette

A 43-year-old man is a long-standing patient in a mental health outpatient clinic. Clinicians note that he is increasingly forgetful. His past psychiatric history is composed of repeated criminal involvement, self-harm, and suicide attempts when he is distressed and unable to cope with disappointments. He is described as quick-tempered and occasionally violent. In a rage, he struck at a store clerk when he was asked to leave. He has a history of substance use disorder but is now sober. His marriage broke down after

6 months because of his temper. He is diagnosed as bipolar and having borderline personality disorder.

This patient illustrates some of the long-term outcomes found in epidemiological studies (e.g., criminal involvement, mental disorder, school failure, dependent living). Figure 2–1 represents the relationship among some of the outcomes of PAE. However, a patient like this man could have all the outcomes and still be cognitively impaired. This calls for a close working relationship between the team of mental health professionals to support the patient. Complicating and contributing aspects of the social determinants of health cut across diagnosis and adverse life outcomes. The confluence of these psychological and social elements results in a complicated negative outcome for the individual with PAE. Prediagnosis, the patient can be misunderstood, and postdiagnosis, the risk factors are cues to the need for extensive and expert involvement of a multidisciplinary team of mental health professionals. Their roles in enhancing resilience are essential for the patient.

International Perspective

In a systematic review of the worldwide prevalence of FASD, the rates of mental disorders were not specifically calculated. Nevertheless, given the relationship between PAE and mental disorders, FASD rates are assumed to be higher based on worldwide estimates (Roozen et al. 2016). Regional differences in rates of FASD were noted but were insufficient to explain the global differences in rates of mental disorders, if any (Popova et al. 2017). The heterogeneity identified was related to geography and ethnicity; for example, rates were much higher in South Africa and Croatia. In a similar study, McQuire et al. (2019) developed a screening tool using a population-based cohort in the United Kingdom. The researchers found that 79% of women reported drinking alcohol during pregnancy, and 6% of the cohort of 13,495 offspring screened positive for ND-PAE/FASD. Additionally, Sayal et al. (2013) used the Strength and Difficulties Questionnaire in the same population-based cohort to determine mental health and learning outcomes among offspring exposed to light drinking during pregnancy. The authors observed that girls at age 11 had more frequent negative outcomes relating to academics. No significant results were found for boys (Sayal et al. 2013).

Low IQ, suggestive of intellectual disability, was overrepresented in a sample of offspring of women who reported drinking more than four drinks per episode during pregnancy (Kesmodel et al. 2012; Popova et al. 2018).

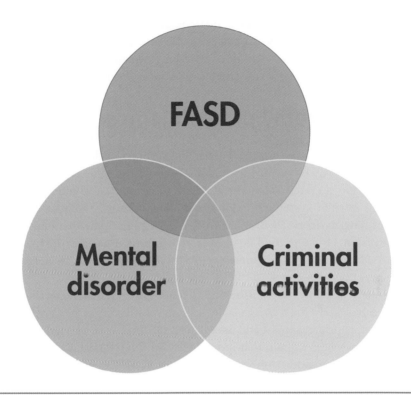

FIGURE 2–1. Confluent relationship of the epidemiologically demonstrated negative outcomes of PAE.

Nevertheless, the authors could not rule out the possible confounding factor of socioeconomic status in this result (Popova et al. 2018). Conduct disorder and behavior problems, borderline personality disorder, and psychotic-like symptoms were overrepresented in representative samples of individuals exposed to heavy alcohol use prenatally. These results suggest a relationship between PAE and mental disorders.

Addiction Services

Many special populations, such as users of alcohol and drug rehabilitation services, have significantly higher rates of ND-PAE/FASD. Nevertheless, researchers have yet to examine this population. Asking individuals who were exposed to alcohol prenatally about their own current alcohol and substance use provides the best source of information about the related rates of ND-PAE/FASD and addiction (Streissguth et al. 2004). On the basis of other interviews and reports of substance use, researchers found that the estimated cost of specialized addiction treatment for patients with ND-PAE/FASD was high (Popova et al. 2013). Self-medication with substances, genetic vulnerability, and increased impulsivity explain the high prevalence of PAE in individuals with substance use disorder (Popova et al. 2013).

Lessons From Epidemiological Findings

Researchers have found that PAE in siblings of probands in studies is related to high rates of various mental disorders in the same siblings. Additionally, Popova et al. (2018) found a high total number of mental health problems in their systematic review and meta-analysis. Their study used samples ranging from 30 to more than 30,000 subjects, with sibling ages ranging from 3 to 26 years. The studies were international, and the findings suggested that family assessment of dysfunction has a role in detecting more patients.

Clinical pathways are outlines that detail how a patient entering the health care system for a particular condition may navigate the system and receive appropriate, timely, and adequately informed care (Anderson et al. 2020). Researchers explain that individuals with ND-PAE/FASD entering mental health and addiction services suffer from inadequate and discriminatory approaches. Stigma, lack of awareness and training, complexity of the systems, and professionals' blind spots with respect to PAE and its associated mental disorders were the main barriers identified in the study of clinical pathways for patients with ND-PAE/FASD navigating the mental health system (Choate and Badry 2019). In the absence of a diagnosable mental disorder, patients are often excluded from services, even when neurocognitive deficits are apparent. Systems that require diagnoses for supports and interventions (i.e., insurer-based systems) often exclude subjects with mere impairments or subthreshold diagnosis. However, people at the interface of PAE and mental disorders rarely have easy and straightforward diagnosable disorders. Unfortunately, complexity in this setting limits diagnosis and emerges as a risk factor for negative outcomes. For patients at this interface, it is therefore challenging to receive a diagnosis and subsequent appropriate support.

Researchers can provide epidemiological data to guide policy that reorients the health care system to focus on professionals' efforts to detect impairment along with diagnosis. Such policies can reduce the burden of care associated with PAE in addition to improving patients' quality of life and health care access. Epidemiological findings that embrace a lifespan perspective have prompted the development of early diagnosis and intervention in mental health treatment. These are essential to appropriately and effectively address behavior management and to support a positive trajectory for individuals with PAE and mental disorders. To manage the multiple diagnoses found in these epidemiological studies, clinicians should target different contributing disorders using evidence available for each disorder. This approach recognizes a relevant interplay between personal and environmental factors that led to the disorders in the first place. Developmentally based treatments thus can remove treatment barriers and facilitate effective interventions through awareness of the patient's early circumstances and their consequent long-term and complex effects.

Vulnerability to ND-PAE/FASD is associated with negative or compromised social determinants of health. As a result, rates of the conditions caused by PAE are higher in high-risk populations, such as children in foster care, individuals involved in the criminal justice system, and those from marginalized communities (Choate and Badry 2019; Popova et al. 2018). Relevant epidemiological factors include poor access to care and insufficient knowledge about the deleterious effect of alcohol use in pregnancy (May et al. 2018). New immigrants and indigenous communities are some examples of marginalized groups with reported higher prevalence rates of ND-PAE/FASD (Hawkins et al. 2008; Lange et al. 2013). Researchers have recommended that these higher rates justify population-based screening to identify affected individuals, which should be followed by activating preventive and interventional strategies (Lange et al. 2013).

Conclusion

Health care policy makers can improve the lives of patients at the interface of mental disorders and ND-PAE/FASD by improving mental health professionals' knowledge about identification and intervention. Integrating the services of separate health care systems serving patients with ND-PAE/FASD and mental disorders could reduce costs and prevent future disability.

CLINICAL PRACTICAL APPLICATIONS

- Because of the sheer numbers of patients with PAE and comorbid mental disorders, mental health professionals should consider the clinical implications of a lack of identification and intervention for their patients.
- Personality disorders, suicidal behaviors, and substance use disorder are significantly elevated in those with PAE; this should inform the assessment and management of cases.

- Taking psychotropic medications, having physical or cognitive impairment, needing special education, and unemployment are potential risk factors for PAE among patients in the mental health system, and evaluation is warranted.

- Siblings of those with PAE have high rates of both PAE and mental disorders that should be considered in clinical settings.

References

Anderson T, Mela M, Stewart MJ: The implementation of the 2012 Mental Health Strategy for Canada through the lens of FASD. Canadian Journal of Community Mental Health 36(special issue):69–81, 2017

Anderson T, Mela M, Rotter T, Poole N: A qualitative investigation into barriers and enablers for the development of a clinical pathway for individuals living with FASD and mental disorder/addictions. Canadian Journal of Community Mental Health 38(3):43-60, 2020

Astley SJ: Profile of the first 1,400 patients receiving diagnostic evaluations for fetal alcohol spectrum disorder at the Washington State Fetal Alcohol Syndrome Diagnostic & Prevention Network. Can J Clin Pharmacol 17(1):e132–e164, 2010

Barr HM, Bookstein FL, O'Malley KD, et al: Binge drinking during pregnancy as a predictor of psychiatric disorders on the Structured Clinical Interview for DSM-IV in young adult offspring. Am J Psychiatry 163(6):1061–1065, 2006

Burd L, Carlson C, Kerbeshian J: Fetal alcohol spectrum disorders and mental illness. Int J Disabil Hum Dev 6(4):383–396, 2007

Chasnoff IJ, Wells AM, King L: Misdiagnosis and missed diagnoses in foster and adopted children with prenatal alcohol exposure. Pediatrics 135(2):264–270, 2015

Choate P, Badry D: Stigma as a dominant discourse in fetal alcohol spectrum disorder. Advances in Dual Diagnosis 12(1/2):36–52, 2019

Clark E, Lutke J, Minnes PM, Ouellette-Kuntz H: Secondary disabilities among adults with fetal alcohol spectrum disorder in British Columbia. J FAS Int 2:e13, 2004

Famy C, Streissguth AP, Unis AS: Mental illness in adults with fetal alcohol syndrome or fetal alcohol effects. Am J Psychiatry 155(4):552–554, 1998

First MB, Gibbon M, Spitzer RL, et al: Structured Clinical Interview for DSM-IV Axis II Personality Disorders (SCID-II). Washington, DC, American Psychiatric Press, 1997a

First MB, Spitzer RL, Gibbon M, Williams JBW: Structured Clinical Interview for DSM-IV Axis I Disorders, Clinician Version (SCID-CV). Washington, DC, American Psychiatric Press, 1997b

Hawkins SS, Lamb K, Cole TJ, et al: Influence of moving to the UK on maternal health behaviours: prospective cohort study. BMJ 336(7652):1052–1055, 2008

Kesmodel US, Eriksen HLF, Underbjerg M, et al: The effect of alcohol binge drinking in early pregnancy on general intelligence in children. BJOG 119(10):1222–1231, 2012

Kessler RC, Barker PR, Colpe LJ, et al: Screening for serious mental illness in the general population. Arch Gen Psychiatry 60(2):184–189, 2003

Lange S, Shield K, Rehm J, Popova S: Prevalence of fetal alcohol spectrum disorders in child care settings: a meta-analysis. Pediatrics 132(4):e980–995, 2013

May PA, Chambers CD, Kalberg WO, et al: Prevalence of fetal alcohol spectrum disorders in 4 US communities. JAMA 319(5):474–482, 2018

McQuire C, Mukherjeer R, Hurt L, et al: Screening prevalence of fetal alcohol spectrum disorders in a region of the United Kingdom: a population-based birth-cohort study. Prev Med 118:344–351, 2019

Mela M, McFarlane A, Sajobi TT, Rajani H: Clinical correlates of fetal alcohol spectrum disorder among diagnosed individuals in a rural diagnostic clinic. J Popul Ther Clin Pharmacol 20(3):e250–e258, 2013

Mukherjee RAS, Cook PA, Norgate SH, Price AD: Neurodevelopmental outcomes in individuals with fetal alcohol spectrum disorder (FASD) with and without exposure to neglect: clinical cohort data from a national FASD diagnostic clinic. Alcohol 76:23–28, 2019

O'Connor MJ, Paley B: Psychiatric conditions associated with prenatal alcohol exposure. Dev Disabil Res Rev 15(3):225–234, 2009

O'Connor MJ, Shah B, Whaley S, et al: Psychiatric illness in a clinical sample of children with prenatal alcohol exposure. Am J Drug Alcohol Abuse 28(4):743–754, 2002

O'Connor MJ, McCracken JT, Best A: Under recognition of prenatal alcohol exposure in a child inpatient psychiatric setting. Mental Health Aspects of Developmental Disabilities 9(4):105–109, 2006

Pei J, Denys K, Hughes J, Rasmussen C: Mental health issues in fetal alcohol spectrum disorder. J Ment Health 20(5):438–448, 2011

Popova S, Lange S, Burd L, et al: Cost of specialized addiction treatment of clients with fetal alcohol spectrum disorder in Canada. BMC Public Health 13:570, 2013

Popova S, Lange S, Probst C, et al: Prevalence of alcohol consumption during pregnancy and fetal alcohol spectrum disorders among the general and aboriginal populations in Canada and the United States. Eur J Med Genet 60(1):32–48, 2017

Popova S, Lange S, Probst C, et al: Global prevalence of alcohol use and binge drinking during pregnancy and fetal alcohol spectrum disorder. Biochem Cell Biol 96(2):237–240, 2018

Rangmar J, Hjern A, Vinnerljung B, et al: Psychosocial outcomes of fetal alcohol syndrome in adulthood. Pediatrics 135(1):e52–e58, 2015

Roozen S, Peters GJY, Kok G, et al: Worldwide prevalence of fetal alcohol spectrum disorders: a systematic literature review including meta-analysis. Alcohol Clin Exp Res 40(1):18–32, 2016

Sayal K, Draper ES, Fraser R, et al: Light drinking in pregnancy and mid-childhood mental health and learning outcomes. Arch Dis Child 98(2):107–111, 2013

Steel Z, Marnane C, Iranpour C, et al: The global prevalence of common mental disorders: a systematic review and meta-analysis 1980–2013. Int J Epidemiol 43(2):476–493, 2014

Streissguth AP, Barr HM, Kogan J, Bookstein FL: Understanding the Occurrence of Secondary Disabilities in Clients with Fetal Alcohol Syndrome (FAS) and Fetal Alcohol Effects (FAE), Final Report to the Centers for Disease Control and Prevention (CDC) (Tech Rep No 96-06). Seattle, University of Washington, Fetal Alcohol and Drug Unit, 1996

Streissguth AP, Bookstein FL, Barr HM, et al: Risk factors for adverse life outcomes in fetal alcohol syndrome and fetal alcohol effects. J Dev Behav Pediatr 25(4):228–238, 2004

Weyrauch D, Schwartz M, Hart B, et al: Comorbid mental disorders in fetal alcohol spectrum disorders: a systematic review. J Dev Behav Pediatr 38(4):283–291, 2017

CHAPTER 3

Prenatal Exposure to Multiple Psychoactive Substances

WHAT TO KNOW

Women using only alcohol during pregnancy is the exception rather than the rule, adding the complexity of sorting out the weight and effect of prenatal exposure to multiple substances.

Pattern of use (consecutive or concurrent) of multiple substances can affect the outcome and clinical presentation of the offspring.

Biological and social factors (e.g., craving, body fat index, and self-medication) combine to predispose women to be more likely than men to experience more complications from polysubstance use.

Specific neurodevelopmental abnormalities are identified for cannabis, tobacco, alcohol, cocaine, and opiate use.

Psychosis in the offspring of a woman using cannabis is more likely with use in early pregnancy and continued use.

Research on the developmental origin of disease and health has identified different sensitive periods during which offending substances cause maximum damage, which explains the continuum on which clinical presentations fall.

Increasingly, researchers have found that fetal outcomes are related to multiple substance[1] exposure. This is thought to be due to the global trend of increasing rates of substance use in the general population as well as factors connected with female empowerment, individual responsibility, and choice (Committee on Addictions of the Group for the Advancement of Psychiatry 2002; McHugh et al. 2014). Emerging policies make access to psychoactive substances easier (Health Canada 2016). Many factors interact during pregnancy to produce differing outcomes. Such is the case when multiple psychoactive substances with teratogenic effects are consumed simultaneously during pregnancy. The direct effect of teratogenic substances may combine with other factors (e.g., heritability, nutritional status, immunity, prenatal care, mental health) to produce the final neurodevelopmental outcome.

The fetal environment is influenced by known and unknown factors. Interested professionals, ultrasonologists, epidemiologists, neonatologists, mental health experts, and pediatricians continue to identify factors affecting fetal development and outcomes (Kinare 2008). Exposure of the developing embryo and fetus to alcohol is rarely the only risk factor occurring during pregnancy. Study findings reflect a high prevalence of polysubstance use in the general population, including among women of childbearing age, which can cause unintentional negative outcomes in offspring (McHugh et al. 2014; Ordean et al. 2017). Predictors of pregnancy-related alcohol and substance use are both unique to individual substances and shared between substances (O'Keeffe et al. 2015). Compared with nonpregnant periods, epidemiological and clinical studies report surprisingly high rates of simultaneous and concurrent alcohol and substance use during pregnancy (Georgieff et al. 2018; Jacobson et al. 2002). This increased likelihood highlights the relevance of multiple fetal exposures.

With high levels of polysubstance use during pregnancy, the factors that can cause adverse effects for the pregnant woman can also negatively affect the fetus. Separating the individual effects and understanding their population, social, individual, and familial implications remains an active area of research. Furthermore, the interactions of these effects with the caregiving environments of children of parents who use multiple substances or are alcohol dependent have long-term biological and psychosocial consequences. Knowledge of these effects is useful for mental health professionals to be effective in their supportive roles.

---

[1]As used in this chapter, "substance(s)" refers to psychoactive substances.

Epidemiology of Multiple Substance Use During Childbearing Age

Exposure to multiple psychoactive substances during pregnancy is best understood as a by-product of rates of polysubstance use in the general population. Researchers have provided rates of prevalence from meta-analyses of rates of combined substance use in the general population. Simultaneous and concurrent use of alcohol among cocaine users, for example, was as high as 74% and 77%, respectively (Liu et al. 2018). However, cannabis use simultaneously and concurrently in the same sample of cocaine users was estimated at 38% and 64%, respectively. Cocaine, cannabis, and alcohol used together can produce additive metabolic and subjective effects. These effects may impact fetal outcomes if this combined use occurred during pregnancy (Liu et al. 2018). In this section, I review evidence for the prevalence of multiple substance use in the general population and identify the relevant risk factors and their consequent effects to provide guidance to identify those at risk. Understanding the mechanism by which neurocognitive damage occurs in exposed individuals can help mental health professionals deliver appropriate interventions. Intervention approaches for pregnant users of multiple substances will differ from approaches used with offspring exposed to multiple substances and will engage other health providers who come in contact with these women.

General Population

Combined alcohol, cigarette, and illicit drug use was estimated in the National Epidemiologic Survey on Alcohol and Related Conditions (NESARC; Hasin et al. 2007). The rates of alcohol use combined with tobacco and those of alcohol combined with another drug in the sample were 21.7% and 5.6%, respectively (Falk et al. 2008). Cannabis is reportedly used by 2.5%–4.9% of the world's population, with few regional variations (Fine et al. 2019). Women generally use less alcohol and fewer drugs than men (11.5% vs. 6.5%) (Fine et al. 2019; Sonon et al. 2016). That gap is narrowing, however, and surveys of lifetime use, previous-year use, and hazardous use associated with having a substance use disorder diagnosis indicate an increasing trend among women (Green 2006). The effect of gender was also related to economic variables. Internationally derived data confirmed the original observations from studies in North America (Carliner et al. 2017; Substance Abuse and Mental Health Services Administration 2013). Annual surveys conducted in the general population indicate that 40%–50% of alcohol users and cigarette smokers are female (Substance Abuse and

Mental Health Services Administration 2013). Compared with men, women are more susceptible to the medical, psychiatric, and social complications and consequences of substance use (Green 2006) and are more likely to self-medicate with a substance and thus transition from use to dependence. They also experience more intense cravings and relapse.

Women of Childbearing Age

Although alcohol is the most studied substance in relation to fetal outcomes, rarely is just alcohol consumed. Evidence of substance use rates in women of childbearing age comes from the NESARC, in which women between the ages of 18 and 24 years reported their combined use of alcohol and tobacco (25.5%) and combined use of alcohol and other drugs (12.5%) (Falk et al. 2008). Similarly, Chen and Maier (2011) studied surveyed nonpregnant women ages 14–44 years and found the following results: Overall, 55% of participants reported drinking alcohol, and 24% reported binge drinking (consuming four or more drinks within 2 hours). The estimated annual and lifetime prevalences of alcohol use disorder were about 5% and 20%, respectively. Comorbidity was common, with 20% of women older than 12 reporting using tobacco products as well. Participants also reported using other illicit drugs (13% annual and 43% lifetime prevalence), of which cannabis was the most prevalent (38.1%), followed by nonmedical use of prescription medications (18.9%), cocaine and hallucinogens (approximately 11% each), inhalants (5.3%), and heroin (1.0%). These rates among women of childbearing age in the United States are similar to those in Canada and other Western societies (Health Canada 2017). In the Canadian Tobacco, Alcohol and Drugs Survey (CTADS; Health Canada 2017), an 11% increase in the use of all drugs (cannabis, cocaine or crack, ecstasy, speed or methamphetamines, hallucinogens, or heroin) occurred over a 2-year period. Ten percent of women of childbearing age reported cannabis use within the past year. Given the prevalent use of drugs and easier access to them, the effect of drug use for women and the combined effect of multiple drugs on the fetus during pregnancy is valuable information for prevention and treatment.

Authors have invoked women's choice, lack of female empowerment, and social disadvantage to explain the trend of increasing substance use (Astley 2010; Singal et al. 2016). The differences in these somewhat contradictory reasons may involve jurisdictional variations and historical factors.

Cannabis Use in Pregnancy Under Review

The outcome of cannabis use during pregnancy is currently undergoing research and review in the scientific as well as public arenas. The driving forces for this review include the increasing numbers of jurisdictions that are legalizing cannabis use, making access to the drug easier. Legalization also could create the illusion that cannabis use is harmless, even in excess. The rates of use among adolescents and women have continued to rise (Ordean et al. 2017). Rates of reported cannabis consumption combined with alcohol, nicotine, and other illicit drugs are also rising (Substance Abuse and Mental Health Services Administration 2017). A recent report showed a 75% jump in the rate of cannabis consumption during pregnancy over a 14-year period (2002–2016) (Health Canada 2017; Jaques et al. 2014). It has become necessary that such an increase be contextualized and understood given the neurodevelopmental damage that is associated with prenatal cannabis use, especially in combination with PAE (K.S. Grant et al. 2018; Volkow et al. 2017).

Rates of exposure to different psychoactive drugs appear to vary by the type of study (surveys, cross-sectional, case control, or cohort). In some studies, the rate of polysubstance use in pregnancy was 50% (Falk et al. 2008). Surveys in the United States in 2012 indicated that 1 million and a one-third of 1 million children were born exposed to nicotine and other illicit drugs, respectively; these estimates were based on national survey results, with 16% and 6% of participants reporting nicotine and illicit substance use, respectively, during pregnancy (Forray et al. 2015). Among subjects seeking treatment in a randomized controlled trial, a high rate of polysubstance use was also reported. Among the 152 women in Forray and colleagues' (2015) study, 96%, 78%, and 73% reported heavy drinking, marijuana, and cocaine use, respectively. Survey and clinic data such as these reveal that the highest rates of polysubstance use come from studies that use self-reported data. Polysubstance use confirmation with urine toxicology also indicates similar rates (Goldschmidt et al. 2004; K.S. Grant et al. 2018).

Fine et al. (2019), in the Adolescent Brain Cognitive Development (ABCD) study, examined the rates of exposure to cannabis in a cohort of 4,316 youth and found that 4.61% had been exposed to cannabis prenatally. In another survey study, 0.1% of pregnant women reported using an opioid in the past month (Sundelin Wahlsten and Sarman 2013). Urine toxicology detection in pregnant women furnished a higher rate (2.6%). Rates of congenital abnormalities associated with opioids were higher in retrospective studies (Sundelin Wahlsten and Sarman 2013). In pregnancy, up to one of every six women were reported to be smoking cigarettes; furthermore, tobacco users often combine cigarette smoking with other substances (Forray et al. 2015; Porath-Waller 2018). Public health campaigns have been successful in reducing general population use of tobacco, which ultimately results in less exposure during pregnancy as well (T.M. Grant et al. 2018; Scherman et al. 2018).

Rates of Comorbid Maternal Substance Use During Pregnancy in Offspring With ND-PAE/FASD

Rates of polysubstance drug use in the mothers of patients with PAE are a proxy measure of the effect of exposure to multiple substances during pregnancy. Current estimates come from a case series in which pregnant women were asked about their substance use (Astley et al. 2000; Porath-Waller 2018). Pregnant women's fear of possible reprisals, including apprehension of the exposed baby, may have decreased the reliability of the self-report data. Compared with information prospectively surveyed, data obtained in clinic settings are accepted as more reflective of the true rate of substance use. In a research context, pregnant mothers may be more likely to limit disclosure. However, when the risk is low, as in when the offspring is at no risk of apprehension, the information may be considered to be more trustworthy. Honest information about substance use is often only obtained within a supportive and therapeutic context, which has led many clinicians to develop patient-centered approaches for obtaining substance use history (Kondracki 2019). An example of a patient-centered approach could include having the health professional (usually an experienced clinic coordinator) first establish and build a positive therapeutic working alliance with the pregnant woman. Then, at an optimal time, the professional can ask about alcohol and substance use, preferably in person (vs. over the phone) so as to observe potential reactions. The expected supportive and therapeutic alliance between the pregnant woman and the clinic coordinator contributes to the reliability of the information. Many clinicians have also developed protocols for interviewing the patient and family that include relationship building to help obtain accurate information (Reid et al. 2008).

Data sets based on clinic-based diagnosis are a more reliable source of clinical information about the rates of comorbid exposure in the fetus (Astley 2010). In a review of approximately 1,400 assessments for the consequences of PAE, information about the mothers and their pregnancies is instructive on this issue. Although only 22% of the mothers attended the clinic for their offsprings' diagnosis, information was corroborated and supported by other reliable sources. Moderate and heavy alcohol use was identified in 44.7% and 54.8%, respectively, of the whole sample. Mothers who reported a diagnosis of alcohol dependence and those who endorsed having an alcohol problem accounted for 79.8% and 91.2%, respectively. It was not surprising, therefore, that 93.3% of the women were reported as having an additional exposure (tobacco 62%; marijuana 36%; cocaine 38%; methamphetamine 7.4%; and hallucinogens 3.4%) (Astley 2010).

Cohort Studies

Cohort studies also provide information about multiple substance use during pregnancy (T.M. Grant et al. 2018). For example, Gunn et al. (2016) reported on a study with a sample of 218 women, including 141 who gave birth to children with PAE. The researchers found that marijuana use in light and heavy quantities was reported by 11% and 16% of the women, respectively. Additional evidence for high rates of comorbid substance use can be found in multicenter and national databases (Gunn et al. 2016). In the Collaborative Initiative on Fetal Alcohol Spectrum Disorders study (Mattson et al. 2010), data were collected on how many pregnant women also reported using illicit drugs. In the Canadian FASD database project (Clarren et al. 2015) that included more than 26 diagnostic clinics, only 40% of the substance use reported during pregnancy was strictly alcohol; the remainder of the sample, reported use of one or more other illicit substances.

PAE is strongly correlated with cigarette smoking and illicit substance (marijuana and cocaine) use. In a case-control clinic-based study, 20% of women who used alcohol during pregnancy also reported daily use of marijuana (T.M. Grant et al. 2018). Another study of substance use in pregnancy (Richardson et al. 2019) reported relatively high rates of cocaine use (14%) and of cocaine use combined with alcohol (7%).

In studies using population cohorts, a large number of women reported using illicit substances (O'Keeffe et al. 2015). In the Avon Longitudinal Study of Parents and Children, up to 31% of women reported exposure to illicit drugs. Smoking during pregnancy was reported by as much as 17% of the approximately 18,000 pregnant women in a combined national longitudinal cohort from Australia, Ireland, New Zealand, and the United Kingdom (O'Keeffe et al. 2015).

Understanding the Effects of Multiple Substance Exposures

Researchers are beginning to determine the exact nature of the damage caused by multiple substance exposure and other factors. A cohort study of more than 4,000 infants in the ABCD study examined the relationship between exposure to multiple substances and psychosis proneness (Fine et al. 2019). Outcome for the offspring was related to the time in the pregnancy when the woman became aware that she was pregnant. Using the Prodromal Questionnaire, proneness to psychosis in offspring was determined to be elevated in infants exposed to cannabis after the mothers became aware of the pregnancy. This suggests that more prolonged use of cannabis during pregnancy, and consequently more exposure, may account for the increased likelihood of developing psychosis later in life. Unfortunately, the timing and exact amount of cannabis use and potential underreporting make it difficult to draw conclusive inferences from this study. Nevertheless, using the Child Behavior Checklist in this cohort, cannabis exposure was not associated with symptoms of attention, internalizing, or externalizing disorders. This study and other emerging findings conclude by recommending that cannabis use be discouraged in pregnancy.

Researchers have repeatedly found that in utero exposure to cannabis increases the risk of that child later becoming a cannabis user at an early age (Zhang et al. 2017). Furthermore, early onset of cannabis use is a significant risk factor for later cannabis use disorders, as well as depression. If, as researchers propose, with the current cannabis legalization policies, cannabis use during pregnancy increases, then increasing rates of cannabis use disorder will result. It is hard to imagine that these outcomes were considered in the debate for legalization, and that is why policies on alcohol and multiple substances should ideally be informed by current evidence.

Pathophysiological Mechanisms

Kinetic changes in the effect of substances used jointly indicate increases in blood levels of alcohol when combined with cannabis. When used in combination, substances can alter the bioavailability of either or both substance or form a metabolite more toxic than either of the parent compounds alone. In a sophisticated animal experiment, cannabis was found to exacerbate the alcohol-related neurocognitive damage by enhancing pharmacodynamic interactions at the neurotransmitter level (Falcão et al. 2018). The highly toxic metabolite cocaethylene, which develops from a combination of cocaine and alcohol, is more potent than either of the original substances alone (Singer et al. 2000). Fetuses exposed to alcohol and cocaine therefore experience adverse effects from both substances and the additional effect of cocaethylene, which is known to have adverse effects on brain development and has been associated with neurobehavioral disorders (Viteri et al. 2015).

Nicotine use in humans decreases blood alcohol concentration, which could be erroneously conceptualized as protective during pregnancy. In contrast, in situations when a pregnant woman desires the euphoric effect of alcohol, a larger quantity of alcohol will be needed and consumed to achieve that effect because smoking reduces the alcohol concentration and effect. The resulting accumulation of the active and toxic metabolite of alcohol causes damage to the fetus. Volume of distribution of the concentrated metabolite acetaldehyde is larger in the pregnant woman. The more concentrated the circulating acetaldehyde is, the more detrimental the effects on the physiology of the fetus and potential organ damage. All these are likely with the occurrence of concurrent use of multiple substances.

The exact mechanisms of the various combinations of drugs used in pregnancy are still being studied. Researchers have hypothesized a few common pathways. Placental insufficiency and growth restriction are the main mechanisms thought to mediate the abnormalities associated with tobacco use (Kawashima et al. 2014). The effects of tobacco use on placental blood flow, leading to reduced growth rate, affect the fetus more directly. Decreased brain glucose metabolism, maternal vascular disruptions, and neurotransmitter abnormalities are among the suspected mechanisms of polydrug-originated fetal organ damage (Thompson et al. 2009). Anemia was overrepresented in mothers reporting cannabis use during pregnancy (Gunn et al. 2016). In addition to low birth weight, some prenatal and perinatal outcomes have been linked to reduced oxygen availability and oxidative stress, which are also linked to the effect of polysubstance drug use. Other obstetrical risks are increased and mediated through the consequences of precipitated labor; this was suggested by the higher rate of placement in the intensive care unit of infants of mothers who used cannabis compared with mothers who did not. Until more information confirms or clarifies the biological mechanism, outcomes are negative enough to inform educational messages against polysubstance drug use (McGowan and Szyf 2010).

Psychosocial Mechanisms of Adverse Outcomes

The role of the psychoactive effects of combined drug use in contributing to negative developmental outcomes is not only biological or molecular. Researchers have found an association between polysubstance drug use and decreased pregnancy planning, which in turn is related to parents' decreased ability to respond to infants' needs (May and Gossage 2011). For instance, Grant et al. (2005) found that cannabis use in the mother was associated with disrupted attachment and mothers' reduced attentiveness to infants' needs. Other indirect negative effects of postnatal cannabis use on the offspring include motor control problems and breastfeeding difficulties. Similar psychosocial consequences have been associated with mothers' postnatal cocaine use. A disadvantageous home environment and other childhood adversities were indicated as contributing to the long-term effect more than the unique effect of the cocaine exposure (Sandtorv et al. 2017).

Although researchers have found that premature birth, stillbirth, and miscarriages are associated with polysubstance drug use, these outcomes and related postnatal variables are more likely in multiple pregnancies in the same woman. In addition to the timing of drug use, potency, and use of other substances, the amount of psychosocial support, whether mothers and infants experience violence, and financial disadvantage after delivery may contribute to adverse outcomes.

Developmental Origins of Disease and Health: Barker Hypothesis

Understanding the long-term outcomes of prenatal exposure to multiple drugs is incomplete without addressing the developmental origins of disease and health. According to the Barker hypothesis, organ development depends on the fetal environment (Georgieff et al. 2018). The presence of essential factors and absence of unwanted factors in this environment determine the outcome of development. By extension, brain development is negatively affected by deficiencies of essential substances and nutrients. Furthermore, the developmental process is disrupted by toxic factors and substances harmful to the brain. From such early exposures, long-term psychopathology develops, with personal, familial, and social consequences. Prenatal exposure to many substances is the norm in the development of ND-PAE/FASD and is related to its varied clinical manifestations and complexity. To more fully understand the longitudinal perspective of multiple substance exposures and their effects, different developmental mechanisms and outcomes of individual drugs are studied in light of the confluent interactions.

Because of the sheer variety of its functions, the brain is not homogeneous in development and interconnections. To function optimally, the gene-environment interaction aspect of the developmental processes must align with a clock-like precision. When these processes happen under adverse conditions in the fetal environment, developmental abnormalities occur. Abnormalities become more prominent when they occur during peak periods of growth and differentiation, migration, and myelination. The stress-diathesis model influences the final outcome of development, which results from the effects of multiple substance exposure combining and interacting with the interplay of predictive genetic expression. Neural circuitry is constructed in an early developmental phase and is affected by exposure to substances in the fetal environment; thus, long-term physical and psychological adult manifestations have their foundation in fetal life. The various mediators include timing and duration of the exposure and region and/or process (migration, myelination, or neurotransmission) affected. Different trajectories have been established for when environmental agents such as alcohol and other toxic substances (e.g., nicotine, cocaine) interfere with the normally developing fetal brain. The abnormality may be permanent, except in cases where the disruptor, if discontinued, produces reversible effects. In other types of environmental exposures, neural plasticity allows for corrective repairs of the architectural and metabolic abnormalities induced by such polysubstance exposure.

The earlier the exposure, the worse the neurotoxic consequences, because the first trimester is characterized by significant neurodevelopment. If, during the postnatal period, the psychosocial demands placed on an infant with neurocognitive deficits due to multiple drug exposure are significant, brain development is further adversely affected. The weight of the psychosocial demands therefore contributes to predicting worse adult outcomes. Each substance produces a particular abnormality and in combination they produce increased risk to the brain.

Association of Multiple Exposures With Mental Health Outcomes

Mental health outcomes are informed by multiple substance exposure interacting with the fetal environment. Infections during intrauterine life, for example, predict several psychopathological conditions. Researchers found that maternal infection during pregnancy, severe infections, and urinary tract infections increased the risk of the offspring acquiring autism and depression (al-Haddad et al. 2019). Infections in the Swedish cohort with more than 1.7 million participants were identified during hospitalization. These were not specific brain-based infections, which led al-Haddad and colleagues (2019) to suggest the role of any inflammation in predicting offspring mental health outcomes. Other relevant conditions relate to exposure to other substances in the fetal environment. For instance, hyperactivity is a well-documented consequence of prenatal exposure to other nonalcoholic substances (Mela et al. 2013; Weyrauch et al. 2017).

Previous follow-up research of exposed offspring almost exclusively examined cannabis exposure alone and found no significant negative outcomes. However, the concentration of tetrahydrocannabinol (THC), the psychoactive substance in cannabis, has steadily increased in the past two decades, necessitating a reevaluation of its effect on the fetus (Jaques et al. 2014; Mehmedic et al. 2010). High concentrations of THC that combine with PAE result in addictive effects on the fetus. In offspring exposed to multiple substances, executive function deficits similar to those delineated in PAE are recognized. The exact mechanism is not yet understood. This field of research, which includes animal models, recognizes the increasing frequency of use and the additive cascading effect of simultaneous cannabis use with alcohol and other substances. Research is expected to correct the previous inference based on lower THC concentration, refine the methodology, and improve studies of the postdelivery outcomes of combined prenatal cannabis, alcohol, and other drug exposure (T.M. Grant et al. 2018).

Data on cannabis use during pregnancy summarized by Porath-Waller (2018) indicated that subtle effects on the offspring include "deficits in memory, verbal, and perceptual skills; impaired performance in oral and quantitative reasoning and short-term memory; and impaired executive functioning, as well as shortfalls in reading, spelling, and academic achievement" (p. 5). Following exposure to heavy maternal cannabis use, hyperactive, inattentive, and impulsive behavior patterns are reported in children (Porath-Waller 2018). The effects of concurrent use of cannabis and alcohol on academic achievement were researched in a cohort study (Goldschmidt et al. 2004). The rates of concurrent cannabis and alcohol use during the first, second, and third trimesters were 14%, 5.3%, and 5%, respectively (Goldschmidt et al. 2004). Among offspring 10 years of age, the combined exposure resulted in reading and academic underachievement. In the same cohort and among 22-year-olds exposed to marijuana during gestation, higher rates were reported for early onset of cannabis use and diagnosis of cannabis use disorder (Richardson et al. 2019).

Long-Term Outcomes of Prenatal Exposure to Illicit Drugs

Data about illicit drug use in pregnancy are indicative of the potential immediate and long-term adverse consequences on the offspring (Table 3–1). Cocaine use in pregnancy can occur alone, but it is mostly used in combination with other psychoactive drugs. Teasing out the specific effect of each drug is particularly challenging (Chen and Maier 2011). Cocaine's ease of crossing the placental barrier is thought to account for the negative fetal consequences of cocaine exposure alone or when used in combination with other substances of abuse. Earlier reports of congenital abnormality, distinct dysmorphology associated with cocaine, were based on case reports (Chasnoff 1992). Other reports described alterations in working memory, attention, and executive function (Uebel et al. 2015). In a study examining the effects of cocaine exposure on 3-year-old toddlers who completed neurocognitive testing, neurocognitive deficits were associated with cocaine use in utero (Farooq et al. 2009). The outcomes were mediated through findings of small head circumference, home environment, and perseverance in a task. In a comparison of exposure with no exposure in a birth cohort, deficits in general knowledge and visuospatial and arithmetic skills were also detected.

TABLE 3–1. Examples of study types and outcomes from a variety of substances used during pregnancy

SUBSTANCE	NUMBER OF SUBJECTS	AGE OF EVALUATION, YEARS	OUTCOME STUDIED	TYPE OF STUDY
Infection	1,791,520	Up to 41	Autism and depression	Cohort (41 years)
Cannabis	606	10	Reading and academic achievement	Clinical cohort
Cannabis	506	22	Early onset of use and depression	Clinical cohort
Cocaine	225	21	Early onset of use, affect dysregulation, conduct disorder	Case control
Opioids (buprenorphine)	28	5–6	Visuomotor and attention problems	Case report

Opioid use in pregnancy takes the form of prescription drug abuse or illicit use. Attempts have been made to replace illicit opioids with methadone and buprenorphine. The long-term effects of this harm reduction method are not fully understood. Methadone use was, however, linked with higher odds of congenital abnormalities such as tetralogy of Fallot, valvular pulmonary stenosis, and hypertrophic obstructive cardiomyopathy. Drawing conclusive inferences from current studies and findings relating to opioid use in pregnancy has proved difficult. This is because multiple variables exist in those studies. The variety of included drugs, their regular availability as prescriptions, their combined use with street drugs, and uncertain quantity used are a few of the variables. As a result, the long-term effects are yet to be determined.

Recently, the world opioid crisis brought to light the need for more research to understand the impact of exposure to these drugs in pregnancy and their long-term effects. An unprecedented number of people are affected by and dying as a result of the intake of fentanyl and other synthetic opioids. The effects of these opioids on pregnant women will not be known for a number of years and until an accurate estimate of socioeconomic consequences has been obtained. The few available studies reported hyperactivity and attention deficits and memory and perceptual problems in older children following opioid exposure during pregnancy.

Amphetamines (methamphetamine, ecstasy, and caffeine) are CNS stimulants. Use of amphetamines in the general population varies from region to region, and epidemic rates have been associated with an increase in psychotic presentations. There is a paucity of evidence-based data regarding fetal amphetamine exposure. Initial findings (cleft lip and cardiovascular and musculoskeletal abnormalities) of the consequences of exposure during pregnancy require more data to draw any conclusions about characteristic patterns. Other longer-term effects reported include poor growth, lower weight, and reduced head circumference in children and low math scores in adolescents.

Findings of congenital abnormalities, nonchromosomal abnormalities, and disorders of cleft lip and palate are replete in the literature. Musculoskeletal (club foot) and cardiovascular disorders were strongly associated with maternal smoking. Even passive smoking increased the risk of abnormalities. In adults, impulsivity, hyperactivity, inattention, and other externalizing behavior problems were the long-term consequences associated with smoking during pregnancy. Language and learning disabilities were equally associated with smoking in pregnancy. Children exposed to multiple substances in utero are at risk for neonatal abstinence syndrome and low IQ. Genetic vulnerability caused by a high level of substance use was also associated with outcomes of mental disorders.

Clinical and Practical Aspects of Multiple Substance Exposure

Compared with control subjects, school-age children exposed to both alcohol and other substances in utero manifested a higher rate of mental health problems. Among the many factors that influence neurodevelopment, the genetic endowment of the offspring is important. Multiple other biological and psychosocial factors exert their effects on this basic building block of epigenetic process. Interactions of risk factors then culminate in the clinical expression of, for example, multiple drug exposure. Reduced birth weight is an example of the common clinical cue. A clinician who notes reduced birth weight is more likely to associate the several causative risk factors with the resulting neurodevelopmental and mental disorder outcomes. These outcomes are also the product of interactions of neurobiological factors, such as cognitive abilities, with the social environment of the child. Clinically identifying the relevant factors therefore depends on the clinician's knowledge of the child's prenatal and postnatal environment. In a practical sense, seeking evidence of factors relevant to prevention, identification, and intervention with respect to the consequences of multiple substance exposure is an essential component of the comprehensive assessments completed by mental health professionals. Clinicians ask questions of patients and caregivers to estimate the quality and adequacy of the nurturing environment and its potentially mitigating influence on the adverse childhood events known to predispose patients to mental health symptoms. In patients with multiple substance exposure, apportioning specific clinical features to individual drugs remains a challenge. With many other nondrug factors contributing to the final outcome, a method to separate these effects is urgently needed.

One such innovative approach to determine the importance of each risk factor is the polygenic risk score. In behavioral genetics, the polygenic risk score, also known as genetic risk score or genome-wide score, provides the best prediction for the overall trait, taking into account multiple genetic variants. It represents a weighted mean number of disorder risk alleles in approximate linkage equilibrium. Risk alleles for different disorders, for example, ADHD and autism spectrum disorder, have been defined. The scores assist in estimating the contributions of multiple exposures. For instance, maternal host factors such as BMI; alcohol, nicotine, and drug exposures; maternal age; and socioeconomic status have all been shown to affect neurodevelopment in the fetus. In multiple exposures, perinatal adversities become important. Immune system–related conditions and nutritional supplementation and deficiency are also important because of their link to neurodevelopmental disorders. These factors are given different weights in their ability to influence neurodevelopment. A large cohort study, for example, examined the relationship between polygenic risk score and childhood outcomes. The polygenic risk score for ADHD was associated with a range of early life exposures linked to neurodevelopmental disorders in offspring (Stergiakouli et al. 2017). This scoring is one way to estimate the weighted contribution of each of the multiple factors and substances in shaping neurodevelopment. This approach should help in determining the additive and synergistic effects of multidrug exposures and related factors in utero.

Risk Factors Associated With Multiple Substance Use and Fetal Exposure to Multiple Substances

Knowing the relevant risk factors that precipitate the use of alcohol and other substances in pregnancy is a significant step toward creating an adequate prevention program. A clinician with this knowledge is able to identify the at-risk population and put into place modifiers of such risk. When the behavioral and situational root causes of alcohol and substance use are identified, target points for prevention are better understood and addressed. Genetic, behavioral, neurochemical, and social explanations about how alcohol and substance use is inherited apply to the pregnant woman. These explanations implicate specific factors that influence women to use alcohol and drugs. Some factors make using substances more likely in the pregnant woman and at the same time increase the risk of developing negative long-term sequelae. Women with histories of sexual abuse, severe prepregnancy substance use, poverty, mental disorder, and poor coping abilities are overrepresented among multiple drug users in pregnancy. Other less direct factors such as socioeconomic inequalities, lack of education, and poor access to health services perpetuate exposure of the fetus to multiple substances.

A growing body of evidence is focusing on translating identified risk factors into actionable strategies of prevention and intervention. Among 80 mothers of individuals diagnosed with ND-PAE/FASD, 86% reported a lifetime history of drug use. At the time of the study, 9% were actively using illicit substances, and 40% indicated that they used substances around the time of birth of the index child. They also endorsed a high lifetime rate of comorbid mental diagnoses and sexual and physical abuse. Lack of social support was an important factor in separating mothers who were not able to abstain from alcohol use from those who abstained (Astley et al. 2000). Similar factors were identified in a systematic review (Gunn et al. 2016) in which polysubstance use was identified as a factor in the agent. A woman's gynecological history, history of depression, and genetic factors also affect the metabolism of or functional sensitivity to alcohol. The risk factors in the host (woman) were differentiated from the agent (the alcohol) and the environment but collectively contributed to the outcome (May and Gossage 2011).

Response to and Intervention for Multiple Substance Use

Treatment Approaches

Clinical Vignette

A young married woman with a 3-year-old child reports to the clinician at the mental health services clinic that she finds planning and accomplishing anything to be daunting and that she spends a lot of time worrying about this. Her other worries include thoughts that she will have a heart attack and that she is not a good mother. Her dysfunction at home creates intense relationship problems with her husband, who usually fulfills many roles in support of her incapacity. The resulting arguments cause her to resort to drinking rum "to steady my nerves." Within a short time, she begins buying benzodiazepines "on the street" and starts using opiates. Because she is not sleeping, she resumes smoking cannabis. Her child has been diagnosed with intellectual disability.

In consultation with the clinician, this patient expresses a desire to have other children. The contact she has with mental health services affords an opportunity for prevention. Being aware of the risk, the clinician will serve the patient better by offering interventions that include detoxification and rehabilitation. Her case illustrates some of the mental health–associated reasons for alcohol and substance use by women during pregnancy. Distress, relationship difficulties, adverse moods, and ignorance about the teratogenic effect of alcohol contribute to drinking. Giving a woman the choice between alcohol use and contraception has been shown to be successful in reducing the risk of PAE in various populations (Floyd et al. 2007; Hanson et al. 2017). Mental health centers focused on intervention, some with special units, have been addressing the problems of women, with the goal of providing care for the mother as a means to preventing PAE in their offspring. This is relevant because having a child with disability is stressful enough to lead to using multiple substances during pregnancy and thus predicts recurrences (Hill et al. 2000). Identification is therefore the first stage in the process of preventing this pattern, and understanding the contributing mental health factors is in achieving this objective.

The goal of identifying pregnant women at increased risk for multiple substance use is to intervene and prevent known negative outcomes. To this end, clinicians should direct their collective efforts to the provision of behavioral and psychosocial interventions. Ensuring access to medical and obstetric services is part of a package addressing social inequalities among high-risk pregnant women. Services should be comprehensive enough to include social amenities such as adequate housing and financial support. Clinical interventions addressing past trauma and current psychological distress are crucial for reducing substance use and supporting positive outcomes for the child.

Residential treatment, as operated in some jurisdictions, provides stability for the pregnant woman (Harvey et al. 2012) and offers relevant medical and mental health services in one place. Services include trauma, violence, and harm reduction interventions, health promotion information, and support for developing parenting skills after delivery. Services are also commonly linked to a mentoring program for mothers with substance exposure during pregnancy. Intuitively, this mode makes sense because of the severe psychopathology associated with multiple drug use, which is a common problem in the population served (Rutman and Hubberstey 2019). Evidently, the comprehensive and multidisciplinary services evaluated in residential treatment centers have shown effective outcomes on current and future pregnancies. The evaluated programs are accessible to vulnerable pregnant women, offer child advocacy, and provide significant benefits from medical services and addiction workers participating in these programs. They fill a prevention gap (Grant et al. 2005).

The Parent-Child Assistance Program is a model with significant positive outcomes (Grant et al. 2005). A home visitation model started during the cocaine epidemic of the 1980s, this program is offered to pregnant women who are using multiple substances. The program encourages recovery from the substance use and supports the well-being of the offspring by linking mothers to community resources that promote healthy and independent living (T.M. Grant et al. 2018).

Results of treatment effectiveness have been reported related to individual drugs. Contingency management, an approach similar to the rehabilitation method of token economy, has been shown to reduce prenatal alcohol use (Finnegan 2013). Other treatments reported as effective for alcohol use include brief intervention, motivational interviewing, counseling, and psychoeducation. For the treatment of nicotine use during pregnancy, data exist about remedial attempts (smoking cessation, pharmacological replacement, and psychotherapy), but none was found to be effective. Moderate gains were reported for nicotine use with contingency management using financial incentives. Similarly, cannabis and cocaine use reduction is reported as an outcome of brief intervention, contingency management, and cognitive-behavioral therapy (Gilinsky et al. 2011). The conclusions reached from these evaluations are not rigorous enough to recommend them outright, however. Opioid replacement therapy with methadone and buprenorphine is showing promising results. At this time, multimodal approach and support are essential (DiClemente et al. 2017).

Clinical Management

Studies of PAE effect and other significant multiple drug exposures identify a drawback in that patients with these conditions are excluded from research participation. As such, there is no robust evidence base of the clinical management of neonates and children exposed to many substances during pregnancy. This important field was recognized during the thalidomide epidemic in the mid-twentieth century and is now increasingly becoming a source for research and clinical management.

The clinical management of a patient known to use multiple psychoactive substances during pregnancy should include an accurate estimation of the various exposures. It should also involve managing the risk of harm to the fetus to reduce long-term negative outcomes. The exact number and quantity of the different substances may be underreported, however. The illicit nature, stigma, and legal consequences of using the drugs limit the reliability of the information. Because the concentrations of active substances keep changing—mostly increasing—underreporting the amount used translates into more risk to the fetus. Patients are also known to conceal their use, go underground, and avoid seeking help.

To improve the quality and accuracy of the information about the number of substances and exposures, mental health clinicians should vet their sources. Direct interviewing demands a sensitive approach. With permission, close family and support persons can be reliable sources of collateral information. Medical, obstetrical, and pediatric records, as well as information from the referring agents, should be reviewed for evidence of a pattern of substance use, including information about past treatments, medical and legal consequences of drug use, and a history of withdrawal symptoms or syndromes. In some situations, clinicians must rely almost exclusively on collateral information, but collateral sources should be devoid of ulterior motives.

It is possible to detect several substances of abuse in body fluids. Opiates, stimulants, hallucinogens, and solvents are identifiable using simple laboratory and, at times, sophisticated assay methods. Hair analysis for multiple substances is more readily available but may require special procedures to transport samples to specialized laboratories.

Presentation is generally more severe in women who use multiple drugs. They may also be treatment resistant. Because single-drug or -substance use is rarer than combined substance use, the effects reported are more commonly related to multiple substances. For example, cases of specific narcotic withdrawal syndrome still include exposure to alcohol and nicotine for the most part. Harm reduction and drug replacement using prescribed substances are usually effective when the patient is supported by a multidisciplinary group of experts. These experts become acquainted with the patient's cycle of relapse and risk factors and respond to those specific clinical needs. They are better placed to detect misuse of prescribed medications usually given as replacements. Management of misuse and diversion includes reduction of the quantity given to take home, urinalysis, and observed administration of the drug in the presence of health personnel, usually a pharmacist.

Management of Neurodevelopmental Outcomes of Multiple Exposures

It is now well established that exposure to multiple drugs is both a sign of significant vulnerability and a contributor to neurodevelopment abnormalities in the offspring. The vulnerable factors interact with the polysubstance exposure to precipitate multiple mental disorders. The exact mechanism for developing consequences of multiple mental disorders is being studied. Knowledge of genetic vulnerability means clinicians must evaluate whether the parents of exposed individuals have additional risk factors for inheritable mental disorders. To effectively manage exposed individuals, clinicians should be aware of other nongenetic factors, such as quality of the caregiving environment, prematurity, and risk and experience of chronic illness. This knowledge is needed to prevent secondary disability, and when the risk factor is corrected or ameliorated, the chances of positive outcomes are increased. Clinicians will then be able to promote protective factors (e.g., better nutrition, reduced stress, improved sleep, enriched environment, physical activity) that will favor normal development. Providing expert assessment of a neonate, educating caregivers about enrichment strategies, and supporting parental training on managing behavior problems are a few of the steps that will eventually support a positive trajectory of development. Overall, this approach reduces the risk of mental disorder.

Experts specializing in caring for exposed offspring and in directed services are important contributors to intentional prevention and intervention approaches. A neonatologist with a long-term perspective should refer cases of neonatal withdrawal syndrome to clinicians with expertise in neonatal care. Infant child psychiatrists and mental health professionals have been developing specialist services in the field. Currently, these services are based in hospitals because mental health problems are prominent among the reasons these patients are rehospitalized after birth. Collaboration between expert clinicians is key to managing patients with multiple exposures.

Types of Established Services

Collaboration between addiction and mental health services using effective evidence-based strategies should improve access and, ultimately, patient outcomes. Pregnant women at risk for alcohol and substance use disorders need concurrent treatment because of a high comorbid presence of other mental disorders. Effective support and engagement of the patient is most likely when professionals share, cooperate, and communicate.

Some services specialized for substance-exposed children are worth emulating more widely. Although these services are well funded, their model can be modified to suit many jurisdictions, even with minimal funding. For instance, Australian studies recognized health service organizations arranged to offer care to pregnant women. Comprehensive and practical advice was contained in the published clinical guidelines for the management of substance use during pregnancy, birth, and the postnatal period. The document also lists the appropriate services needed to cater to the unmet needs of the population of women (white and aboriginal) to facilitate patient management (Harvey et al. 2012).

Haukeland University Hospital in Bergen, Norway, takes referrals of patients with developmental impairment exposed to nonalcoholic substances. Referrals to the hospital come from health care providers, social workers, and physicians in primary health care, as well as pediatric units and child psychiatric units. Services include specialized assessment, professional consultation, family therapy, and a host of parent-child interventions. This family-centered and rehabilitation-based approach allows researchers to refine approaches and examine the targets of normal development and function.

The Emory Healthcare Brain Health Center also conducts assessment for a large catchment area supported by government funds. The center depends on the expertise of a number of professionals to support families of children exposed to multiple substances. The clinician researchers identify individuals exposed early, collaborate with other experts, and work with agencies to ensure success. Mental health, social, educational, and legal services are integral to the work of the center. The goals of prevention and intervention are central to the work there.

Another example of an established service is the neonatal intensive care unit of University Hospital Rainbow Babies and Children's Hospital in Ohio. The family-centered innovative program engages the services of a part-time consultation-liaison psychiatrist. The need was clearly evident from the evaluation of the first 150 mothers referred when their child was in the neonatal intensive care unit. The reasons for referrals, inability to cope with the child's hospitalization, very low birth weight, and symptoms of mental disorder aligned with multiple substance exposure. Studies of the center's assessments and interventions show positive outcomes. The level of acceptance was good, and satisfaction with the service was high. The durations of consultation and interventions were shortened, suggesting the high value of engaging and caring for whole families.

Such services are very much in need given the increasing rates of substance use in women of childbearing age and the potential of legalization supporting use of marijuana during pregnancy. Prevention efforts should be enhanced given that current efforts have yet to reduce the rates of prenatal exposure to multiple substances. Services incorporating rehabilitation for substance-using mothers, integrating trauma-informed approaches, will address the needs of these patients. Reducing the trauma associated with a poor environment ameliorates the escalating risk factors and could positively improve development. Research is needed given initial results from environment-enhancing strategies.

In a review of the available programs targeting women with substance use, researchers used mixed methods to evaluate the components and benefits of such programs. The eight programs in the Canadian context helped women access better prenatal care and reduced substance use among them. The study identified the following program elements: additional help in developing social support, friendship, and parenting skills and advocating for the children to remain with their mothers (Rutman and Hubberstey 2019). Commenting on the essential components of the programs, Rutman and Hubberstey (2019) characterized these to employ non-judgmental, relationship-based, trauma-informed and harm reduction approaches and that also understand and seek to remove social environmental barriers to participation, such as transportation, child care, meals, stigma, and fear of child removal, have been found to be most effective in reaching vulnerable pregnant and parenting women with substance use issues (p. 17).

The future of psychiatry and mental health care should involve preventive mental health practices. Exposure to substances, developmental impairment, cognitive delay, unstable home life, trauma, and early behavioral problems collectively predispose the exposed to high rates of mental illness.

These disorders can be successfully prevented if the infant develops in an environment where strategies and interventions are implemented that recognize the period of infancy and early childhood development as critical. Negative influences will be reduced, and positive factors of development will be enhanced. By promoting mental health in infants, toddlers, preschoolers, and their families, the infant and child psychiatrist is rightly placed to impact long-term outcomes. Overseeing the contributions of genes, neighborhood, trauma, adversity, and substances, experienced infant and child psychiatrists can chart a new trajectory for individuals exposed to multiple substances and prevent negative mental health outcomes. Such outcomes are premised on taking advantage of interventions that capitalize on the plasticity of the brain at such a period of malleability in the neonate, infant, and young child. The full range of biopsychosocial interventions focus on family and interrelationships using multidisciplinary teams offering the different components of care needed. Selecting high-risk families allows for a more significant impact on the disparities and disadvantages. The families can be taught about the risk of symptoms likely to emerge in individuals exposed to substances and learn how to manage them. Early mental health assessment can be facilitated by raising the level of awareness among caregivers who refer to the services. Early child psychiatry practice can mitigate the social and economic risk factors of multiple substance exposure and the consequent outcome of mental health problems.

Conclusion

Mental health professionals are expected to play an important role in recognizing those affected by alcohol and psychoactive substances, either directly as patients or indirectly as patients' offspring. Clinicians should endeavor to elicit the many relevant environmental and biopsychosocial risk factors in exposed individuals, which will then inform the interventions necessary for the mother–offspring pair. Greater and more severe adverse effects are positively associated with cumulative consequences of multiple risk factors. Heavy polysubstance users are an important clinical group. Clinicians should recognize that these patients are at an increased risk of using larger amounts of substances during pregnancy and will require support throughout pregnancy and beyond. The experts' level of suspicion should be high, given that trauma and maltreatment as well as behavioral problems are commonly associated with substance-exposed children. A preventive perspective should guide programs directed at helping addicted parents and exposed offspring and supporting families. Intervention directed toward mothers serves to reduce harm in exposed offspring, who are at a greater risk of negative outcomes. The same intervention serves to prevent exposure in future pregnancies. Intervention directed at mothers necessitates an understanding of what brought about and perpetuates the substance use, including understanding and empathizing with the multiple negative life circumstances patients contend with. Blaming women for polysubstance drug use is an ineffective approach in reducing use and preventing the outcomes of exposure.

CLINICAL PRACTICAL APPLICATIONS

- A high index of suspicion should prompt clinicians to inquire about polysubstance use in all women during antenatal care.

- Legalization and other social policies interfere with known patterns of use. Clinicians should be current about what is happening in the general population to understand what the prenatal period may entail.

- Obtaining reliable and trustworthy information about substance use in pregnancy relies on the clinician's ability to establish and maintain a therapeutic alliance with the pregnant patient.

- A pregnant woman who smokes may consume more alcohol because nicotine reduces blood alcohol concentration.

- Professionals involved in health education and prevention efforts should explain that the concentration of tetrahydrocannabinol in cannabis products is higher than previously thought.

- It is important to improve access to care in which stigma and the illicit nature of drug use in pregnancy are understood.

- Multiple substance use in pregnancy may indicate failures in the clinical course of care and necessitates management approaches applicable for those with treatment resistance.

- A responsive service for women with mental disorder and substance use concerns should address the dual diagnoses concurrently.

References

al-Haddad BJS, Jacobsson B, Chabra S, et al: Long-term risk of neuropsychiatric disease after exposure to infection in utero. JAMA Psychiatry 76(6):594–602, 2019

Astley SJ: Profile of the first 1,400 patients receiving diagnostic evaluations for fetal alcohol spectrum disorder at the Washington State Fetal Alcohol Syndrome Diagnostic & Prevention Network. Can J Clin Pharmacol 17(1):e132–e164, 2010

Astley SJ, Bailey D, Talbot C, Clarren SK: Fetal alcohol syndrome (FAS) primary prevention through FAS diagnosis: II: a comprehensive profile of 80 birth mothers of children with FAS. Alcohol Alcohol 35(5):509–519, 2000

Carliner H, Mauro PM, Brown QL, et al: The widening gender gap in marijuana use prevalence in the U.S. during a period of economic change, 2002-2014. Drug Alcohol Depend 170:51–58, 2017

Chasnoff IJ: Cocaine, pregnancy, and the growing child. Curr Probl Pediatr 22(7):302–321, 1992

Chen WA, Maier SE: Combination drug use and risk for fetal harm. Alcohol Res Health 34(1):27–28, 2011

Clarren S, Halliwell CI, Werk CM, et al: Using a common form for consistent collection and reporting of FASD data from across Canada: a feasibility study. J Popul Ther Clin Pharmacol 22(3):e211–e28, 2015

Committee on Addictions of the Group for the Advancement of Psychiatry: Responsibility and choice in addiction. Psychiatr Serv 53(6):707–713, 2002

DiClemente CC, Corno CM, Graydon MM, et al: Motivational interviewing, enhancement, and brief interventions over the last decade: a review of reviews of efficacy and effectiveness. Psychol Addict Behav 31(8):862, 2017

Falcão MAP, de Souza LS, Dolabella SS, et al: Zebrafish as an alternative method for determining the embryo toxicity of plant products: a systematic review. Environ Sci Pollut Res Int 25(35):35,015–35,026, 2018

Falk D, Yi HY, Hiller-Sturmhöfel S: An epidemiologic analysis of co-occurring alcohol and drug use and disorders: findings from the National Epidemiologic Survey of Alcohol and Related Conditions (NESARC). Alcohol Res Health 31(2):100–110, 2008

Farooq MU, Bhatt A, Patel M: Neurotoxic and cardiotoxic effects of cocaine and ethanol. J Med Toxicol 5(3):134–138, 2009

Fine JD, Moreau AL, Karcher NR, et al: Association of prenatal cannabis exposure with psychosis proneness among children in the Adolescent Brain Cognitive Development (ABCD) study. JAMA Psychiatry 76(7):762–764, 2019

Finnegan L: Substance Abuse in Canada: Licit and Illicit Drug Use During Pregnancy: Maternal, Neonatal and Early Childhood Consequences. Ottawa, ON, Canadian Centre on Substance Abuse, 2013. Available at: https://ccsa.ca/sites/default/files/2019-04/CCSA-Drug-Use-during-Pregnancy-Report-2013-en.pdf Accessed October 1st, 2020

Floyd RL, Sobell M, Velasquez MM, et al: Preventing alcohol-exposed pregnancies: a randomized controlled trial. Am J Prev Med 32(1):1–10, 2007

Forray A, Merry B, Lin H, et al: Perinatal substance use: a prospective evaluation of abstinence and relapse. Drug Alcohol Depend 150:147–155, 2015

Georgieff MK, Tran PV, Carlson ES: Atypical fetal development: fetal alcohol syndrome, nutritional deprivation, teratogens, and risk for neurodevelopmental disorders and psychopathology. Dev Psychopathol 30(3):1063–1086, 2018

Gilinsky A, Swanson V, Power K: Interventions delivered during antenatal care to reduce alcohol consumption during pregnancy: a systematic review. Addiction Research and Theory 19:235–250, 2011

Goldschmidt L, Richardson GA, Cornelius MD, Day NL: Prenatal marijuana and alcohol exposure and academic achievement at age 10. Neurotoxicol Teratol 26(4):521–532, 2004

Grant KS, Petroff R, Isoherranen N, et al: Cannabis use during pregnancy: pharmacokinetics and effects on child development. Pharmacol Ther 182:133–151, 2018

Grant TM, Ernst CC, Streissguth A, Stark K: Preventing alcohol and drug exposed births in Washington State: intervention findings from three Parent-Child Assistance Program sites. Am J Drug Alcohol Abuse 31(3):471–490, 2005

Grant TM, Graham JC, Carlini BH, et al: Use of marijuana and other substances among pregnant and parenting women with substance use disorders: changes in Washington State after marijuana legalization. J Stud Alcohol Drugs 79(1):88–95, 2018

Green CA: Gender and use of substance abuse treatment services. Alcohol Res Health 29(1):55–62, 2006

Gunn JKL, Rosales CB, Center KE, et al: Prenatal exposure to cannabis and maternal and child health outcomes: a systematic review and meta-analysis. BMJ Open 6(4):e009986, 2016

Hanson JD, Nelson ME, Jensen JL, et al: Impact of the CHOICES intervention in preventing alcohol-exposed pregnancies in American Indian women. Alcohol Clin Exp Res 41(4):828–835, 2017

Harvey SR, Schmied V, Nicholls D, Dahlen H: Key components of a service model providing early childhood support for women attending opioid treatment clinics: an Australian state health service review. J Clin Nurs 21(17-18):2528–2537, 2012

Hasin DS, Stinson FS, Ogburn E, Grant BF: Prevalence, correlates, disability, and comorbidity of DSM-IV alcohol abuse and dependence in the United States: results from the National Epidemiologic Survey on Alcohol and Related Conditions. Arch Gen Psychiatry 64(7):830–842, 2007

Health Canada: A Framework for the Legalization and Regulation of Cannabis in Canada: The Final Report of the Task Force on Cannabis Legalization and Regulation. Ottawa, ON, Health Canada, 2016. Available at: http://healthycanadians.gc.ca/task-force-marijuana-groupe-etude/framework-cadre/alt/framework-cadre-eng.pdf. Accessed October 2, 2020.

Health Canada: Canadian Tobacco Alcohol and Drugs (CTADS): 2015 Summary. Ottawa, ON, Health Canada, 2017. Available at: https://www.canada.ca/en/health-canada/services/canadian-tobacco-alcohol-drugs-survey/2015-summary.html. Accessed October 1, 2020.

Hill SY, Lowers L, Locke-Wellman J, Shen SA: Maternal smoking and drinking during pregnancy and the risk for child and adolescent psychiatric disorders. J Stud Alcohol 61(5):661–668, 2000

Jacobson SW, Chiodo LM, Sokol RJ, Jacobson JL: Validity of maternal report of prenatal alcohol, cocaine, and smoking in relation to neurobehavioral outcome. Pediatrics 109(5):815–825, 2002

Jaques SC, Kingsbury A, Henshcke P, et al: Cannabis, the pregnant woman and her child: weeding out the myths. J Perinatol 34(6):417–424, 2014

Kawashima A, Koide K, Ventura W, et al: Effects of maternal smoking on the placental expression of genes related to angiogenesis and apoptosis during the first trimester. PLoS One 9(8):e106140, 2014

Kinare A: Fetal environment. Indian J Radiol Imaging 18(4):326–344, 2008

Kondracki AJ: Prevalence and patterns of cigarette smoking before and during early and late pregnancy according to maternal characteristics: the first national data based on the 2003 birth certificate revision, United States, 2016. Reprod Health 16(1):142, 2019

Liu Y, Williamson V, Setlow B, et al: The importance of considering polysubstance use: lessons from cocaine research. Drug Alcohol Depend 192:16–28, 2018

Mattson SN, Foroud T, Sowell ER, et al: Collaborative Initiative on Fetal Alcohol Spectrum Disorders: methodology of clinical projects. Alcohol 44(7-8):635–641, 2010

May PA, Gossage JP: Maternal risk factors for fetal alcohol spectrum disorders: not as simple as it might seem. Alcohol Res Health 34(1):15–26, 2011

McGowan PO, Szyf M: The epigenetics of social adversity in early life: implications for mental health outcomes. Neurobiol Dis 39(1):66–72, 2010

McHugh RK, Wigderson S, Greenfield SF: Epidemiology of substance use in re-productive-age women. Obstet Gynecol Clin North Am 41(2):177–189, 2014

Mehmedic Z, Chandra S, Slade D, et al: Potency trends of Δ9-THC and other can-nabinoids in confiscated cannabis preparations from 1993 to 2008. J Forensic Sci 55(5):1209–1217, 2010

Mela M, McFarlane A, Sajobi TT, Rajani H: Clinical correlates of fetal alcohol spectrum disorder among diagnosed individuals in a rural diagnostic clinic. J Popul Ther Clin Pharmacol 20(3):e250–e258, 2013

O'Keeffe LM, Kearney PM, McCarthy FP, et al: Prevalence and predictors of al-cohol use during pregnancy: findings from international multicentre cohort studies. BMJ open 5(7):e006323, 2015

Ordean A, Graves L, Chisamore B, et al: Prevalence and consequences of perinatal sub-stance use—growing worldwide concerns. Subst Abuse 11:1178221817704692, 2017

Porath-Waller AJ: Clearing the Smoke on Cannabis: Maternal Cannabis Use During Pregnancy—An Update. Canadian Centre on Substance Abuse, 2018

Reid C, Greaves L, Poole N: Good, bad, thwarted or addicted? Discourses of sub-stance-using mothers. Crit Soc Policy 28(2):211–234, 2008

Richardson GA, De Genna NM, Goldschmidt L, et al: Prenatal cocaine exposure: direct and indirect associations with 21-year-old offspring substance use and behavior problems. Drug Alcohol Depend 195:121–131, 2019

Rutman D, Hubberstey C: National evaluation of Canadian multi-service FASD prevention programs: interim findings from the Co-Creating Evidence study. Int J Environ Res Public Health 16(10):E1767, 2019

Sandtorv LB, Hysing M, Rognlid M, et al: Mental health in school-aged children prenatally exposed to alcohol and other substances. Subst Abuse 11:1178221817718160, 2017

Scherman A, Tolosa JE, McEvoy C: Smoking cessation in pregnancy: a continuing challenge in the United States. Ther Adv Drug Safe 9(8):457–474, 2018

Singal D, Brownell M, Hanlon-Dearman A, et al: Manitoba mothers and fetal alcohol spectrum disorders study (MBMomsFASD): protocol for a population-based co-hort study using linked administrative data. BMJ Open 6(9):e013330, 2016

Singer LT, Arendt R, Minnes S, et al: Neurobehavioral outcomes of cocaine-exposed infants. Neurotoxicol Teratol 22(5):653–666, 2000

Sonon K, Richardson GA, Cornelius J, et al: Developmental pathways from prenatal marijuana exposure to cannabis use disorder in young adulthood. Neurotoxicol Teratol 58:46–52, 2016

Stergiakouli E, Martin J, Hamshere ML, et al: Association between polygenic risk scores for attention-deficit hyperactivity disorder and educational and cognitive outcomes in the general population. Int J Epidemiol 46(2):421–428, 2017

Substance Abuse and Mental Health Services Administration: Results from the 2012 National Survey on Drug Use and Health: Summary of National Findings (NSDUH Series H-46, HHS Publ No SMA 13-4795). Rockville, MD, Substance Abuse and Mental Health Services Administration, 2013

Substance Abuse and Mental Health Services Administration: Reports and Detailed Tables From the 2016 National Survey on Drug Use and Health (NSDUH). Rockville, MD, Substance Abuse and Mental Health Services Administration, 2017. Available from: https://www.samhsa.gov/data/sites/default/files/cbhsq-reports/NSDUHDetailedTabs2017/NSDUHDetailedTabs2017.pdf. Accessed October 2, 2020

Sundelin Wahlsten V, Sarman I: Neurobehavioural development of preschool-age children born to addicted mothers given opiate maintenance treatment with buprenorphine during pregnancy. Acta Paediatr 102(5):544–549, 2013

Thompson BL, Levitt P, Stanwood GD: Prenatal exposure to drugs: effects on brain development and implications for policy and education. Nat Rev Neurosci 10(4):303–312, 2009

Uebel H, Wright IM, Burns L, et al: Reasons for rehospitalization in children who had neonatal abstinence syndrome. Pediatrics 136(4):e811–e820, 2015

Viteri OA, Soto EE, Bahado-Singh RO, et al: Fetal anomalies and long-term effects associated with substance abuse in pregnancy: a literature review. Am J Perinatol 32(5):405–416, 2015

Volkow ND, Compton WM, Wargo EM: The risks of marijuana use during pregnancy. JAMA 317(2):129–130, 2017

Weyrauch D, Schwartz M, Hart B, et al: Comorbid mental disorders in fetal alcohol spectrum disorders: a systematic review. J Dev Behav Pediatr 38(4):283–291, 2017

Zhang A, Marshall R, Kelsberg G, Safranek S: What effects – if any – does marijuana use during pregnancy have on the fetus or child? J Fam Pract 66(7):462–466, 2017

PART II

Etiology

Etiology

CHAPTER 4

Understanding Etiological Mechanisms

<u>WHAT TO KNOW</u>

The varying degrees of severity of fetal damage due to substance exposure are a product of the timing of that exposure, which can disrupt particular phases of fetal development.

The overwhelming evidence on the outcome of PAE involves the interaction of genetic variables and environmental factors.

Social and health inequalities are a common denominator for PAE, the negative outcomes of PAE, and mental disorders.

Oxidative stress (excess of free radicals versus antioxidants in the body) is one mechanism that explains PAE-related neurocognitive deficits.

DSM criteria for ND-PAE mirror the Institute of Medicine criteria for alcohol-related neurodevelopmental disorder.

DNA methylation and other biological indices are heralded as potential biomarkers for PAE and its consequences.

WHAT TO KNOW

The more subtle the manifestation of damage in the substance-exposed offspring is, the more likely the exposure was minimal and in the later part of pregnancy.

The quest to understand how ingested alcohol exerts negative effects on the fetus has occupied the minds of investigators for years. Its beginnings coincided with the period of scientific inquiry that emphasized the roles of nature and nurture in causing those effects. Study of the outcomes of specific structural dysmorphias and abnormal behaviors found in the offspring of women who drank alcohol during pregnancy helped researchers. It was established that fetal damage occurred because alcohol permeated the placenta. Historically, PAE was given a major role in understanding the postnatal effect and consequences observed in the neonate. The question researchers battled with was whether these outcomes were hereditary. Animal studies conducted at the time attempted to separate the direct prenatal insult of alcohol on a developing fetus (nonhereditary) from a purely hereditary explanation. In the latter, parental alcohol use was linked to generational degradation in the offspring. Current concepts of the etiology, led by the questions raised to clarify the mechanisms of consequences associated with PAE, are more nuanced than those previous simple conceptualizations. In this chapter, I review current understanding of etiology, its relevance to the pathophysiology of mental disorder, and practical application of the knowledge in supporting patients with PAE and its mental disorder sequelae.

The construction of neural circuits can be disrupted when essential factors necessary for normal development are missing. Similarly, abnormal neural circuitry can result from developmental processes in which factors that negatively affect neural tissue development are introduced during prenatal life. These effects are time dependent. The disruptive events and insults of substance exposure can occur early or late in fetal life, producing consequences of varying degrees of severity. Significant cell migration and neuron formation occur in the first 8 weeks of pregnancy. As such, developmental disruption in this early period results in severe structural abnormalities. Events occurring in the second and third trimesters are associated with more subtle effects, becoming only clinically relevant in adult life. Still, they serve as a recognized risk of symptom development later in life.[1]

---

[1] *Interface* is used often in this chapter; see "Introduction" for clarification of meaning.

Gene Environment and Etiology of ND-PAE/FASD

Genetic factors play a role in the etiology of ND-PAE/FASD, expressed through the mechanisms of the variants of alcohol-metabolizing enzymes. These different enzymes interact with the ingested alcohol to produce different outcomes, one of which affects the offspring's IQ. The effect the enzymes exert intersects with the different time course of alcohol metabolism. Alcohol dehydrogenase enzymes catalyze the oxidation of alcohol to the corresponding aldehyde or ketone. Therefore, the metabolic process of alcohol breakdown is genetically determined. Found clustered on chromosome 4, the genetic variation leads to differences in the enzymes' ability to metabolize alcohol (Georgieff et al. 2018). This difference manifests as variable alcohol concentration and outcome effects in the fetus. If the alleles contribute to fast metabolism, the alcohol levels are lower and short lived. Thus, the fetus of a fast metabolizer is less vulnerable to the harmful effects of PAE compared with the offspring of a slow metabolizer. Using a large cohort, Bale et al. (2010) established four different variants of alcohol dehydrogenase that influenced the IQ status of the offspring, but only when the mother drank alcohol during pregnancy. This is an example of the interaction between genes and the environment. In this study, different compositions of genes are recognized, and the interaction explains the origins of the IQ differences in individuals with PAE.

Because alcohol is noted to cross the placenta and influence development, the search for the mechanism responsible began. The final developmental outcome depends on the PAE effect mediated by early fetal programming. The interplay of the effect of the PAE effect on fetal programming in the fetal environment is understood to play a role in organ damage in the offspring. Potential mechanisms related to this process include disruption to placental function, as well as exposure to anoxia, maternal cortisol, and environmental toxins. Additional early fetal programming effects are also mediated by epigenetic changes. These noninherited changes to the genome provide the basis for a strong hypothesis for the development of both mental disorder and consequences of PAE (ND-PAE/FASD). A comparable maternal-child genome-sharing environment occurs in the hypothesis of causation of mental disorders. Important risk factors include malnutrition, stress, smoking, and PAE, and these factors are important prenatally in epigenesis (Paintner et al. 2012). The relevant postnatal factors that contribute to the final negative outcome include neonatal and childhood adversity, impoverished living environment, low socioeconomic status, and poor parenting style.

Relevant Factors in the Etiology of ND-PAE/FASD

Alcohol use is a significant and necessary piece of the puzzle; however, alone it is not sufficient to account for the outcomes of many mental disorders found in individuals with PAE. Even when quantity, frequency, and timing of alcohol use are accounted for, alcohol use fails to be the sole etiological factor, considering the wider epidemiological, clinical, and prognostic implications. Other factors related to the fetal environment (mother or host) that affect outcomes include the number of previous pregnancies, the mother's overall health status, and the mother's age. Additionally, a number of postnatal risk factors have been identified, such as childrearing practices, secure attachment, nurturing, and home stability.

Role of Social Inequalities in Etiological Mechanisms

Consequences of PAE commonly manifest in the form of externalizing (disruptive, hyperactive, and aggressive) behaviors. Especially prevalent in children, these are also prominent in settings where the social determinants of health are unsatisfactory. Mental disorder is similarly overrepresented in the same types of social contexts. It has been proposed that social inequalities may be why high rates of comorbid externalizing disorders, mental disorders, and FASD coexist (Badry and Felske 2013; Lange et al. 2017). With the recognition of the combined effect of the damage from PAE and the socioeconomic environment of adversity, poor parent-child interaction was postulated as the essential process that informs the adverse outcomes. Poor quality of maternal caregiving and the all too common experience of unstable foster care placement combine to explain the increased vulnerability to externalizing disorders in FASD.

Many host and environmental factors contribute to aggravating or ameliorating the impact of the original brain injury in FASD. As noted, these factors on their own do not constitute the whole explanation of the mechanisms by which FASD develops. The importance of host and environmental factors lies in guiding clinicians to understand the mechanism of damage and its outcomes. With that knowledge, clinicians work to prevent FASD and other consequences of PAE by enhancing the environment in which the child is raised. For exposed children, adequate nutrition, home stability, appropriate parenting style, and an enriched environment modify the outcomes for mental disorder and the negative outcomes of PAE. Access to services for diagnosis and early intervention are important for their long-term survival. Psychosocial factors, including social and financial support, have been associated with more positive outcomes. In the absence of these protective factors, FASD and negative consequences result. These factors mitigate those long-term outcomes as shown in a very early study. Streissguth et al. (1996) identified diagnosis before the age of 6 years, a stable and nurturing home environment, fulfillment of basic needs, and the absence of experienced violence as protective against the negative outcomes of PAE. Herein lies the importance of monitoring and modifying the social determinants of health.

Clinical Vignette

The adoptive parents of a 7-year-old patient request an appointment on behalf of their daughter, who was recently diagnosed with ND-PAE. Both parents are university lecturers. Their daughter was adopted from Romania. The parents are concerned because they do not know anything about the negative consequences of PAE. Their daughter is quick-tempered; aggressive with property, including her dolls; sleeps poorly; and sometimes oppositional. The adoption papers were recently mailed to them, and the papers revealed that their daughter's biological mother used alcohol and other drugs during her pregnancy. The couple is determined to raise their daughter, and they want some explanation of the behavioral manifestations they witness. They have questions about the mechanism by which the damage could have occurred and want to know if there is anything they can do to foster a more positive trajectory for their daughter.

The consultation should allow parents to voice their concerns, ask questions, and receive additional helpful information. More than one appointment may be necessary, especially when parents feel overwhelmed about the prospect of raising a child with a disability. The clinician should provide a list of and contact information for resources available for the patient and her parents, including support groups found through the National Organization on Fetal Alcohol Syndrome. Parents can provide positive prospective social determinants of health, such as a nurturing environment and good nutrition, and with effort can foster the child's sense of secure attachment. This concerted support can make a difference. Protective actions can mitigate damage. Conversely, identified risk factors such as malnutrition, adverse childhood experiences, and poor attachment aggravate the brain dysfunction. It is important that parents be well informed about the burden of care, which is known to be high with chronic disorders. They should be aware of the transitions (such as starting school or finishing school and beginning friendships), sources of support, and available treatment proven to be helpful.

Role of Etiological Factors in Understanding Other Mental Disorders

Over the past three decades, significant progress has been made in understanding the multiple factors that contribute to mental disorder. Previous binary and simple models of psychic conflict interacting with the parenting environment have given way to more nuanced biopsychosocial approaches. Knowing the risk factors is essential in a pursuit to target treatment to specific symptoms and contributory factors and thereby improve patient outcomes. Recent advances in technology, innovations in genetics through the Human Genome Project, and analysis of large referent data have led to improved knowledge about the causes of mental disorder. The significant contributions of various etiological factors to mental disorder are beginning to be recognized. This is the case for disorders with a high heritability: velocardiofacial syndrome associated with psychotic disorders; a specific genetic contribution to narcolepsy and its psychiatric manifestation; and the imbalance of hormones that contributes to the experience and expression of sexual deviation or mood conditions. The exact weight of the contribution of each factor continues to be researched. Already these discoveries have made it into the respective mental disorder classification systems, signifying how important these high-heritability factors are in disorder criteria (American Psychiatric Association 2013).

The concept of trauma as a cause for PTSD can shed light on how to estimate the weight contributed by certain etiological factors of mental disorder. Exposure to significant trauma, which leads to PTSD in 20% of women and 8% of men, does not mean that it is the only relevant etiological reason for the diagnosis. PTSD research identified other relevant factors that contribute significantly to the development of PTSD even after a serious traumatic event. History of sexual abuse, other related past trauma, and genetic predisposition are considered risk factors and provide additional information for the explanatory mechanisms. Some factors are major contributors, and others are minor risk or prognostic factors for PTSD (Shalev 2001). Understanding this concept of major and minor contributions can assist in understanding the mechanisms for the acquisition of FASD and, by extension, of associated mental disorder sequelae of PAE. The genetic composition of the mother and the fetus, quantity and timing of alcohol exposure, and postnatal factors all contribute to the PAE outcome, albeit with differential weights for each component. Another paradigm involves the etiological role of chromosome 22. If detected, its presence elevates the diagnosis of a psychotic disorder (O'Rourke and Murphy 2019). Similarly, PAE should assist clinicians in attributing causality to the symptoms of neurocognitive deficit present in patients. Consideration of these deficit symptoms allows the consequences of PAE and mental disorder outcomes to be linked. Doing so ascribes a certain weight of PAE to the specific outcome under consideration.

Understanding the etiology of a disorder informs many clinical applications. One function is employing an etiological framework to classifying categories of mental disorder. Conceptualized as a risk and prognostic factor among many other factors, PAE is recognized as making a minor contribution to DSM-5 diagnoses and conditions. PAE's role is noted in various sections of DSM-5, including under developmental coordination disorder, autism spectrum disorder, and ADHD. In those disorders, PAE plays a limited role, but PAE is etiologically a major contributor to ND-PAE (see DSM-5 Section III, "Conditions for Further Study" [American Psychiatric Association 2013]). It is curious, and likely a product of differential scholarship, that the same contributor (PAE) is given such dissimilar weight when considering etiology; etiology continues to be considered separately for individuals with FASD and those with other diagnosed mental disorders. For the mental health professional, early identification is favored for individuals with PAE to prevent worse outcomes (Streissguth et al. 2004). Clinicians who have advanced knowledge of the PAE–mental disorder mechanism of etiology are better able to identify clinical cases in which PAE is closely related to mental disorder. That awareness informs the comprehensive care that facilitates access to appropriate treatment and support for patients. Apart from the explanations of DSM-5 in apportioning differential weights to the PAE-related disorders, the relationship between mental disorder and PAE outcomes shares relevant cardinal features and a few superficial differences.

Among differences noted for those with FASD/ND-PAE, they have been identified distinctly by a history of binge drinking, alcohol dehydrogenase genetic polymorphism, abnormalities of DNA methylation, and, for the most part, a larger etiological effect of PAE (Lewis et al. 2012). Additionally, a subset of this population is distinguished by unique pathognomonic facial dysmorphia and growth retardation. Neurocognitively, a specific characteristic pattern of sluggish cognitive tempo associated with executive functioning deficits is an exclusive finding in individuals with PAE (Graham et al. 2013). Although a specific neuropsychological profile has been elusive, there may yet be unique neurocognitive and neuroanatomical differences ascribed to PAE damage (Kodituwakku and Kodituwakku 2014). On the basis of the sheer number of medical comorbidities associated with PAE, whole-body disorder is the current term used to describe the observable physical manifestations. Their specificity has not yet been subjected to scientific rigor and etiological hypothesis.

In individuals with mental disorder, current explanations implicate the gene-environment interaction in etiology. Furthermore, rather than a single big factor of etiology, it is postulated that multiple factors add cumulative small effects to produce the final outcome. Prevention is a major theme in the treatment of PAE and the resulting diagnostic outcomes. Using preventive strategies to address mental disorder is still at a level best described as emerging. Mental disorder and treatment approaches have long been subjected to rigorous evaluations. A wide range of research is available, and there are particular treatment protocols and specific indications for the biopsychosocial treatment of patients with mental disorder. These treatment programs are better described as evidence-based programs. Treatment for individuals with PAE and its outcomes is still in its infancy and not as readily available; at best, there exist promising practices.

Despite the differences between individuals with PAE and those with mental disorders, some similarities still make distinguishing them challenging. Both populations share a high rate of family history of mental disorders and overall low IQs. (It is worth noting that a wide range of IQs has been reported in both PAE outcomes and mental disorder, including superior intelligence [Quattlebaum and O'Connor 2013].) There are common explanatory models for affect regulation difficulties experienced by individuals with PAE and those without PAE who have other mood and anxiety disorders. Abnormalities associated with the hypothalamic-pituitary-adrenal axis manifest as lack of moderation of affect, and this connection appears to be true for patients at the interface of PAE and mental disorder. Consequences of both conditions manifest common features of conduct disorder, externalizing and internalizing disorders, hyperactivity, impulsivity, and criminality; comorbidity with multiple diagnoses is the norm, and distinguishing categorical and dimensional models of taxonomy bedevils the fields of etiology and diagnosis. Figure 4–1 demonstrates the various factors at play in the understanding of the mechanisms of damage.

Understanding the Mechanisms for Coexisting ND-PAE/FASD and Mental Disorder

One possible explanation of the relationship between FASD and comorbid mental disorders is etiological. Patients with ND-PAE/FASD and those with other mental disorders share similar findings of hyperreactivity to stress, brain alterations in neuroimaging, and electrophysiological changes. Another etiological implication is the high rates of comorbid disorders in

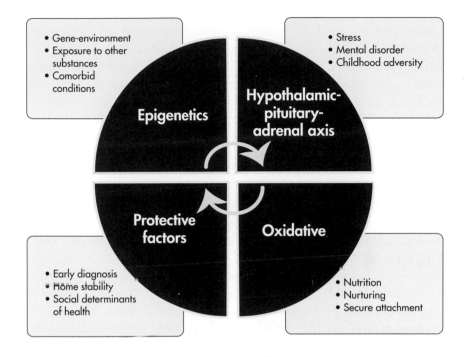

FIGURE 4–1. Interaction of suspected etiological mechanisms of PAE and factors associated with the mechanisms.

patients with ND-PAE/FASD and those with mental disorder. Additionally, mental disorder and ND-PAE/FASD have in common similar treatment approaches, suggesting an intricate relationship. Despite these similarities, the interface of these conditions is still riddled with unexplained relationships and enmeshed mechanisms that are responsible for developing each disorder or both in persons affected.

Phenomenology of Pathophysiology and Etiological Mechanisms

The first label given to the abnormality associated with PAE was FAS. Attaching the agent, alcohol, to the name implied a causative role. This label informed models subsequently developed to understand the etiology and pathophysiology of the damage resulting from PAE. Consequently, alcohol as a teratogen received significant weight in explaining the latter manifestations of the damage to the fetus. Although the exact molecular etiology is not completely understood, some hypotheses were only possible because of studying the teratogenic effect of alcohol. Currently, alcohol is proposed to induce apoptotic cell death at the molecular level, causing damage as it acts on the fetal brain. The agreed mechanisms that facilitate apoptosis include increase in oxidative stress, decrease in nerve growth factors, and damage to neurotransmitters. Additional factors that have been identified as having possible implications include cell signaling defects, changes in gene expression, and deficiencies of essential nutrients such as iron, choline, folic acid, and vitamins. Historically, these different mechanisms were presented linearly, with alcohol as the most significant agent of damage. However, more recently, it has been noted that it is likely these mechanisms or potential pathways interact with one another.

ND-PAE is designated as a condition for further study in DSM-5; this allows for original comparative studies in mental health patients (American Psychiatric Association 2013). So far, research has indicated that the DSM criteria for ND-PAE are reliable and valid (Kable and Coles 2018). Additional research is needed to refine the weight of factors that intersect or differentiate ND-PAE from other mental disorders. Current evidence suggests that multiple factors contribute to individual effects that combine to cause mental disorder. In a large cohort study, consumption by the mother of >21 units of alcohol per week, especially in the first trimester, was significantly associated with the presence of psychotic-like symptoms in the 12-year-old offspring (Zammit et al. 2009). These associations were found to likely reflect genetic vulnerabilities and shared familial mechanisms.

This etiological role ascribed to alcohol is not sufficient to lay to rest the search for explanatory models for how mental disorder and outcomes of PAE actually relate. There is reason for optimism in studying the importance of phenomenology and disease classification. Now introduced into the classification system, ND-PAE becomes an entity available for research. Focusing the search of the available evidence and new research on the etiological classification of the diagnostic categories should illuminate new insights. Research should endeavor to recognize and isolate contributing factors that have etiological relevance. For example, recognition of the 30-fold risk of schizophrenia and psychosis in people with 22q11.2 deletion syndrome (O'Rourke and Murphy 2019) aligns with efforts to identify etiological factors of schizophrenia. The chromosomal abnormality assumes a large effect in schizophrenia causation.

Acknowledgment of 22q11.2 deletion has both a classification and etiological significance and can be applied to PAE's role in causation. Through the mechanism of heritability, PAE contributes to an etiological understanding of alcohol and substance use (addiction) disorders and other externalizing and neurodevelopmental disorders. Specifically, PAE was shown to predict alcohol use disorder better than a family history of alcohol and substance use. The value of PAE in the etiology of mental disorder was further teased out when PAE among adoptees predicted early onset of mental disorder and use of multiple substances (nicotine, drugs, and alcohol) (Grant et al. 2013; Yates et al. 1998). Through more research in phenomenology, the etiological role of PAE in other mental disorders will be better recognized and understood in the future. DSM-5 has already included PAE as a predictive risk factor in ADHD and developmental coordination disorder (Harris et al. 2015).

To comprehend the etiology of disorders at the interface of PAE and its outcomes, nurture and nature paradigms should be embraced. Symptom consistency across ages is a parameter used to establish the etiological origin of a disorder such as ND-PAE. This is because the neural underpinnings of the disorder are inferred from a large proportion of subjects who retain the same diagnosis over time once it is made. The changes noted in other inconsistent evaluations were associated with shifting diagnostic classification and not etiological error. Consistent diagnostic and symptom patterns were achieved when 3- to 10-year-old children diagnosed with ND-PAE were evaluated (Kable and Coles 2018). The children responded to questions regarding the different factors that influenced their symptoms. Environmental factors did not affect symptom endorsement. ND-PAE symptoms were highly consistent and did not vary by age. In another study, researchers found that DSM-5 ND-PAE criteria accurately described 89.5% of subjects previously diagnosed with alcohol-related neurodevelopmental disorder (Johnson et al. 2018). Coherence and confluence of the two diagnostic systems were therefore evident. This means that even mental health professionals with different backgrounds, mainly psychiatrists and psychologists, are able to diagnose the consequences of PAE using the diagnostic frameworks with which they are comfortable. To ensure the etiological role of PAE is scientifically sound, diagnosis of ND-PAE/FASD should be valid and reliable. It can then be inferred that an entity like ND-PAE/FASD can be measured and quantified. There are still limitations to the rigor expected of the diagnostic process. Pathophysiology and etiology are not necessarily dependent on diagnostic criteria and are not the only reason for using DSM. DSM's other equally important purposes are ensuring consistent communication among clinicians, easing access to health care treatment for people with a specific diagnosis, and providing recognizable coding required for qualifying for health insurance benefits. The advantages of diagnosing ND-PAE/FASD include improving access to diagnostic services, fostering communication between professionals, calculating prevalence of the disease, and by having a diagnostic system, those at risk are not misdiagnosed (Cook et al. 2018). It is important to realize that some jurisdictions provide access to care services based on measured level of impairment and not diagnosis.

In such jurisdictions, the diagnostic process and efforts provide no advantage to the person seeking services.

The field of epigenetics is providing a more cogent understanding of the significance of PAE, which is known to cause widespread changes in gene expression with relevance to etiology (Lussier et al. 2017). DNA methylation changes, as identified in the hypothalamus in an animal model, have emerged as potential mediators and biomarkers for neurodevelopmental and mental disorders because they share numerous phenotypes and comorbidities. Through the link between the genome, environmental conditions, and neurodevelopmental outcomes, epigenetics explains reprogramming of the neurobiological systems (Lussier et al. 2018). Two recent human studies confirm the role of DNA methylation in the pathophysiological explanation of PAE-induced damage; thus, DNA methylation changes are potential biomarkers for PAE (Lussier et al. 2018).

Neurocognitive Features of the Etiological Mechanisms

Neurocognitive development is essentially a fetal process with postnatal modifications. Several conditions with developmental origins (schizophrenia, autism, anxiety/mood disorders, learning disabilities, and intellectual disability) share similar processes. Clinical reports of patients assessed for an FASD diagnosis commonly identify previously diagnosed mental disorder (Bertrand et al. 2004). Researchers and clinicians explain this finding differently. When two separate disorders are diagnosed in one person, some refer to this as a misdiagnosis, whereas others use the concepts of dual diagnosis or comorbid diagnosis. The coexistence of diagnoses is particularly common and challenges basic assumptions about patients with PAE. There is no unique pattern of neurocognitive features for these individuals. Patients with PAE and its consequences have multiple diagnoses, which, at times, change with age and the clinical orientation used to understand their etiology. When comparing the common features in patients with PAE and those with different DSM diagnoses, similarities were found for virtually all the clinical features, a finding that cut across age groups (children, adolescents, and adults).

Interrupting or intruding behavior in children occurs as a consequence of PAE; disorders with similar symptom effects include autism, ADHD, bipolar disorder, and depression. The inability to consider consequences is a well-known symptom of PAE that is also attributed to sensory integration disability, autism, and bipolar disorder. Mood swings are a neurocognitive manifestation of PAE typically also found as sequelae to trauma, oppositional defiant disorder (ODD), depression, reactive attachment disorder, bipolar disorder, and ADHD. These overlapping symptoms bring together co-occurring disorders, which could be the ultimate expression of misdiagnosis or misattribution of neurocognitive symptoms. It is entirely possible that comorbidity is to be expected in patients with PAE, given its ubiquitous etiology and pathophysiology similar to mental disorders.

Hyperactive, inattentive, and impulsive symptoms, for instance, are likely the shared symptoms most frequently seen in the diagnoses of FASD and ADHD. Conduct disorder, ADHD, attachment disorder, and ODD were reported as the most prevalent comorbid DSM diagnoses among individuals with PAE (Weyrauch et al. 2017). As in symptom manifestation, the diagnostic consequences of PAE exist along a continuum of various diagnostic criteria. Comorbid explanations may have etiological relevance and are based on the pathophysiological similarities of PAE and other mental disorders. It is likely that a few patients at the interface will have a comorbid or dual diagnosis. Other patients at the interface have clearly been misdiagnosed, as evidenced by several streams of research. Research has found unusually high rates of misdiagnosis. ND-PAE/FASD was commonly misdiagnosed as the DSM diagnoses of adjustment disorder, reactive attachment disorder, ADHD, or PTSD (Chasnoff et al. 2015). If misdiagnosed, inappropriate support and misdirected intervention mean that clinical distress and dysfunction are prolonged; this compounds the complexity of the manifestation. The diagnoses found to be comorbid with FASD are the same conditions that are easily misdiagnosed instead of FASD. Individuals with FASD are frequently misdiagnosed, and their deficits have been noted as a misattribution of the neurocognitive deficits caused by PAE. This confusion of symptoms and diagnoses calls for a better understanding of the unique features of the consequences of PAE and, more relevantly, the formulation of a comprehensive diagnosis. One way to improve identification is to adopt more parsimonious bases for these common diagnoses (Glass and Mattson 2017). Still, a more comprehensive assessment is needed to explain causation in line with the neurocognitive deficits of ND-PAE/FASD.

To explain how such misattribution complicates the clinical picture of patients with FASD, some authors focused their attention on two disorders: reactive attachment disorder and autism spectrum disorder, based on the common social skills impairment. Expressing social impairment is integral to the neurocognitive abnormalities resulting from PAE. A distinct lack of understanding of social cues and indiscriminate social behavior makes communicating in social contexts difficult for patients with FASD (Streissguth 1997). Social skills deficits have been shown to occur in both adolescents and adults (Olson et al. 1998) with PAE. These can easily be confused with lack of inhibition, withdrawal, intentional inappropriate approaches, and unsafe involvement with strangers. These behaviors are also common manifesting features of reactive attachment disorder and autism spectrum disorder; similar neurocognitive manifestations are found in various forms of DSM attachment disorders (American Psychiatric Association 2013). Sorting out the different diagnoses requires a careful, prudent approach and substantial knowledge of FASD from mental health professionals.

Researchers who adhere to a hierarchical model adopting the most parsimonious principle (De Jong et al. 1984; McKenzie et al. 1993) prefer to see the neurocognitive deficits of PAE as foundational to the emergence and temporal nature of DSM comorbid disorders. Knowing the neurocognitive differences in the spectrum of disorders helps identify the most responsible diagnosis.

Contribution of Treatment to the Etiological Mechanisms

Given the multiple genetic and environmental factors at play in the phenotypic manifestations of PAE and mental disorder, potential interventions depend on the contribution of each factor. Certain aspects of the treatment of patients with PAE share similar properties with the more standardized and established treatment for mental disorders. The biopsychosocial treatment approach is used for mental disorder and ND-PAE/FASD, albeit with few modifications. The genetic and environmental similarities provide further explanation of how the damage of PAE occurs, which may suggest comparable or complementary targets for treatment, similar to the biopsychosocial approach of mental disorder. For instance, PAE-induced neurotransmitter damage, which informs treatment with specific ligands, forms a common treatment pathway for both PAE and its consequences and mental disorder and its pathogenesis. Stimulants, antipsychotics, and antidepressants are widely used in the treatment of ND-PAE/FASD, suggesting these medications, which are used to treat many mental disorders, may be acting on targets akin to those of mental disorders (Petrenko and Alto 2017). Evidence is being sought on the effectiveness of psychotropic medications that act on adrenergic, dopaminergic, and serotonergic pathways (Mela et al. 2018; O'Malley and Nanson, 2002). Treatment of neurocognitive deficits in PAE and mental disorder should have common pathways, given the profile similarities at the PAE–mental disorder interface. Approaches used for intellectual disability with neurocognitive deficits have not been widely applied to the consequences of PAE. Cognitive remediation is an up-and-coming practice with growing and promising evidence for mental disorders characterized by neurocognitive deficits in executive function, attention, memory, and intellect; a similar approach may be successful for treatment of ND-PAE/FASD. The future understanding of etiology will benefit from comparing treatment outcomes of individuals at the interface to identify shared treatment pathways. Until then, prevention remains a discipline where approaches with effective outcomes may be shared to reduce the negative consequences of PAE and related mental disorders.

Application of Knowledge to the Etiological Mechanisms

There are benefits to knowing how a patient's symptoms came to be from an etiological perspective. First, treatments are informed by knowledge of the pathophysiology. When the etiology is fully understood, treatments are more targeted. Second, given the stigma associated with PAE, explanation about the comprehensiveness of causation educates patients on why they are the way they are. Such knowledge can help relieve shame and guilt, empowering the affected person. If this explanation is provided in a supportive manner, it is liberating and fundamental to the patient's motivation and to enhancement of treatment adherence. This was shown to be true in severely ill patients with schizophrenia, and there is every reason to apply similar approaches to patients with ND-PAE/FASD and related disorders (Bäuml et al. 2016; Petrenko and Alto 2017).

Relatives are better able to process the patient's behaviors through an etiological lens and to shift their belief that the behaviors are due to bad parenting. Recognizing the importance of etiological mechanisms, a number of training and intervention programs were developed with parents in mind. Because nurturing and good-quality caregiving are consistent with the protective factors of positive outcomes, parental education and training flowed automatically to address these same etiological factors. Programs such as Breaking the Cycle and Coaching Families as well as parent training workshops provide FASD education and use approaches geared toward correcting etiological factors. These programs all seem to produce positive benefits (see Figure 14–1 in Chapter 14, "Psychological Treatment"). An indirect benefit is reduced burden of care, which is typically high in caregivers. Under the care of well-informed clinicians, patients who are known to have specific deficits enjoy the holistic approach to care. These clinicians know that the whole body is possibly affected, and thus, they do not only attend to the manifesting complaints; they avoid compartmentalizing the symptoms.

Through the life trajectory of patients affected by PAE, a common experience is that they have to navigate many systems within the health and social sectors. Professionals in these sectors unknowingly approach patients with deficits as though they were competent (Grant et al. 2013, 2014). Under such assumptions, and without the knowledge of the cause and origin of the damage, they use traditional approaches (screening, assessment, diagnosis, treatment, prevention, and prognostication) for these patients, and the result is either ineffectual or even harmful. Therefore, knowledge of neurocognitive deficits is essential for mental health professionals in these sectors to modify their approach to these patients (Grant et al. 2013). This knowledge is also beneficial in a social environment. An employer is better able to place a neurocognitively impaired person in a position in which his or her strengths are maximized. By adjusting the workplace environment, the employer ensures responsivity to the style of learning and facilitates support of observed weaknesses of a person who was prenatally exposed to alcohol. Support in the long run may help ensure a stable work environment; it enhances self-confidence and productivity. In court and criminal and civil justice systems, individuals are better protected if their caregivers and administrators are conversant with the FASD-related deficits in people encountering the system (Fast et al. 1999). Therefore, teachers, social workers, justice officials, corrections workers, and mental health frontline workers need information about the weaknesses and strengths of the people with whom they interact. This knowledge is informed by an understanding of the mechanisms involved in acquiring the consequences of PAE. The same information can be used to advocate for insurance, housing, employment, and educational support. That is the value of a comprehensive assessment, which is an integral process in diagnosing patients with PAE and its sequelae. Without such assessment results, suffering is perpetuated and negative outcomes are perpetuated.

The plethora of factors that combine to produce the negative outcomes of PAE imply that if corrected and modified, the same factors could be protective. The mother–child relationship serves as a model for building resilience; the opportunity to develop a healthy attachment with an adult mitigates a chaotic upbringing environment. Other stable persons and consistent adults in the life of the offspring with PAE provide models for secure attachment. This has protective value. Attempts to correct an impoverished environment, provide a nourishing diet, and eliminate abuse serve to increase resilience. Ensuring that the offspring is kept in stable housing and receives consistent care has been shown to enhance positive outcomes. These care strategies are informed by knowledge of the relevant factors that guide professionals and family members to understand the etiology of PAE outcomes.

Advocating for cognitively impaired patients not only engages these patients but also provides policymakers with important information for improving services. Previously, mental health and social services were not responsive to the needs of patients specifically identified as affected by PAE. Positive indices of social return on investment have been reported in jurisdictions where policies developed in response to such advocacy were reviewed and evaluated (Jonsson et al. 2018). The primary explanation was a change in policy as a result of understanding the etiology and the basic mechanisms involved in FASD (Jonsson 2019). On the basis of this knowledge, innovative programs can target PAE-related deficits, expand the diagnostic services, and emphasize well-informed prevention programs. Therefore, enhanced support is essential for the full and complete understanding of the mechanisms of causation to have a holistic impact on all systems of care, systems in which professionals regularly come in contact with someone with PAE.

Conclusion

More nuanced explanation of the outcomes of PAE implicates gene expression, the social determinants of health and mental health, and the complex interaction of PAE and other causes of mental disorder. The developmental origin of disease and health is the leading concept in acknowledging how fetal programming is affected by PAE. Alcohol is a necessary, heavily weighted factor—yet by itself an insufficient factor—in the pathophysiology of PAE outcomes. Interacting factors in the mother, the fetus, and the environment determine outcome in the offspring. Some of these factors, such as nutrition, stress, mood disorder, use of other substances, and genetic predisposition, help align the consequences of PAE and other mental disorders. Postdelivery, protective factors may include a nurturing environment, secure attachment, early access to diagnosis and care, and prevention of adverse childhood experiences. The value of this knowledge about etiological mechanisms lies in the recognition of factors amenable to efforts directed toward prevention and intervention. Clinically, mental health professionals target trauma and integrate strategies to apportion variable weights to etiological factors. They attempt to separate misdiagnosed patients from those manifesting comorbidity. The requisite skills, which stem from knowledge of the mechanisms involved in the development of ND-PAE/FASD with or without other mental disorders, inform patient care.

CLINICAL PRACTICAL APPLICATIONS

- Because no safe limits have been established, abstinence from alcohol and substances during pregnancy is recommended.

- Prevention of adverse outcomes of PAE should address childhood adversity, quality of attachment and parenting practices, residential stability, nutrition, and education.

- Early intervention, which engages multiple and well-informed professionals with the patient, is preferable.

- Because family history of mental disorder and lower IQ are shared by patients with PAE and those with mental disorder, this should be explored.

- Mental health professionals' clinical use of the DSM-5 diagnostic criteria can contribute to the refinement of the diagnostic criteria of ND-PAE.

- Cognitive remediation may benefit a certain group of patients with specific neurocognitive deficits of ND-PAE/FASD.

- Patient and social justice advocacy remains a strong tool for clinicians hoping to improve health outcomes in their patients with ND-PAE/ FASD.

References

American Psychiatric Association: Diagnostic and Statistical Manual of Mental Disorders, 5th Edition. Arlington, VA, American Psychiatric Association, 2013

Badry D, Felske AW: An examination of the social determinants of health as factors related to health, healing and prevention of foetal alcohol spectrum disorder in a northern context: the Brightening Our Home Fires Project, Northwest Territories, Canada. Int J Circumpolar health 72, 2013

Bale TL, Baram TZ, Brown AS, et al: Early life programming and neurodevelopmental disorders. Biol Psychiatry 68(4):314–319, 2010

Bäuml J, Pitschel-Walz G, Volz A, et al: Psychoeducation improves compliance and outcome in schizophrenia without an increase of adverse side effects: a 7-year follow-up of the Munich PIP-Study. Schizophr Bull 42 (suppl 1):S62–S70, 2016

Bertrand J, Floyd RL, Weber MK, et al: Fetal Alcohol Syndrome: Guidelines for Referral and Diagnosis. Atlanta, GA, Centers for Disease Control and Prevention, National Center on Birth Defects and Developmental Disabilities, 2004

Chasnoff IJ, Wells AM, King L: Misdiagnosis and missed diagnoses in foster and adopted children with prenatal alcohol exposure. Pediatrics 135(2):264–270, 2015

Cook JL, Green CR, Lilley C, et al: Response to "A critique for the new Canadian FASD diagnostic guidelines." J Can Acad Child Adolesc Psychiatry 27(2):83–87, 2018

De Jong A, Giel R, Lindeboom EG, et al: Foulds' hierarchical model of psychiatric illness in a Dutch cohort: a re-evaluation. Psychol Med 14(3):647–654, 1984

Fast DK, Conry J, Loock CA: Identifying fetal alcohol syndrome among youth in the criminal justice system. J Dev Behav Pediatr 20(5):370–372, 1999

Georgieff MK, Tran PV, Carlson ES: Atypical fetal development: fetal alcohol syndrome, nutritional deprivation, teratogens, and risk for neurodevelopmental disorders and psychopathology. Dev Psychopathol 30(3):1063–1086, 2018

Glass L, Mattson SN: Fetal alcohol spectrum disorders: a case study. J Pediatr Neuropsychol 3(2):114–135, 2017

Graham DM, Crocker N, Deweese BN, et al: Prenatal alcohol exposure, attention-deficit/hyperactivity disorder, and sluggish cognitive tempo. Alcohol Clin Exp Res 37 (suppl 1):E338–E346, 2013

Grant TM, Brown NN, Graham JC, et al: Screening in treatment programs for fetal alcohol spectrum disorders that could affect therapeutic progress. Int J Alcohol Drug Res 2(3):37–49, 2013

Grant TM, Brown NN, Graham JC, Ernst CC: Substance abuse treatment outcomes in women with fetal alcohol spectrum disorder. Int J Alcohol Drug Res 3(1):43–49, 2014

Harris SR, Mickelson ECR, Zwicker JG: Diagnosis and management of developmental coordination disorder. CMAJ 187(9):659–665, 2015

Johnson S, Moyer CL, Klug MG, Burd L: Comparison of alcohol-related neurodevelopmental disorders and neurodevelopmental disorders associated with prenatal alcohol exposure diagnostic criteria. J Dev Behav Pediatr 39(2):163–167, 2018

Jonsson E: Fetal alcohol spectrum disorders (FASD): a policy perspective. Can J Psychiatry 64(3):161–163, 2019

Jonsson E, Clarren S, Binnie I (eds.): Ethical and Legal Perspectives in Fetal Alcohol Spectrum Disorders (FASD): Foundational Issues (International Library of Ethics, Law, and the New Medicine, Vol 75). Cham, Switzerland, Springer, 2018

Kable JA, Coles CD: Evidence supporting the internal validity of the proposed ND-PAE disorder. Child Psychiatry Hum Dev 49(2):163–175, 2018

Kodituwakku P, Kodituwakku E: Cognitive and behavioral profiles of children with fetal alcohol spectrum disorders. Curr Dev Disord Rep 1:149–160, 2014

Lange S, Rovet J, Rehm J, et al: Neurodevelopmental profile of fetal alcohol spectrum disorder: a systematic review. BMC Psychol 5:22, 2017

Lewis SJ, Zuccolo L, Smith GD, et al: Fetal alcohol exposure and IQ at age 8: evidence from a population-based birth-cohort study. PLoS One 7(11):e49407, 2012

Lussier AA, Weinberg J, Kobor MS: Epigenetics studies of fetal alcohol spectrum disorder: where are we now? Epigenomics 9(3):291–311, 2017

Lussier AA, Morin AM, MacIsaac JL, et al: DNA methylation as a predictor of fetal alcohol spectrum disorder. Clin Epigenetics 10:5, 2018

McKenzie DP, McGorry PD, Wallace CS, et al: Constructing a minimal diagnostic decision tree. Methods Inf Med 32(2):161–166, 1993

Mela M, Okpalauwaekwe U, Anderson T, et al: The utility of psychotropic drugs on patients with fetal alcohol spectrum disorder (FASD): a systematic review. Psychiatry and Clinical Psychopharmacology 28(4):436–445, 2018

Olson HC, Morse BA, Huffine C: Development and psychopathology: fetal alcohol syndrome and related conditions. Semin Clin Neuropsychiatry 3(4):262–284, 1998

O'Malley KD, Nanson J: Clinical implications of a link between fetal alcohol spectrum disorder and attention-deficit hyperactivity disorder. Can J Psychiatry 47(4):349–354, 2002

O'Rourke L, Murphy KC: Recent developments in understanding the relationship between 22q11.2 deletion syndrome and psychosis. Curr Opin Psychiatry 32(2):67–72, 2019

Paintner A, Williams AD, Burd L: Fetal alcohol spectrum disorders: implications for child neurology, part 1: prenatal exposure and dosimetry. J Child Neurol 27(2):258–263, 2012

Petrenko CL, Alto ME: Interventions in fetal alcohol spectrum disorders: an international perspective. Eur J Med Genet 60(1):79–91, 2017

Quattlebaum JL, O'Connor MJ: Higher functioning children with prenatal alcohol exposure: is there a specific neurocognitive profile? Child Neuropsychol 19(6):561–578, 2013

Shalev AY: Review: 14 risk factors for post-traumatic stress disorder include childhood abuse and family psychiatric history. Evid Based Ment Health 4(2):61, 2001

Streissguth A: Fetal Alcohol Syndrome: A Guide for Families and Communities. Baltimore, MD, Paul Brooks, 1997

Streissguth AP, Barr HM, Kogan J, Bookstein FL: Understanding the Occurrence of Secondary Disabilities in Clients with Fetal Alcohol Syndrome (FAS) and Fetal Alcohol Effects (FAE). Final Report to the Centers for Disease Control and Prevention (CDC), August, 1996 (Tech Rep No 96-06). Seattle, WA, University of Washington, Fetal Alcohol & Drug Unit, 1996. Available at: http://lib.adai.uw.edu/pubs/bk2698.pdf. Accessed October 2, 2020.

Streissguth AP, Bookstein FL, Barr HM, et al: Risk factors for adverse life outcomes in fetal alcohol syndrome and fetal alcohol effects. J Dev Behav Pediatr 25(4):228–238, 2004

Weyrauch D, Schwartz M, Hart B, et al: Comorbid mental disorders in fetal alcohol spectrum disorders: a systematic review. J Dev Behav Pediatr 38(4):283–291, 2017

Yates WR, Cadoret RJ, Troughton EP, et al: Effect of fetal alcohol exposure on adult symptoms of nicotine, alcohol, and drug dependence. Alcohol Clin Exp Res 22(4):914–920, 1998

Zammit S, Thomas K, Thompson A, et al: Maternal tobacco, cannabis and alcohol use during pregnancy and risk of adolescent psychotic symptoms in offspring. Br J Psychiatry 195(4):294–300, 2009

CHAPTER 5

Neurocognitive Mechanisms

WHAT TO KNOW

Neuroimaging and neuropsychological assessment provide the best evidence available for complementing our understanding of the clinical manifestation of neural circuit development adversely affected by PAE.

Diffuse brain damage refers to the ubiquitous nature of brain abnormality evident in white and grey matter attributed to PAE.

The specific mechanisms associated with PAE-related deficits include its role in causing epigenetic modifications, interfering with neuronal migration, and inhibiting proliferation of astrocytes and thus disrupting the architecture and connectivity of grey and white matter.

Significant damage results if PAE coincides with a period of rapid growth in astrocytes and other components of neural circuitry.

Alcohol exposure during gestation is a significant factor in the development of neurocognitive deficits in offspring. A variety of deficits result from the combined effects of the interaction of PAE and conditions that either aggravate or mitigate the outcomes. It is still too early to pinpoint all the specific mechanisms that precipitate the outcomes of mental disorder as the sequelae to PAE. In this chapter, I propose mechanisms that are, first, important for explaining the behaviors and clinical manifestations of ND-PAE/FASD. Second, these mechanisms constitute pragmatic models with supporting evidence, thus serving to inform the types and potential benefits of current effective interventions. Unanswered questions about the current neurocognitive mechanisms include the effect of age of development and the weight of influence of PAE when considered singly or in combination with other etiologies. In addition, and important to mental health professionals, research is still required to establish how knowledge of the neurocognitive mechanisms informs prevention of disorders that are associated with the burden of sociobehavioral and cognitive dysfunction. Clinicians are particularly interested in these types of questions because they have a direct bearing on supporting positive outcomes in their patients.

Neural correlates of PAE are objectively assessed by neuroimaging techniques or neuropsychological testing. These neural correlates can be inferred from the clinical and social behavior of the impaired person. However, at the most basic level, knowing how these neural effects occur is important to explain obvious and observable clinical presentations. The relevance of the process is appreciated when multiple outcomes are primarily PAE related but even more so when PAE outcomes exist in combination with other physical and mental disorders. For instance, a patient with schizophrenia and ND-PAE/FASD may present with the inability to form relationships, behave in a socially appropriate way, or make socially acceptable statements. Deficits in frontotemporal neural integrity, social cognition, and executive function provide the obvious explanation for such inabilities from a neurocognitive perspective. As such, the relevant neural correlates of this interface are assumed. It remains to be determined if these correlates, as expressed by their interaction in the two comorbid conditions (mental disorder and ND-PAE/FASD), can be separated from the contextual environmental and sociocultural predisposing factors. Factors such as trauma, adversity, social determinants of health, and conditions of upbringing exert their influence on neurocognitive development directly. They also interact with biological etiological factors to indirectly influence multiple outcomes. The same interactions are recognized in the etiology of both psychotic disorders and ND-PAE/FASD. Separating the individual effects still requires an in-depth knowledge of how neural circuitry develops from gene-environment interaction at a molecular level.

Biological Origin and Contribution of the Neurocognitive Mechanisms

Information about the structural brain abnormalities attributed to PAE, which comes from autopsies of brains of patients with FASD, has been supported by neuroimaging studies. Changes in white matter, shown by diffusion tensor imaging, and grey matter, shown by MRI, point to the abnormalities linked to PAE. Recognized as ubiquitous, the brain damage aligns with expected neurocognitive mechanisms associated with the clinical picture. Jones et al. (1973) described the observed CNS disorganization as made of "errors in neuronal migration, neuroglial heterotopias, microcephaly, and abnormalities of the brainstem, cerebellum, basal ganglia, hippocampus and corpus callosum, pituitary gland and optic nerve" (quoted in Wilhelm and Guizzetti 2016, p. 1). In addition to the diffuse brain abnormalities associated with PAE, ventricular abnormalities have been confirmed. Abnormalities of the frontotemporal area (Jones and Smith 1975) and corpus callosum have been demonstrated according to diffusion tensor imaging findings (Ma et al. 2005; Wozniak et al. 2006). These abnormalities are postulated to involve various mechanisms, such as epigenetic modification, neural crest cell migration interference, and inappropriate activation of microglia (Jarmasz et al. 2017).

Clinically relevant impairment in those presenting with PAE and its mental disorder sequelae are thought to be as a result of structural, functional, and metabolic brain abnormalities. These abnormalities are frequently noted to include reduced brain volume, abnormalities in the corpus callosum, and other deficits in neurometabolic profiles in the frontal and parietal cortex, thalamus, and dentate nuclei (Donald et al. 2015). As noted, neuroimaging studies point to abnormalities in both grey and white matter. Specific structural abnormalities associated with PAE include reduced brain size, reduced cerebrum and basal ganglia volume, and limbic and grey matter asymmetry (Gautam et al. 2015). Others include hypoplasia and disrupted architecture and connectivity in the white matter. These abnormalities are related to consequences of PAE on glial cells of all kinds (Wilhelm and Guizzetti 2016). The PAE effect on altered development and function of glial cells results from abnormalities of neuronal migration and formation. When alcohol exposure coincides with the growth spurt period, astrocytes fail to proliferate and mature accordingly. Microcephaly, a common occurrence of PAE associated with such critical periods, reflects the reduced amount of astrocytes, because they do not survive. Glial cells such as oligodendrocytes and microglia support myelination, synaptic pruning, and neural plasticity (Wilhelm and Guizzetti 2016). PAE disrupts such developmental processes and has been associated with neural cell death, apoptosis. The resulting neural abnormalities lay the foundation for the mechanisms of neurocognitive deficits.

Clinical Relevance of Neurocognitive Mechanisms

Some clinicians take the view that treatments should be standardized for all patients. Although this is an efficient approach, it is not better than the colloquial one-size-fits-all approach. Patients with neurocognitive deficits face challenges in the clinical setting. Those with executive function deficits are unable to take information learned in one setting and apply it in another context. Frustrated clinicians have used the phrase "they just don't get it" to describe this deficiency. Understanding the clinical implications of neurocognitive mechanisms of damage is highly recommended if clinical outcomes are to be improved. Consider the level of expectation by a clinician who is unaware of the disability resulting from PAE. Clinical encounters in which a patient repeatedly fails to generalize information and strategies create friction spots, especially when that patient professes understanding of the concepts taught by the clinician.

Circumstances known to demand cognitive ability are associated with dysfunction in these patients. Life transitions, stressful life events, and physical ailments are examples of such demanding situations. Dysfunction follows an increase in stress response. Clinicians should anticipate and plan for such critical periods. Subjects with neurocognitive deficits engage in high-risk behaviors such as self-harm, antisocial behavior, and repeated noncompliance. These behaviors can be understood by realizing that in a higher-stress situation, affected persons have limited ability to consider cause and effect. Because these negative behaviors are often not recognized as arising from PAE, clinicians may not expect this. In a more distressed state, patients will be expected to transfer certain knowledge and apply it in a different setting, which could result in harmful interactions. Patients may incorrectly be considered capable of handling risky situations. Their inability to recognize risk and follow through with their naïve clinicians' instructions leads to negative outcomes. Patients may be thought of as oppositional, and risky actions may be considered deliberate. Knowledge of the frontotemporal brain area and its effect on executive function mediating some cause and effect considerations is useful to clinicians in supporting patients rather than harming them.

The exposure of a developing fetus to alcohol affects the various brain areas differently. The timing of exposure with developmentally critical periods is important in understanding the specific neurocognitive outcomes. This in turn informs the clinical manifestations. Memory, language, and executive function have different developmental trajectories. For instance, patients may appear fluent and yet lack comprehension and show poor judgment. This is feasible if the exposure skipped the earlier critical period of hippocampal and temporal lobe development but occurred and affected the developmental phase of the dorsolateral prefrontal cortex. Consequently, the rather inconsistent clinical picture can be explained by exposure at different critical periods of brain development (Georgieff et al. 2018). Individuals with language deficits misunderstand speech in clinical settings. Thus, they appear noncompliant because on the surface they seem to be agreeing that they not only understand what is said to them but that they will follow the instructions given to them.

Further complications of the neurocognitive deficits occur in interpersonal and clinical interactions wherein individuals lack appropriate social cognition. Cues for socially appropriate interactions are missing, leading to misunderstanding and, in certain situations, boundary violations. Coupled with insecure or inappropriate attachment, patients with such cognitive deficits have been sanctioned in clinical settings as being intrusive and invading others' personal space. A chain of negative events can be expected when attempts are made to process such violations and inappropriateness from a normative cognitive perspective. A similar challenge occurs when a therapist who is unaware of patients' neurocognitive deficits, uses insight-oriented approaches with PAE-affected persons. The patients' inability to assimilate these techniques can be understood only if their neurocognitive deficits are initially recognized. Rather than viewing patients' behaviors as treatment interfering, it is more prudent to consider the neurocognitive mechanisms associated with such behaviors. Clinically, brain-based behaviors serve as pointers or red flags to guide assessment and treatment.

Neural Links to Neurocognitive Mechanisms

Advances in neuroimaging allow noninvasive study of the structural and functional abnormalities induced by PAE. Using group averages, neuroimaging studies (structural and functional) have provided a distinct comparison between patients with PAE and those without. Abnormalities of the frontal lobe have been associated with neuropsychological impairment of attention, working memory, and executive function (Nuñez et al. 2011). Increased cortical thickness in the right ventral and inferolateral frontal lobe, findings in both those with dysmorphic and nondysmorphic types of FASD, suggest that PAE is responsible. In subjects with PAE and related impairment in visuospatial functioning, grey and white matter volume reductions were reported in the left parietal lobe. Abnormalities in subcortical areas, the cerebellum, and corpus callosum have been mapped and linked in several studies to memory, cerebellum-dependent verbal learning, and verbal learning performance respective to the brain regions (Moore et al. 2014). Because no clear neuropsychological profile can yet be attributed to PAE, advances in the diagnostic utility of neurocognitive mechanisms are becoming informative. A potential diagnostic formula was recently proposed that combined neurocognitive correlates, clinical features, and neuroimaging (Suttie et al. 2018). Although this may not yet be ready for clinical use, the need for valid diagnosis based on a simplified neurocognitive profile will likely depend on a solid understanding of neurocognitive mechanisms.

Substance Use Disorder and Neurobiology

The duration of adolescence appears more protracted or delayed in those with ND-PAE/FASD. Risk taking, including indiscriminate sexual activity, aggression, and criminal and antisocial activities may continue into their early and late twenties. How this changes in the fourth or fifth decades of life is now an area of research interest. Substance use is a challenging outcome of the impulsivity, sensation-seeking, and risk-taking domains of FASD. As long as substance use lasts, so do its negative consequences. Risk-taking is now understood as allowing the adolescent to explore adult behavior and privilege and accomplish normal tasks of development, mastery, and improved self-esteem. Understanding substance use can serve as a guide to understanding FASD; substance use is based on disturbances of neural circuits. The preoccupation and anticipation stage of craving, for instance, is based on abnormalities of corticostriatal glutamate projections in the prefrontal cortex (Koob and Volkow 2016). The addicted person also has a deficient reward system mediated through cue-induced incentive. The combined interaction produces the basis for the positive and negative reinforcement associated with drug-seeking behavior. Determination of reinforcements depends on epigenetic changes mediated at the molecular level, which in turn create neural circuits with significant vulnerability. This type of understanding is required to be in tune with the clinical picture and helps guide future development of effective interventions.

Neurocognitive Mechanisms: Lessons From Animal Models

One of the mechanisms contributing to neurocognitive deficits is based on the increase in oxidative stress by prenatal alcohol brain-derived neurotrophic factor (BDNF) expression in the hippocampus. This effect is mapped to the long-lasting learning and memory problems detected in behavioral experiments. Similar to these studies, research on humans found that serotonin transporter and monoamine oxidase A activity and a variant of BDNF interact to confer heritable qualities that predict the outcome of PAE (Gorlyn et al. 2008; Schmidt et al. 2007). Specific cortical and subcortical structures are altered in animals that resemble the neuropathological changes identified in human studies (Jarmasz et al. 2017).

Understanding Neurocognitive Mechanisms and Treatment

A common clinical requirement for intervention is understanding the origin and pattern of symptoms. Treatment modes vary in their response to neurocognitive deficits. In most instances, the attitude of caregivers needs to change. Given past repeated failures and disappointment of their attempts to intervene, along with their lack of awareness of the neurocognitive basis of the problems, relatives may react negatively. These reactions can hardly support the patients' treatment and rehabilitation. To facilitate the requisite compassion shown to affected persons, treatments should be modified to account for these deficits. Caregiving within a family setting can be stressful; appropriate intervention reduces caregivers' stress and burden. Patients also feel engaged when services are modified in response to their needs. Individuals with executive function problems exhibit more social skills deficits, which affect their social interactions in many contexts—with family, at work, and in therapeutic settings. A review of social skills deficits in individuals with FASD implicated abnormalities in executive function, sensory processing, and communication (Kully-Martens et al. 2012; Schonfeld et al. 2006). Knowledge of the neurocognitive mechanism of deficits in behavior is of value to both those affected and those involved in care and therapy. This awareness can help identify potential routes for intervention to improve social skills.

Clinical Vignette

The adoptive parents of a 13-year-old boy consult the local chapter of the National Organization on Fetal Alcohol Syndrome. The boy was adopted from a Romanian orphanage and was subsequently diagnosed with alcohol-related neurodevelopmental disorder. The parents are concerned about their son's behavior in the past 6 months since he changed schools. He was suspended for disrupting class and throwing a pen at his teacher because he was frustrated with questions asked of him when he was not paying attention in the class. His parents report that he is lying and stealing and has run away from home, staying away overnight. He is not kind to his younger sister and is quick to anger when he is corrected or does not get his way. The parents say they are experienced in administering behavior modification techniques, but they cannot get that approach to work with him, even when it is about developing and sticking to simple sleeping rituals.

As the organization's expert, the clinician is asked to explain how different the boy with ND-PAE/FASD could be and why it will be so difficult for such experienced parents to manage him. Here, knowledge of the neurocognitive mechanisms will prove useful. The problematic behaviors should be anchored to the neural correlates associated with the psychological assessment test results specific to deficits in the neurocognitive domains. Lying is a common complaint of caregivers about those with ND-PAE/FASD (Rasmussen et al. 2008). Individuals with memory problems attempt to fill in the blanks by creating stories, appearing to be deliberately wanting to deceive. Failure of cause and effect thinking associated with poor inhibitory control contributes to such behaviors. Hippocampal and prefrontal cortex damage found in PAE-affected individuals explains the foundation of such recall and inhibitory deficits. If this boy's cognitive domains are deficient, his ability to register, store, and recall information is impaired because his information processing speed is slow. Stealing is explained by the executive function deficit of impaired abstraction and an inability to understand ownership. The parents can be supported by explaining that with executive function deficits come concrete thinking and impulsive activity, and these are recognized as PAE-related prefrontal cortex damage. We can turn to the concept of default mode network abnormality and its role in inattention to understand the behavior disorder displayed in the classroom by the boy. Classroom behavioral disorder can fit the default mode network abnormality from inattention. The boy's behavior is explainable if inattention and the speed of delivery of class material leave him frustrated. The quickness to anger at home and school is linked to a disturbance of affect regulation, located in the hypothalamic-pituitary-adrenal axis, a finding supported by animal studies and studies of human anxiety and depression in PAE sequelae (Hellemans et al. 2010; Price et al. 2017).

Neurocognitive mechanisms not only explain the observable "tip of the iceberg" behaviors (Table 5–1), they inform the therapeutic advice and support the clinician will give parents and caregivers. In line with the neurocognitive findings and aligning with specific strategies, certain training programs are designed with these deficits in mind. Affect regulation, improvement in attention, and specific executive function strategies find expression in the GoFAR (focus and plan, act, and reflect), MILE (Math Interactive Learning Experience), and Alert programs (Coles et al. 2018;

Reid and Petrenko 2018). Parents' and caregivers' experience and courage should be validated. They should be encouraged to try slowing down the speed of information coming in, check for full and true understanding in conversation, elicit triggers from recent changes and aspects of a new school and people, and teach the concept of ownership. Changes in school can be better managed if transitions are recognized and verbalized before they happen. Parents and caregivers can advocate for special accommodations in the school. These efforts are better supported with the understanding of neurocognitive mechanisms.

TABLE 5–1. Proposed neurocognitive mechanisms that explain observable behavior disturbance ("tip of the iceberg")

TIP OF THE ICEBERG BEHAVIOR	NEUROCOGNITIVE BASIS
Frustration from lack of attention	Default mode network dysfunction
Social skills, social cognition, and executive function missteps	Damage to frontotemporal neural integrity
Frustration from slow speed of information processing	Disruption of architectural connectivity of white matter
Lying manifesting from memory and cause and effect deficits	Oxidative stress damage and brain-derived neurotrophic factor deficit
	Hippocampal damage and grey matter reduction in prefrontal cortex
Anger at home and classroom disturbance resulting from poor affect regulation and impulse control	Impaired hypothalamic-pituitary-adrenal axis and executive function

Neurodevelopmental disorders become more complex and clinically demanding when comorbid with other mental disorders or medical conditions. Down syndrome and autism spectrum disorder, for instance, do not cease to exist nor are they subsumed or replaced by comorbid anxiety, depression, or even psychotic disorder when an individual has an additional or multiple disorders. Instead, by nature of their developmental origins, these disorders occupy relevant foci for understanding etiology, pathophysiology, and a foundation for intervention. It is therefore helpful to conceptualize FASD in the same way. The neurocognitive deficits associated with PAE resemble identified deficits in many mental disorders. Executive dysfunction, for instance, occurs in as many as two-thirds of those diagnosed with FASD. This may be part of, or the full explanation of, the executive function deficits in those with FASD comorbid with depression or psychotic disorder. Understood in this way, the etiology and mechanisms of the comorbidity become clearer. Treatment and helpful strategies are better aligned with such understanding. For instance, Gorlyn et al. (2008) reported that subtle prefrontal dysfunction identified through executive dysfunction was responsible for nonresponse to fluoxetine treatment for major depressive disorder. Not recognizing such developmental and etiological connections risks the exclusion of patients from appropriate and needed services. Recognition of the same clinical trajectory from the developmental phase serves to initiate intervention and prevention for both FASD and mental disorder broadly.

Conclusion

Similar factors of trauma, adversity, social determinants of health, and access to care are important in understanding the clinical features of those with PAE who also have mental disorder. The mechanisms underlying the manifested clinical features of PAE damage have roots in the effect of alcohol on neural circuitry. Identifying affected individuals has the advantage of facilitating understanding of their behavior, aligning intervention to their needs, and supporting those who care for them. Frontline staff and caregivers often experience frustrating moments; recognizing that negative behaviors are caused by brain-based deficits can potentially promote better care and outcomes.

CLINICAL PRACTICAL APPLICATIONS

- From clinical understanding of the implications of the neurocognitive mechanisms of damage flows awareness of the uniqueness of each patient and the need for individualized treatment to improve outcomes.

- The diathesis-stress model identifies increased demand on deficient neurocognitive function (e.g., life transitions, stress, physical ailment) as a direct precipitant of inability to cope (e.g., which underlies risky and noncompliant behaviors).

- Because cognitive functions (memory, language, and executive function) are achieved differentially at specific critical periods, the patient's inconsistent presentation is perfectly consistent with the effect PAE exerts on this continuum of developmental trajectories.

- A patient with neurocognitive deficits and noted as intrusive and culpable of boundary violations in the clinical setting should be considered for a full psychiatric and neurocognitive assessment.

- Refining diagnostic categorization will require a combination and clustering of clinical, neuroimaging, and neurocognitive correlates to understand different types of patients.

- Educating caregivers and frontline staff about the mechanisms of neurocognitive damage encourages a response of empathy, compassion, and understanding toward the patient.

References

Coles CD, Kable JA, Taddeo E, Strickland D: GoFAR: improving attention, behavior and adaptive functioning in children with fetal alcohol spectrum disorders: brief report. Dev Neurorehabil 21(5):345–349, 2018

Donald KA, Eastman E, Howells FM, et al: Neuroimaging effects of prenatal alcohol exposure on the developing human brain: a magnetic resonance imaging review. Acta Neuropsychiatr 27(5):251–269, 2015

Gautam P, Lebel C, Narr KL, et al: Volume changes and brain-behavior relationships in white matter and subcortical gray matter in children with prenatal alcohol exposure. Human Brain Mapping 36(6):2318–2329, 2015

Georgieff MK, Tran PV, Carlson ES: Atypical fetal development: fetal alcohol syndrome, nutritional deprivation, teratogens, and risk for neurodevelopmental disorders and psychopathology. Dev Psychopathol 30(3):1063–1086, 2018

Gorlyn M, Keilp JG, Grunebaum MF, et al: Neuropsychological characteristics as predictors of SSRI treatment response in depressed subjects. J Neural Transm (Vienna) 115(8):1213–1219, 2008

Hellemans KG, Sliwowska JH, Verma P, Weinberg J: Prenatal alcohol exposure: fetal programming and later life vulnerability to stress, depression and anxiety disorders. Neurosci Biobehav Rev 34(6):791–807, 2010

Jarmasz JS, Basalah DA, Chudley AE, Del Bigio MR: Human brain abnormalities associated with prenatal alcohol exposure and fetal alcohol spectrum disorder. J Neuropath Exp Neurol 76(9):813–833, 2017

Jones KL, Smith DW: The fetal alcohol syndrome. Teratology 12(1):1–10, 1975

Jones KL, Smith DW, Ulleland CN, Streissguth P: Pattern of malformation in offspring of chronic alcoholic mothers. Lancet 1:1267–1271, 1973

Koob GF, Volkow ND: Neurobiology of addiction: a neurocircuitry analysis. Lancet Psychiatry 3(8):760–773, 2016

Kully-Martens K, Denys K, Treit S, et al: A review of social skills deficits in individuals with fetal alcohol spectrum disorders and prenatal alcohol exposure: profiles, mechanisms, and interventions. Alcohol Clin Exp Res 36(4):568–576, 2012

Ma X, Coles CD, Lynch ME, et al: Evaluation of corpus callosum anisotropy in young adults with fetal alcohol syndrome according to diffusion tensor imaging. Alcohol Clin Exp Res 29(7):1214–1222, 2005

Moore EM, Migliorini R, Infante MA, Riley EP: Fetal alcohol spectrum disorders: recent neuroimaging findings. Curr Dev Disord Rep 1(3):161–172, 2014

Nuñez SC, Roussotte F, Sowell ER: Focus on: structural and functional brain abnormalities in fetal alcohol spectrum disorders. Alcohol Res Health 34(1):121–131, 2011

Price A, Cook PA, Norgate S, Mukherjee R: Prenatal alcohol exposure and traumatic childhood experiences: a systematic review. Neurosci Biobehav Rev 80:89–98, 2017

Rasmussen C, Talwar V, Loomes C, Andrew G: Brief report: lie-telling in children with fetal alcohol spectrum disorder. J Pediatr Psychol 33(2):220–225 2008

Reid N, Petrenko CLM: Applying a developmental framework to the self-regulatory difficulties of young children with prenatal alcohol exposure: a review. Alcohol Clin Exp Res 42(6):987–1005, 2018

Schmidt LA, Fox NA, Hamer DH: Evidence for a gene–gene interaction in predicting children's behavior problems: association of serotonin transporter short and dopamine receptor D4 long genotypes with internalizing and externalizing behaviors in typically developing 7-year-olds. Dev Psychopathol 19(4):1105–1116, 2007

Schonfeld AM, Paley B, Frankel F, O'Connor MJ: Executive functioning predicts social skills following prenatal alcohol exposure. Child Neuropsychol 12(6):439–452, 2006

Suttie M, Wozniak JR, Parnell SE, et al: Combined face-brain morphology and associated neurocognitive correlates in fetal alcohol spectrum disorders. Alcohol Clin Exp Res 42(9):1769–1782, 2018

Wilhelm CJ, Guizzetti M: Fetal alcohol spectrum disorders: an overview from the glia perspective. Front Integr Neurosci 9:65, 2016

Wozniak JR, Mueller BA, Chang PN, et al: Diffusion tensor imaging in children with fetal alcohol spectrum disorders. Alcohol Clin Exp Res 30(10):1799–1806, 2006

PART III

Presentation

CHAPTER 6

Clinical Presentation

WHAT TO KNOW

One out of every 10 people exposed to alcohol prenatally has the distinctive dysmorphic facial features that originate when alcohol is consumed at the particular period of the pregnancy when facial structures are being formed.

Although there are many physical facial and nonfacial abnormalities in individuals with ND-PAE/FASD, the most constant features include the shortened palpebral fissure lengths, flattened or smooth philtrum, and thin upper lip.

Confirming the sentinel facial features is pathognomonic of PAE and serves as a biomarker of the disorder.

FASD is referred to as a whole-body disorder because of its pervasive nature, affecting all bodily organs through PAE, thought to be inflammation and hormone mediated.

Better outcomes were seen in patients with physically recognizable features than in those with the invisible form of the disorder. This emphasizes the need for a functional assessment component in the diagnostic process.

Adaptive dysfunction, affect dysregulation, hyperarousal problems, cognitive inflexibility, and hyperactivity are the expression of the most severe neurocognitive deficits of memory, language, and executive function.

Individuals affected with the consequences of PAE experience a wide range of medical, psychiatric, social, and physical symptoms. They have unique physical features and other general nonspecific features common in other clinical syndromes and disorders. Patients with the features of PAE present in a variety of clinical settings, and a range of clinical skills is required for accurate identification of these features, which vary by age, context, and severity at the time the person meets with a clinician. When patients are encountered, their concerns could stem from non-PAE-related matters, and thus, PAE may not be the clinician's immediate consideration. It is important, given its ubiquitous manifestation, that mental health professionals are sensitized to the possibility of encountering patients with PAE and its adverse consequences. The features presented in this chapter involve the unique physical characteristics, behavioral aspects, and medical symptoms and signs, as well as the wider clinical warning signs of PAE.

A mental health professional employs pattern recognition to identify essential features and organize them around an understandably defined clinical entity. By so doing, clinical encounters are concerned with the roles and utilities of diagnosis. The diagnosis may be the only unifying concept for a wide variety of symptoms in the case of individuals with PAE who are navigating the mental health system.

Clinical Vignette

A 24-year-old man attending an outpatient clinic complains of anger toward his father. Superficially, such a complaint may not trigger considerations of PAE. However, a closer look at the clinical picture leads the clinician to identify features of the history that suggest the contribution of PAE. The patient provides additional history, so much so that the process of diagnosis could be conceptualized as a form of intervention. As a 5-year-old boy, the patient was "run over by a vehicle." As a result, he spent about 36 months (6 of these in coma) in the hospital for several corrective surgeries to repair his fractured rib cage and skull and to remove an injured kidney (nephrectomy). The patient describes an inability to sleep without medication and a long-standing history of significant alcohol and stimulant drug use. Up until this moment, the role of the significant traumatic events and head injury stemming from the accident constitute the major foci of the intervention considered.

However, information about the death of the patient's mother 2 years earlier introduces a new dimension—or alternative consideration. She had a history of persistent alcohol use disorder and died from chronic liver disease. The patient was raised by his maternal grandfather, who taught him about indigenous spiritual ceremonies. Because of the patient's own struggle with alcohol and substances, and in keeping with traditional expectations, he was not able to participate in and benefit from the available spiritual activities and ceremonies. He was in a special education program but dropped out of school in grade seven. He has more than four dozen convictions, mostly breaches of conditions of supervision and property offenses. He is repeatedly unemployed and is dependent on social and disability financial support. The patient's previous contacts with mental health services led to multiple diagnoses, which in turn led to the prescription of multiple psychotropic drugs.

Through a systematic approach and with collateral information, some warning signs of PAE and mental disorder sequelae become obvious. The formulation of the case could be conceptualized primarily from a PAE perspective or from a combined PAE and traumatic brain injury perspective. The approach that is utilized has important outcome implications. In this chapter, I describe common examples of comorbid cases and the means of identifying physical, medical, social, and mental presentations of patients. Clinicians are advised to investigate services in their jurisdiction that cater for the needs of those with neurocognitive deficits. Online training programs exist that range from simple to advance knowledge of FASD (e.g., https://canfasd.ca/online-learners/).. It is hoped that some will be encouraged to seek out more training opportunities or at the very least to engage a referral system that links the patients they suspect of PAE with proper diagnostic assessment.

The following scenario may appear to be more PAE related and yet still be comorbid with other mood, perceptual, anxiety, and personality disorders. Substance use and impulse control disorders are frequent in patients with the effects of PAE. Being aware of this is important, as shown in the vignette:

Clinical Vignette

After losing seven jobs within a 2-year period, a 45-year-old divorced man visits a mental health clinic and asks to be assessed because "I want to know what is wrong." He struggles to organize his daily schedule. He describes a pattern of running out of money long before the next payday. As a result, he resorts to selling household goods and property at very cheap rates to obtain cash. Members of his family have begun to avoid him because of his excessive alcohol consumption, which usually results in embarrassing and agitated behavior. He was involved in an industrial accident in which a number of his coworkers died; he observed some of the events and felt helpless to rescue his colleagues. He reported that he experiences disturbing dreams about the incident three to five times a week.

It is important that clinicians know the diagnostic criteria for ND-PAE/FASD and how to clinically assess for each. For each diagnostic criterion, there appears to be an inverse relationship between the ease of obtaining the information and its lifelong relevance for patients. For instance, measuring the deficit associated with growth is easy enough, but its relevance for long-term outcome is low (Table 6–1). The converse is true for neurocognitive deficits, on which so much of the clinical picture depends; neurocognitive testing is the most strenuous and demanding of resources. Clinicians should be aware of this and should allocate efforts in a reasonable way to diagnose and support patients.

TABLE 6–1.   Criteria for ND-PAE and FASD diagnosis: ease and diagnostic relevance of the component domains

DIAGNOSTIC FEATURE	EASE OF DIAGNOSIS	CLINICAL RELEVANCE
Growth deficit	Very high	Low
Dysmorphic facial features	High	Moderate
Prenatal alcohol exposure	Moderate	High
Neuropsychological deficits	Low	Very high

Note. FASD=fetal alcohol spectrum disorder; ND-PAE=neurobehavioral disorder associated with prenatal alcohol exposure.

Dysmorphic and Physical Signs of PAE

In about one-tenth of individuals exposed to alcohol prenatally, unique and pathognomonic dysmorphic facial features are clinically identifiable. Alcohol consumed at a circumscribed period of gestation, critical to the development of the structures of the face, gives rise to these sentinel facial features (Cook et al. 2016). At the outset, clinicians treating FAS recognized the existence of several clinical signs: micrognathia, flat midface, ptosis of the eyelids, epicanthal folds, and upturned nose with a flat nasal bridge. Other nonfacial physical abnormalities are a curved fifth finger (clinodactyly) and an upper palmar crease that widens and ends between the second and third fingers (hockey-stick crease) (Wattendorf and Muenke 2005) (Figure 6–1). An underdeveloped upper part of the ear parallel to the ear crease, which gives a track (railroad track) appearance was also noted in those with PAE (Figure 6–2). These abnormalities have been depicted in Wattendorf and Muenke's 2005 article in the journal of the *American Family Physician* (www.aafp.org/afp/2005/0715/p279.html). Microcephaly was also recognized as a clinical feature in those with ND-PAE/FASD. Although these physical signs were present in patients exposed to alcohol, they were neither prerequisite for diagnosis nor specific to PAE.

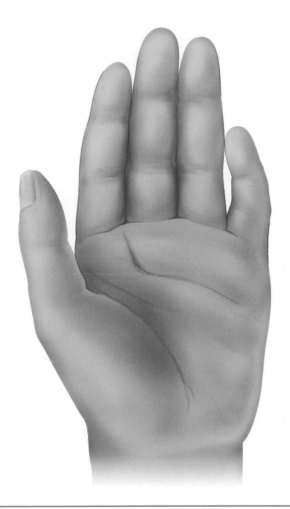

FIGURE 6–1. Curved little finger (clinodactyly), called hockey stick finger and hockey stick palmar crease.

Source. Image: Darryl Leja, National Human Genome Research Institute, National Institutes of Health, Bethesda, Maryland.

However, three dysmorphic features were singled out as most constant and have now been included as criteria in the various diagnostic schemes. The *palpebral fissure length* (PFL; horizontal distance from the endocanthion to the exocanthion for each eye in millimeters) in people with FASD is characteristically shortened. The criterion is established when the measured horizontal distance is converted to percentiles or compared with the expected mean using norm-referenced charts. Differences of one and one half to two standard deviations below the population mean is accepted as

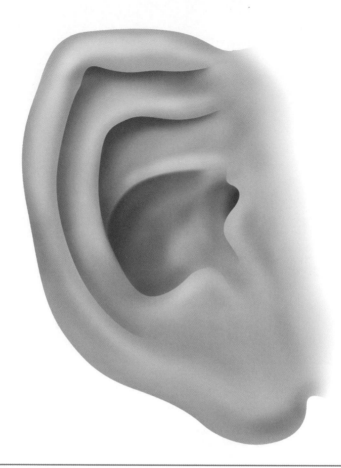

FIGURE 6–2.   Underdeveloped upper part of ear parallel to the ear crease resembles railroad tracks.

Source.   Image: Darryl Leja, National Human Genome Research Institute, National Institutes of Health, Bethesda, Maryland.

significant (Cook et al. 2016). This is counted as meeting one criterion among the three dysmorphic features. The *philtrum* is the groove that runs from the center root of the septum of the nose to the border of the upper lip. Known as the infranasal depression, the ridge of the philtrum is affected by alcohol's neurotoxic effect during its formation, said to be around the twenty-first day of gestation. In FASD, the philtrum is classified based on its smoothness or fullness. It is smoothest in the disorders associated with significant PAE. The third feature is based on the thinness or thickness of the upper lip. In individuals with FASD, the upper lip is thinned out. The philtrum and upper lip are rated on a Likert scale of the Washington Lip-Philtrum Guides to complete criteria for FASD (Astley and Clarren 2001).

To determine the presence or absence of the three dysmorphic facial features, individuals with overlapping epicanthal folds, surgery for cleft lip or palate, thick moustache, facial injury or surgery, and muscle loss associated with aging and those who are edentulous should be examined carefully (Wattendorf and Muenke 2005). Because these can obscure the facial features, individuals may need to be reexamined at a later date. These features, if present, are especially specific to PAE and support a diagnosis of ND-PAE/FASD even when a history of PAE cannot be reliably confirmed. When present, the dysmorphic features almost exclude other conditions not associated with PAE. Norms (PFL, philtrum, and upper lip measures) were developed from an ethnically diverse group of subjects. These norms are frequently referred to as the gold standard (Astley 2004; Astley and Clarren 2000; Clarren et al. 2010). The facial features are affected by several factors, and the fullness of the philtrum and the thinness of the upper lip have interracial variation such that the scales used to measure them accommodate those differences (Moore et al. 2007). Unlike the many features identified in PAE, these three specific facial features are more stable throughout the lifespan, but they can be affected by physical distortion due to injury or surgical manipulation as in repair of cleft palate abnormality (Clarren et al. 2010). Refining methods for facial measurements is necessary to elevate the identification of clinical features relevant to diagnosis (Fang et al. 2008; Moore et al. 2007).

Expertise in Facial Measurements

Training programs equip clinicians with the requisite skills to measure, estimate, and confirm the dysmorphic facial features associated with PAE. The facial features are documented using basic measurement instruments such as calipers or a plastic ruler and the Washington Lip-Philtrum Guide. Software for facial photographic analysis is an alternative tool available for use by clinicians.

A Likert scale of pictures used to compare philtrum and upper lip have been normed for interracial groups. Sample photographs of nonsmiling persons are used to compare with the patient's nonsmiling still face. The philtrum and lip are observed and compared with the criterion-normed standard pictures arranged as a Likert scale. This guide developed by researchers at the University of Washington in Seattle recognizes the racial difference in the composition of the lip and philtrum. Guides for white and African American patients are available for use.

To ensure accurate measurement of the facial features, unhindered by deep angle perception, the patient's middle ear and the angle of the eye should be parallel and align with those of the clinician. This is best achieved with the clinician sitting face to face with the patient, with the height of the chairs adjusted to align the said parallel line of the patient and clinician on a plane (Figure 6–3). Mental health professionals specializing in the field have successfully been trained and demonstrate expertise in facial measurements.

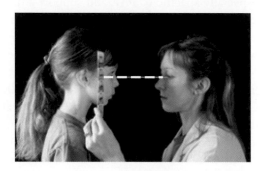

FIGURE 6–3. Clinical position to assess lip and philtrum using the Frankfort horizontal plane.

The Frankfort horizontal plane is defined by a line (*dashed line*) that passes through the patient's external auditory canal and the lowest border of the bony orbital rim. The physician's eyes (or camera lens) should be directly in line with this plane. If the physician stands above this plane looking down on the patient, the patient's upper lip could appear thinner than it truly is. An animation demonstrating how the clinician should align himself or herself in the patient's Frankfort horizontal plane is available at http://depts.washington.edu/fasdpn/htmls/fas-tutor.htm#frankfort.

Source. Copyright © 2020, Susan (Astley) Hemingway, Ph.D., University of Washington. Used with permission.

The use of photographic analysis is limited for epicanthal folds; they should be maneuvered manually to expose the exact spot for measurement when using a ruler or caliper. Figure 6–4 depicts use of a plastic ruler. The PFL can be measured as a horizontal distance. Gently moving the skin is preferred to guessing the point of measurement under the skin. The person being examined may need an elevated seat to align with the clinician. Children or shorter individuals require such adjustment to enhance accurate measurement. Looking straight over the clinician's head into the distance, patients should be instructed to open their eyes as widely as possible. This process effectively exposes the endocanthion to facilitate the measurement of the PFL. To maintain that uncomfortable posture long enough, the patient is prewarned about the discomfort of having a ruler or caliper so close to the eye. It is best to measure the PFL last if the patient is not overly restless at the beginning of the examination (Wattendorf and Muenke 2005). Repeated encouraging comments allow the process of measurement to go unhindered, except for a few moments when blinking is unavoidable. Up to 1 mm difference in PFL between the eyes is possible and acceptable. The normed data should be region specific because ethnic differences in PFL and their distribution across the world ranges widely (Clarren et al. 2010).

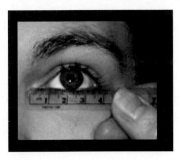

FIGURE 6–4.   Palpebral fissure length (the distance from the inner corner to outer corner of the eye) measured with a small plastic ruler.
Source.   Copyright © 2020, Susan (Astley) Hemingway, Ph.D., University of Washington. Used with permission.

Computer-based photographic analysis compares a patient's facial photograph with standardized computer lengths and distances that equate to the set criteria. Photographic facial analysis was developed as an alternative method described in a few FASD diagnostic schemes (Astley 2015; Astley and Clarren 2000; Mutsvangwa et al. 2010). Three pictures (front, angle, and side views) of the nonsmiling face are taken. The person is instructed to remain still so that an imaginary line can be drawn through the ear canal from a line just below the eyes. A software program analyzes specific locations on the still-face image and compares them with a picture with normed standard measurements. The PFL, philtrum, and upper lip are traced and outlined, and the computer-generated figures provide a four-point Likert scale to use to rate the range of dysmorphic facial features. This Likert scale is based on the four-digit code diagnostic system (Astley and Clarren 2000).

Medical Examination

It is important that patients are examined medically and, if indicated, by a geneticist. A family history of genetic disorders and atypical physical and psychological manifestations are indicators to consider in genetic consultation. The purpose of this consultation is to explore potential differential diagnosis of genetic conditions and provide treatment of common conditions comorbid with PAE. The examination should focus on indicia of common disorders comorbid with ND-PAE/FASD. These include thyroid insufficiency and iron and protein deficiency, which are regularly encountered and can be corrected. If indicated, laboratory investigations should be ordered and reviewed to address any important findings (see Chapter 11, "Laboratory Testing"). In the event that a clinician is not set up to conduct physical examinations, the patient should be referred to a colleague capable of helping. So often, medical conditions are neglected. Current findings of multiple organ damage should influence the assessment and care patients with ND-PAE/FASD receive.

Specifically, alcohol affects the fetus so much so that disease states have been associated with virtually all organs of the body. In a systematic review of comorbid medical conditions in those with FASD, the sheer frequency of ocular, renal, cardiac, musculoskeletal, and hepatic disorders revealed significant impairment (Popova et al. 2016). Although these are not essential for diagnosis, when present, they are important in identifying the clinical manifestation. Several physiological changes across the whole body are commonplace in those with PAE (Shelton et al. 2018). Because medical symptoms and diagnoses are common in those with a history of PAE, the term *whole-body disorder* was coined to apply to the multiple conditions of FASD. The inadequate fetal environment in which offspring exposed to alcohol develop increases their susceptibility to chronic health problems. Markers of inflammation and hormonal alterations are now thought to be fundamental features of PAE. This then increases the risk associated with later development of medical disorders in the exposed person. The symptoms of heart, kidney, and liver disease serve as telltale signs of PAE and should be evaluated during comprehensive assessment.

Unique to PAE are the effects on the growth of the offspring. Weight, height, and head circumference are measured to establish deviations from the norm. Low weight and height become relevant to the diagnosis when they fall below the tenth percentile. These signs are important and should be evaluated, especially given the metabolic problems common in endocrine disorders and PAE's close association with several endocrine problems. Weight, BMI, and indicia of common PAE-induced physical disorders are easy to evaluate and should form part of a prudent assessment.

Psychological and Behavioral Presentation

CNS dysfunction and behavioral sequelae are the most devastating of the deleterious effects of PAE. Functional changes associated with brain abnormalities exert the greatest impact on the lives of those with ND-PAE/FASD. Because the most notable facial dysmorphic features only occur in a small percentage of exposed individuals, clinical recognition of functional deficits is of utmost importance. Many patients will be misclassified if clinicians only depend on physical features for detection of ND-PAE/FASD. This is particularly relevant for preventing negative outcomes in those without the characteristic facial features who are not so easily recognized. Studies show that long-term outcomes were better in patients with easily identifiable facial markers than in those with the invisible disorder (Rasmussen et al. 2008; Streissguth et al. 2004). Mental health practitioners ascribe patients' neurocognitive dysfunctions to other diagnoses, neglecting the contribution of PAE in precipitating the manifesting deficits and clinical features.

The presentation of these negative outcomes is identified clinically. Subjects exposed to alcohol and followed up were shown to exhibit maladaptive behaviors such as impulsivity, teasing/bullying, dishonesty (lying, cheating, and stealing), avoiding school or work, intentional destruction of property, sexual inappropriateness, physical aggression, and self-injury (Bodnarchuk et al. 2006; LaDue et al. 1992). Age-related manifestations are influenced by developmental age, expectations, and how late the person presents to services. Chapter 16 ("Special Issues in Children and Adolescents [the Young]"), Chapter 17 ("Special Issues in the Elderly"), and Chapter 18 ("Special Issues in Forensic Mental Health") present the more subtle features of special populations.

Studies with reported high rates of mental health symptoms imply that those symptoms are useful for identifying those with PAE. Girls with PAE as young as 6 years were reported to have significant features indicative of depression. Thus, clinicians' level of suspicion should be aroused by symptoms of mood disorder, OCD, PTSD, panic disorder, and alcohol use disorders (O'Connor et al. 2002; Weyrauch et al. 2017). Many mental disorders are comorbid with the consequences of PAE. ND-PAE/FASD is easily misdiagnosed as many other mental disorders. Common misdiagnoses include reactive attachment disorder, pervasive developmental disorder, anxiety disorder, mood disorder, personality disorder, and alcohol and substance use disorders. Symptoms of these mental disorders should be carefully evaluated and, when present, serve as identifying clinical features to be ruled out.

The close link between ADHD and FASD also means that hyperactivity, impulsivity, and inattention should raise the suspicion of ND-PAE/FASD. The relative risk of FASD in patients with ADHD was estimated as 7.6 and the attributable risk as 87% (Burd 2016). These risk estimates are even higher for ADHD in patients with FASD (13.28 and 92.5%). This fact is strengthened by research comparing three populations (patients with FASD, ADHD, and ADHD/FASD; $N=164$). The behavioral and cognitive profiles of those with FASD were poorer than those with ADHD alone or in combination with FASD. Subjects with FASD also had worse deficits in full-scale IQ, perceptual reasoning, verbal comprehension, and working memory compared with those with ADHD; individuals with FASD exhibited weaker verbal comprehension when joined with ADHD. The researchers suggested that those findings could serve as red flags for clinicians to trigger more comprehensive assessments (Raldiris et al. 2018). Additionally, to differentiate between ADHD and FASD, the researchers found differences in externalizing behavior, hyperactivity, higher levels of atypicality, and aggression. These are also helpful identifiable clinical features.

Suicidal Behavior as Clinical Presentation

Suicidal behavior is a prominent clinical presentation among those with ND-PAE/FASD. In a longitudinal follow-up, patients diagnosed with FASD were five times more likely to attempt suicide than the general population (Streissguth et al. 1996). Compared with individuals with intellectual disability, in whom 11% were known to have attempted suicide, those with PAE were 2.5 times more likely to attempt suicide (Lunsky 2004). The reasons for the high prevalence of suicide ideation (more than 30% of those with PAE), suicide attempt, and completed suicide demand the attention of the mental health professional. Arguably, suicide is catastrophic, and the most devastating consequence of mental disorder. Suicidal behavior is an important clinical manifestation and arouses suspicion in the mental health professional who adopts a PAE lens.

Sensory integration occurs when the brain processes sensory information from the different senses. Disorders of sensory processing, which manifest as hypersensitivity or hyposensitivity to sensory stimuli, are common in individuals with PAE. As a result, they become easily overwhelmed and experience clinical inability to focus attention. Specific to suicide attempts in those with PAE, the individuals overreact to stimuli. Coupled with their tendency to be cognitively inflexible, experiencing difficulties means they are not able to generate options or problem solve those difficulties. The suicide attempt is an expression of the neurocognitive deficits of specific executive functioning. Poor impulse control and difficulties with estimating cause and effect combine with disorders of affect regulation to propagate increased suicidal behaviors.

Additionally, suicide risk is elevated in those with PAE because they disproportionately experience more adversity than the average person. Studies of the relationship between adverse childhood experiences (ACEs) and suicide reveal that the greater the number of adverse events per person, the more the likelihood of attempting suicide. For instance, children and adults with seven or more adverse events were found to have a 51-fold and 30-fold risk of suicide attempt, respectively, compared with those with no such adverse events (Dube et al. 2001). Because PAE is strongly associated with ACEs, the increased suicide risk is understandable. Studies of those with PAE confirm that they are four times more likely to be affected with ACEs than the general non-PAE population (Lebel et al. 2019; Price et al. 2017). This high risk is prominent in those with substance use, low self-esteem, and depression, which are by their nature common findings in people with PAE. Among the plethora of cumulative risk factors, increased suicide risk is an important clinical red flag for PAE and should be a focus of FASD-informed interventions, considering the alarmingly high rate of suicide in those with PAE. Suicide was the leading external cause of death in a mortality study of those with FAS. This contributed to the low life expectancy in those with PAE (Thanh and Jonsson 2016).

Informed care for individuals at risk of suicide includes enhancing protective factors. Youth do better when they are socially connected with positive support from family and friends (Breen and Burns 2012). Those with social support from cultural, religious, or spiritual groups also report positive outcomes. Care should recognize the effect of trauma, and patients should be counseled about the negative effects of adversity. Approaches that support resilience and foster hope and well-being should be used to mitigate the complex relationship between suicide and PAE. Positive recreational activities and a focus on regulating biological systems are part of the care approach with the best potential to reverse negative outcomes.

Self-harm was reported in subjects with FASD as a reaction to stress and a result of poor coping skills. Therefore, PAE and its consequences should be considered in those with repeated incidents of self-harm, suicidal behavior, and associated risk unawareness. Because these patients visit the emergency room repeatedly, they should be directed to have a full and comprehensive assessment. Otherwise, negative outcomes and costly health care services are inevitable.

Symptoms Associated With DSM-5 Diagnosis of ND-PAE

The characteristic symptoms of ND-PAE are organized around the neurocognitive deficits of three clusters of symptoms. Although standardized psychometric tests are ideal in establishing the deviation of a person's score compared with the norm, this is not always possible for clinicians. DSM-5 generally emphasizes the practical and clinical evaluation of deficits. As the criteria are set for further study, no specific process or cutoffs have been established. This calls for proficiency in recognizing the common patterns that an individual presents. Current research shows that those diagnosed with FASD using a multidisciplinary team approach may not always be identified using the criteria for ND-PAE. The neurocognitive domains are identical, but the criteria applied and the variance of clinical versus standardized testing deductions are at odds (Sanders et al. 2017). Certain populations were also determined to be at an increased risk of PAE, prompting the recommendation for screening such populations (Bell 2016). Additional studies showed that when diagnosing patients, the nondysmorphic form of PAE and DSM-5 ND-PAE were indistinguishable. ND-PAE is credited with an acceptable internal validity, supporting the use of its descriptive clinical features in identifying those with PAE (Kable and Coles 2018). Until the threshold for diagnosis is validated and the criteria documented in DSM, the manifested symptoms help clinicians identify and intervene with those with PAE. This section therefore follows the DSM criteria aligned with the identified patient presentation by a team of experts (Hagan et al. 2016).

Cluster of Neurocognitive Symptoms

With some variations in age, the essential neurocognitive domains represented are executive function, memory, cognition, and learning. Impairment in these domains produces long-term deficits. Patients present with the inability to apply learning in different settings where it is needed. School, employment, and social contexts reveal that they struggle to learn new material, forget information, and learn less if experiencing anxiety. Executive dysfunction is indicated when patients cannot learn a sequence of events and cannot plan. Such patients are likely to show evidence of cognitive inflexibility, which manifests as an incessant inability to adjust to changes and new schedules. Individuals appear to be stuck; they engage in repetitive actions, even if those are harmful. Repeated self-harm is one of the actions they may perform, although other neurobehavioral explanations (sensory processing, hypersensitivity of the hypothalamic-pituitary-adrenal axis, and affect dysregulation) are also part of that complex behavior. Patients with deficits in the neurocognitive domain demonstrate poor academic abilities, exhibiting learning problems, especially in math. They regularly list a number of subject failures or evidence of attending special education programs. Their behaviors, usually a reaction to the learning problem and the resulting effort used to cover the learning deficits, create new symptoms. The patients may have been suspended or even expelled from school.

Patients seem to have problems registering information in their long-term memory; they forget personal information and lose or misplace personal possessions easily. Visuospatial processing is also said to be deficient in those with PAE. This is manifested in challenges with finding and following directions and applying diagrammatic representations and interpretations. For example, solving puzzles and reading maps are not the patient's favorite pastimes.

Cluster of Self-Regulation Symptoms

From an early age, self-regulation problems are identified: sleep difficulties, irritable mood, inability to self-sooth, or becoming easily overwhelmed and frustrated. These symptoms continue to be prominent even in adult life, albeit with age-related variation. Temper tantrums become difficulties handling stress and frustration in older patients. At an earlier stage, the inability to keep emotions in check manifests as angry outbursts, short temper, and intense disposition; these become more prominent later. Individuals affected by PAE display a series of actions that suggest they do not act in their own long-term best interests, evidenced by the inability to resist impulses. They also demonstrate that they cannot talk themselves out of negative emotions.

Attention problems are common in this cluster, and certain features set these apart as unique. The attention issues associated with PAE are characterized by difficulty sustaining attention, encoding problems, and slow cognitive tempo. Patients are easily distracted and fight against any activity that exerts demands on their cognitive capacity. Patients show disorganized play, with trouble playing quietly. They have trouble waiting their turn, show poor impulse control and impatience, and regularly interrupt others. They cannot maintain their focus enough to finish tasks, which causes secondary effects; perpetual awareness of never finishing tasks, combined with others' diminished expectations and critical comments, leads to anxiety and low self-esteem. School children and adolescents may daydream, and adults commonly procrastinate. Consequently, patients present clinically with anxiety and behavioral and attention difficulties in school, home, and social contexts. Other consequences such as law breaking, misconduct, aggression, and mood swings have their origins in these complex interactions of neurocognitive deficits with the developmental environment of the individual with PAE.

Cluster of Adaptive Functioning Symptoms

Assessment of functional impairment across a broad range of domains is used not only for diagnosis but also to select the appropriate intervention. The relevant elements of adaptive function involve communication, social and motor skills, and activities of daily living. The goal of treatment is interdependence or independence that promotes agency in the individual. Patients may talk a lot and show superior verbal fluency but have difficulty with receptive language. This disconnect is a risk factor because professionals assume wrongly that the patients actually understand speech when they acquiesce to what is said.

Individuals with PAE have problems with visual motor integration and gross motor abnormalities. They are also known to be clumsy and poorly coordinated. Deficits in motor skills are more frequently assessed in younger patients. Current research shows that PAE is significantly associated with difficulties with fine motor skills, visual motor integration, and balance (Safe et al. 2018). If adequately examined, these abnormalities are recognized as persisting in older persons with a history of PAE. The manifestation may be through academic performance. Inability to copy diagrams, writing deficiency, and motor coordination problems characterize these individuals' school records.

Socially, several deficient areas exist. Individuals with PAE are known to be gullible and poor in estimating risk. They lack appropriate social skills; they are either hostile and suspicious or overfamiliar, friendly, and jovial. At times, they appear as overfriendly and generous even to their own disadvantage. They are unable to read social cues, which leads to boundary violations. This can lead to sexual inappropriateness in some patients. Thus, these patients need a lot of supervision, especially when they are seemingly unaware of the effect of their negative actions on others.

Because concepts of money, time, and space are challenging, those with PAE misunderstand others' points of view. Consequently, they fail in completing activities of daily living. The second vignette described earlier illustrates the challenges of one who is unable to organize his time to make appointments, cannot maintain employment, and gets into financial trouble easily. People with PAE are very suggestible and can be victimized and taken advantage of.

The proportion of people with PAE who have an IQ <70 is high; the average IQ ranges between 65 and 85 (Streissguth et al. 2004). This means that poor intellectual prowess, along with its varied manifestations (e.g., lack of awareness, poor coping skills, and learning disability), is a clinically important domain. In a study of young adults, being vulnerable to manipulation was reported in 92% of those with FASD. Not only were those with FASD noted to be victims of violent offenses (87%), as many as 77% reported sexual and/or physical abuse (Flannigan et al. 2018; Rasmussen et al. 2008). Identifying those with significant trauma is a high priority. Symptoms and sequelae of trauma are essential features to watch out for in those with ND-PAE/FASD.

It is crucially important to understand and unique to the neurodevelopmental origins of ND-PAE/FASD that patients' abilities are not consistent with their developmental stage. When misaligned with the patient's age, these symptoms are misinterpreted and labeled with negative connotations. Consequently, manifesting these "misaligned" symptoms has led to the application of many averse and harmful approaches to patients with ND-PAE/FASD. In a description of a patient with PAE, comprehension and social maturity appear to be the least developed, followed by social skills and concepts of money and time. Patients' capacities do not reflect to any degree the patients' physical age. Because these patients have fully developed expressive language skills, physicians may believe they comprehend and can follow instructions and thus may blame them for failure to follow through. Mental health professionals must understand the origins of and contextualize the patient's symptoms. Otherwise, the symptoms will be misconstrued, and the patient will not receive the appropriate care.

Internalizing and externalizing symptoms of conditions commonly comorbid with ND-PAE/FASD are also important clinical cues to assess. Many studies identify high rates of anxiety-, depression-, personality-, and trauma-related disorders (Barr et al. 2006; Clark et al. 2004; O'Connor et al. 2002). Both children and adults with PAE were classified either as having a comorbid disorder or exhibiting significant traits of several disorders (Baer et al. 2003). Adults presenting with a history of special education, multiple psychiatric disorders, frequent unemployment, dependence on a disability pension for financial support, and prescription of multiple psychotropic medications (Rangmar et al. 2015) display the classical adaptive function deficits.

Practical Use of Identified Symptoms

The diagnostic categories and labels a clinician applies to a group of clinical symptoms depend on the available diagnostic classification and the clinician's training and perspective. During clinical encounters, professionals identify the manifesting symptoms and ascribe them to relevant diagnoses. It is conceivable that two professionals with different training (one in mental disorder and the other in developmental disability disorder) could identify symptoms and classify the same symptoms as different diagnostic entities. PAE intricately produces many psychological, neurological, and functional symptoms, and various conditions can be inferred from the clinical manifestation of its consequences. The wider implications of correctly diagnosing an exposed individual include the provision of relevant support to the person diagnosed. Given that symptoms arising from PAE span a range of diagnostic entities, clinical benefits are best when symptoms are correctly apprehended and classified. This is dependent on the skills and expertise of the professional. Pertinent to ND-PAE/FASD, the right care also prevents longer-term adverse outcomes and issues (previously termed secondary disabilities). Clinically identifying manifesting symptoms and their associated factors helps to ascribe accurate diagnostic significance to the symptoms. The following vignette should guide clinicians in how to apportion symptoms.

Clinical Vignette

A 40-year-old woman attempted suicide after the recent firing from her job as a cashier in a fast food restaurant. The clinical consultation reveals that she recently experienced increased stress on account of the high volume of customers during the school holidays. The demand for her attention was too high, and she was distracted by the large volume of orders. Working at the register was a promotion for her; she had worked successfully for about 11 years in the kitchen of the same restaurant. The stress continued to affect her, and she experienced a lot of anxiety at work. She made mistakes at the register. She felt ashamed to ask for help in managing herself and the job. For a period of more than 4 weeks, she describes disturbed sleep and reduced appetite. She "went off social media for 2 weeks" before the suicide attempt.

On further questioning, she indicates how sad she feels, blaming herself for "not being there for my brother." She acknowledges he had a hard life. Her brother was apparently killed in gang-related violence, and she believes he was diagnosed with FASD. She attended her brother's funeral in an adjoining town. She was thinking about her brother's death in addition to the loss of her job over the previous several days. When she was driving one day, she immediately had an impulse and swerved the car off the road to kill herself. When the car stopped, she called an ambulance and was transported to the emergency room.

She describes how she feels easily overwhelmed with everything happening to her, including some relationship problems with her coworkers. She has a history of social anxiety disorder but no alcohol or substance use history. She struggled with learning in school. As part of the school's services for academic struggles, she was referred to a mental health clinic for assessment. She was told there was "nothing wrong" with her. She was advised to work harder to achieve good grades. She was able to obtain her high school equivalency certificate.

Additional information reveals that after about nine different foster and group home placements, she was adopted with her brother and was supported by her now aged parents. She provides no history of experiencing emotional, sexual, or physical abuse but recalls fun family holidays when she was growing up with her adoptive family.

Red Flags: What Else Could It Be?

The following are indicators of maladaptive function that should raise suspicion of a disability. The patient, even with a history of job stability, became easily overwhelmed and displayed a lack of problem-solving ability. Stressed by the grief and loss of her brother, her experience of anxiety and distress worsened her coping ability. The challenges of managing the cash register could be related to difficulties comprehending orders, poor math skills, increased distractibility, and deficits in executive function (Koditu-wakku 2009). As noted, individuals with PAE easily feel overwhelmed but more so when stressed and anxious. This means she would be unable to or-ganize, plan, sequence, and complete tasks associated with the role of a ca-shier. Additional information about a sibling with FASD reinforces the possibility of her also experiencing PAE. This will need to be confirmed when she is assessed.

A previous assessment of "nothing wrong" or no mental disorder is a recognized red flag for PAE when the clinical picture shows as much dys-function as depicted in the vignette. Patients surveyed after diagnosis of ND-PAE/FASD not only report being disqualified for treatment by the mental health system, they indicate that they were previously assessed as normal or "cleared mentally" (Anderson et al. 2020; Choate and Badry 2018). This assertion makes clinical sense when those diagnosed with ND-PAE/FASD only become aware of the deficits long after they were labeled with other diagnoses. In a study of foster and adopted children, 86.5% of the clinical sample were misdiagnosed or had never been diagnosed (Chas-noff et al. 2015). Similar high rates are reported in research studies using a case ascertainment approach (Fast et al. 1999). As counterintuitive as it may sound, a patient with plenty of symptoms of dysfunction at the point of care who reveals a previous finding of normality should arouse suspicion of PAE. Although not definite as a red flag, it cues clinicians to seek out other more definite features to warrant a more comprehensive evaluation.

The patient's poor coping and stress-induced suicidal behavior are in keeping with the suspicion of PAE. Those with PAE are significantly at a higher risk of impulsive behaviors. With her mood instability, refusal to ask for help, and evidence of poor cognitive ability to resolve problems, she demonstrated the pattern reported in self-harming patients with PAE. Such red flags signal the need for further evaluation.

Cases similar to that in the vignette "Identifying Risk Factors" provide few definite indicators of PAE. Only the presence of the sentinel facial fea-tures is pathognomonic. For that reason, the value of risk factors or red flags lies in comprehensive assessments to determine if a diagnosis can be made. Current evidence in this vignette, such as having a sibling with a di-agnosis and the patient's unstable living circumstances (being in many fos-ter and group homes), implicates PAE. The rate of FAS in the offspring of a woman who already has given birth to a child with FAS was estimated at 771 per 1,000 births (Huebert and Raftis 1996). Having a sibling with PAE remains a strong predictor of ND-PAE/FASD and is an item in several screening instruments relevant as clinical tools. Multiple broken placements are almost characteristic of PAE. The mean number of placements (foster homes, group homes, and adoptive family placements) is high (Streissguth et al. 1996). A high percentage of those with FASD are removed from their biological homes, are not placed with immediate family, and are relocated several times before adolescence. Studies show an overrepresentation of ND-PAE/FASD in the child welfare system, with a pooled 6% rate in a recent meta-analysis (Lange et al. 2017). Youth with FASD are frequently moved from home to home. Those experiences seem to predict worse outcomes, such as school failure, criminal activities, and mental health adversity (Streissguth et al. 1996).

Clinically, suggestions of lower intellectual prowess and executive dysfunction are indicators of PAE (Kodituwakku 2009). Clinical research has found that 86% of patients with any of the FASD symptoms have an IQ in the low average or borderline ranges (Streissguth et al. 1996). Complete neuropsychological profiles of those with PAE indicate high rates of deficits in executive function. These deficits translate to adaptive dysfunctions that represent red flags, which should be sought out during the clinical encounter. The vignette patient therefore qualifies to be more comprehensively evaluated, preferably by a multidisciplinary team with expertise in PAE evaluation.

The question that is regularly asked is what difference does noting red flags (potential low intellect, sibling with FASD, evidence of impulsivity, poor coping, multiple foster care placements, and a history of service exclusion) make in the conceptualization and management of the case? The quality of the assessment is enhanced because it is more focused to elicit the necessary diagnostic criteria for ND-PAE/FASD. Both limited teams and multidisciplinary professional teams should confirm these identified risks.

ND-PAE–Focused Evaluation

In evaluation for ND-PAE, information on maternal health and disease is sought. Efforts are made to identify the presence or absence of chronic liver disease; successful and specifically unsuccessful participation and involvement with alcohol treatment and rehabilitation; history of depression, especially in the perinatal period; and experience of abuse in multiple ways. Personality disorders and a history of incarceration are important in associating PAE with offspring. Childhood abuse, domestic violence, and sexual victimization as an adult were all reported as exceptionally high in mothers who gave birth to children with PAE and its associated consequences (Astley et al. 2000). Mothers who gave birth to children diagnosed with FASD had relative risk of 12.65 and 12.93 for having a substance use disorder and personality disorder, respectively. This fact should prompt clinicians to inquire of such diagnoses during the diagnostic process (Singal et al. 2017). Relative risk (~12) of pre and post substance use disorders and personality disorders in mothers with prenatal alcohol use call for a specific review of family history of mental disorder, especially in the mothers (Singal et al. 2017). In addition, close examination of the pregnancy may reveal a higher and substantial level of psychological distress (Singal et al. 2017).

Additional information about family members may reveal a sibling diagnosed with ND-PAE/FASD or other neurodevelopmental disorders. The patient's life trajectory should be reviewed with a focus on the type or level of education completed; special versus regular education, specific learning problems (e.g., math, spelling, writing, reading), conduct problems suggesting difficult externalizing behaviors, hyperactivity, and disciplinary actions (suspension or expulsion) are strong factors to be assessed. Patients' experience with ACEs and unsuccessful residential placements are also highly indicative of PAE. Patients with PAE and resulting negative outcomes of alcohol and substance use, as well as criminal behavior, have a characteristically early age of onset for these behaviors. Coupled with behavior, showing poor recognition of risk and gullibility should be evaluated thoroughly (Greenspan and Driscoll 2016; Gudjonsson and Clare 1995). These methods of pursuing likely clinical features assist in full assessment, especially when the processes have to be truncated because of poor resources. Efforts should still be made to adhere to rigorous and valid diagnostic process.

A critical aspect of identifying red flags is ordering assessment to confirm the suspicion of PAE and its consequences. The policies and procedures of the existing health care system in any jurisdiction determine how to access such an assessment. Assessments properly conducted identify deficits, which in turn inform modifications in treatment approach necessary to enhance functioning and provide support for the patient. The expression of poor coping and depressive symptoms is understood as affect dysregulation, common in those with PAE (Cook et al. 2016). These symptoms may require specific interventions using guidelines for the treatment of mood disorders or modified approaches that recognize PAE-induced deficits (Kennedy et al. 2016; Mela et al. 2018). The patient's employment success should now be fostered by modified and realistic expectations and accommodation for whatever deficits the assessment identifies. Coaching, mentoring, change of pace, and even return to the previously successful kitchen work for the patient in the vignette are options to consider.

Lessons From Age-Related Clinical Presentations

Psychopathology associated with PAE occurs with or without intellectual disability. Identifying the features assists in providing a neurodevelopmental trajectory in children. For instance, internalizing, externalizing, sleep, stereotypy, and behavioral disturbances are frequently characterized in those with ND-PAE/FASD. Adult manifestations support the notion that the psychopathology persists and may evolve but, more importantly, may develop and only become obvious after a period of subtle or no childhood manifestation. Features noted in adults include psychotic, mood, personality, alcohol, and substance use disorders (Leibson et al. 2014). Higher rates of eating disorders, ADHD, and autism cut across the age trajectory. Among the neurocognitive deficits common in many mental disorders, executive function (e.g., difficulties with set shifting, planning, fluency) deficits are the most prevalent in those with PAE. In addition to executive function deficits, manifestations of difficulties with working memory, mathematical ability, processing speed, cognition, and interhemispheric transfer should cue clinicians to ND-PAE/FASD.

Other Research-Based Clinical Indices of PAE

In some cases, the complaints of and phrases used by caregivers provide a clue to deficits associated with PAE. Parents and caregivers report patients as lying for no good reason and stealing without covering their acts or trying to avoid detection; they accuse patients of being silly. Owing to deficits in boundary awareness, patients are also described as "liking to poke the bear" or gravitating toward younger people in relationships. Descriptions such as "hyperactive, disruptive, impulsive, or delinquent" are common with ADHD but should be red flags in ND-PAE/FASD (Mattson and Riley 2000; Roebuck et al. 1998). Certain features should lead clinicians to ascribe PAE to the patient. Terms or phrases used to convey how the patient is easily overwhelmed and that coping resources are quickly depleted include "My voices are acting up," "I am bugging out," and "I can't explain it," and for the desperate or suicidal patient, "I feel I should slash up," and "I can't cope with this."

After many years of failed services, patients begin to use terms referent to their deficits. It is important to scrutinize how patients with ND-PAE/FASD are referred to by their family, front line staff, and other preceding professionals, especially those not consciously aware of the person's PAE-related deficits. Patients are referred to as deliberately missing appointments and being aggressive, dishonest, unreasonable, or antisocial. Viewed through the lens of PAE, these behaviors are seen as the result of forgetfulness, cognitive inflexibility, impulse control problems, concrete thinking, and hypersensitivity to sensory stimuli. As a result, some experts, usually well-meaning yet ill-equipped staff, coined the acronym NURMU (noncompliant, uncooperative, resistant, manipulative, and unmotivated) to characterize patients. It is known that even patients start to view themselves in those terms and consider themselves bad and stupid (Substance Abuse and Mental Health Services Administration 2014). These terms and labels allow the astute clinician to note the gaps and cracks in the patient's service trajectory and develop new approaches to correct them. The status quo only perpetuates negative stereotypes and outcomes.

Specific Diagnostic Features

During the patient interview, common features of ND-PAE/FASD should be evaluated. Patients are usually born small for their age and experience repeated ear infections (otitis media) that require insertion of tubes in their ears. Asking about a history of and surgery related to cleft lip or palate is appropriate. From repeated findings in populations of those with PAE, the rates of ACEs are about fourfold higher than that of the general population. Interviewers should determine if there is an indication of abuse (emotional, sexual, neglect, or physical). Evidence of early behavioral problems or diagnosis of oppositional defiant disorder, conduct disorder, ADHD, or autism spectrum disorder should not only serve as a red flag but should direct the line of clinical inquiry. Thus, it is important to evaluate this during the clinical encounter.

For the adult person, adaptive problems of self-care and dependent living have repeatedly been identified in research and should be explored. Research also suggests that adults with FASD become involved in crime, and their age of onset for criminal activity occurs between 12 and 14 years or even younger. The offenses are repeated, unnecessary, and impulsive. These individuals also show a significant level of easy manipulation as well as risk unawareness. Some data exist that show people with neurocognitive deficits from PAE in the criminal justice system have long records of criminal involvement. Their offenses were notably those of habitual breaches of release conditions (Brintnell et al. 2019). It has been suggested that these offenses are due to deficits in impulse control, memory, and organization and mental disorder, which jointly or singly contribute to ongoing offending (Byrne 2002; Kodituwakku, 2009).

Clinical Interview With a Purpose

A clinician who encounters a patient with several indicators suggestive of neurocognitive deficits has different options. Focus can be diverted to eliciting more complete prenatal and perinatal accounts of the patient's birth history. Adopting a PAE lens, certain questions ideal for the child and adolescent patient may yield less clinical information for the adult patient. Eliciting helpful information about possible etiology, development, functioning, previous treatment, and prognosis should guide the questioning.

Estimating the likelihood of PAE generally is more successful for patients in the younger age group. Caregivers are more readily available, and when approached by clinicians with sensitivity and tact, they are able to reveal confirming histories of preconception adversity, trauma, and alcohol or substance use. Clinicians should inquire about adequacy and appropriateness of prenatal care and the methods and outcomes of delivery. Developmental milestones, achieved or delayed, provide clinically useful guides to how the patient functioned, which impacts trajectories in the educational, social, and employment realms. Indices or behaviors associated with difficulties of temperament, emotional regulation, and the rhythmic system that controls the biological clock should be inquired about. Evidence of disruptive childhood experiences and expressions (internalizing and externalizing) should be sought. The advantage of younger patient assessment is that caregiver information recall is better closer to the time of birth and information is more recent and reliable. Moreover, the required confirmation of maternal substance or alcohol use is more likely because the chances of the birth mother being alive are higher.

Screening tools used during pregnancy can detect alcohol use in women but have been developed with little or no relationship-building techniques. A *therapeutic working alliance* is a relationship between the clinician and the patient that yields beneficial change. Importantly, the change flows from clinician–patient engagement, characterized by a trusting bond. This is the platform for sensitively and tactfully obtaining information with a negative connotation. Confirming PAE falls into that realm and calls not only for appropriate questioning but careful timing. Recent surveys employ questions that are not critical of the woman but supportive. They also point the respondent to sources of help, especially if she will become pregnant in the future. Compared with previous tools for inquiring about maternal use of alcohol, a maternal history checklist developed for postpregnancy mothers incorporates the appropriate items in a more nonjudgmental way. A few areas of inquiry are noted in Table 6–2.

In the assessment of the adult patient, a third-party concept is adopted. Information about the birth mother's life before and after pregnancy relies on the

TABLE 6–2. Areas of inquiry for birth mother

DESCRIBE THE FOLLOWING ENCOUNTERS AND EXPERIENCES DURING YOUR PREGNANCY WITH THE PATIENT:
Whole duration of gestation
Mood and behavior changes
Nutrition and healthy behaviors
Strategies to positively influence pregnancy outcome
Things avoided during pregnancy
Negative influences you could not avoid
Sources of support and help during pregnancy

patient's awareness of discussions about prenatal and perinatal life. Indicators common in PAE include relevant factors that make maternal alcohol consumption during pregnancy likely. Social disadvantage, stressful life circumstances, unawareness or ignorance about the danger of prenatal alcohol use, mental and substance use diagnoses, and having a sibling with alcohol-related developmental problems are helpful clues. Others, such as child welfare involvement, residential instability, ACEs, and several foster and group home placements, have been strongly associated with PAE. The adult's functioning in educational, employment, legal, and social contexts are also instructive.

Reviewing past records for adaptive, psychoeducational, and cognitive scales is clinically important. All successful and unsuccessful treatments and outcomes should be investigated.

Addressing Diagnostic Capacity in the Mental Health System

Multidisciplinary teams are not new in the mental health and addiction systems. What is new is the skill required to complete a comprehensive assessment of individuals with ND-PAE/FASD. It goes without saying that a screening method will help facilitate the identification of potential candidates for full assessments. If effective, such a tool will be highly sought because it presents the best cost-effective means of identifying people in the mental health system who could also have ND-PAE/FASD. No such tool currently exists. Tools in existence have not been designed for use by mental health professionals. However, some approaches are worth mentioning. The older a patient being assessed is, the more difficult it is to confirm PAE. A set of criteria were developed that are thought to represent direct and indirect indications that characterize women more likely to have consumed alcohol during pregnancy (Brown et al. 2015). These criteria can be applied in the absence of a confirmed maternal history of alcohol use. Maternal alcohol use cannot be confirmed in the event the mother is dead, not accessible, or declines contact on account of guilt, shame, or blame or if the patient was adopted or fostered and the records are missing or incomplete. Some patients deliberately isolate themselves; refusing to contact their mother is their way of trying to resolve the anger associated with abandonment.

Professionals should be aware of these circumstances and adopt processes that are nonjudgmental and supportive (Table 6–3). Supportive interviewing techniques should be used with both the patients and their mothers (biological and alternate caregivers). Frontline staff of group homes should also be trained in supportive communication techniques.

TABLE 6–3.   Characteristic features arousing clinical suspicion of PAE in the mother

PAE IS HIGHLY SUSPECTED IF THE OFFSPRING'S MOTHER DISPLAYS CERTAIN CHARACTERISTICS/EXPERIENCES:
Maternal risk indicators*
Physical, sexual, or emotional abuse
Alcohol and substance use disorder
Major depressive disorder
Suicidal ideation and attempts
Birth of another offspring with ND-PAE/FASD
Domestic violence
Diagnosis of personality disorder
History of incarceration

*Alcohol dehydrogenase polymorphism, heavy drinking spouse/partner, family history of alcoholism, high rates of stillbirths

Screening: Identifying Those Likely to Present to Mental Health Systems With Consequences of PAE

Attempts to develop screening tools have existed for as long as patients suspected of manifesting the consequences of PAE have presented to clinicians. This is especially the case for mental health professionals because the symptoms of their traditional patients need to be distinguished from the frequently occurring clinical manifestation of those with PAE. Some tools are in use to screen for evidence of maternal drinking, dysmorphic features, and behavioral and social profiles. None of these have formally and systematically been introduced in the mental health system. The call for such a screening process, however, is supported by the high rates of FASD in the mental health system and the need to reduce complications from inappropriate care and support. To be ethically and clinically sound, the tools developed should be easy for busy clinicians to use, reliable, valid, and context specific. Relevant characteristics of populations for screening range from age groups to those receiving mental health services in which there is an overrepresentation of patients with the consequences of PAE. Patients receiving clinical services for mental disorder or alcohol and substance use disorder and patients receiving child and adolescent, forensic, or geriatric services are a natural fit for these types of tools. Nonclinical populations with an overrepresentation of ND-PAE/FASD, such as those in foster care and the child welfare system, would also benefit from screening.

The idea for screening is laudable; however, the task of creating a screen is daunting because it seems unlikely that one screening method will suffice and be applicable to different clinical and nonclinical populations. For mental health professionals, ethical screening involves acquiring the necessary competence to easily administer the tool and intervene with effective treatments. This is the basis of the modifications now incorporated in several screening and substance use treatments (Grant et al. 2013).

Current screening tools and programs for PAE were developed differently and without patients in the mental health system in mind. Questionnaires preferentially used in screening programs suffer from the problem of untested validity. In certain situations, eliciting a history of prenatal alcohol use has been wrongly equated with FASD. Behavioral and developmental patterns of behavior can be put together to develop a profile and can be used as a screening tool. The assay of meconium to detect free fatty acid ethyl ester levels can be used in the postnatal period. However, this biological test is not yet available in most centers.

Common Clinical Presentation

Those with neurocognitive deficits and sequelae of PAE present clinically with a host of issues and difficulties. Research on the reasons for referral is instructive. Behavioral control problems and inattention were noted as the most prevalent reasons among children. Hyperactivity is a more common reason for referral among children than adults.

Guideline recommendations regarding reasons for referral recognize the importance of varying threshold levels. Specifically, the threshold is lower for those in foster care, in adoptive families, with a history of a sibling with FASD, with criminal involvement, and with maternal history of alcohol-related disorders. It has also been suggested that those living in a community with a known higher rate of alcohol consumption should be included in the low-threshold referral category. Research found that communities with a high per-capita consumption of alcohol also had a high rate of ND-PAE/FASD (Bell 2014, 2016).

These features are not surprising given the direct consequences of PAE and those observed with careful study. The deficits associated with cognitive dysfunction manifest as problems with impulse control, attention, and executive function. These impact behavior control and are distressing, especially to family members and teachers. Lack of recognition of the underlying deficits and progression of untreated behavior result in worse outcomes in the adolescent and adult patient. Patients show disruptive and aggressive behaviors that can easily be confused with individual or collective signs and symptoms of mental disorder. Deficits in social function emerge as difficulties in communication skills, as well as impaired recognition of social cues, and create relationship difficulties. School functioning and socialization, which depend on effective social function, are critically hampered by these difficulties in children and youth. These deficits disturb functioning and can lead to misunderstanding, exploitation, invasion of privacy and boundary violations, and criminal behavior in adolescents and adults (Brown et al. 2018).

One common, yet unique, difficulty manifesting in patients with FASD is adaptive dysfunction, which is so critical that it is a major diagnostic criterion. Those identified usually present with poor problem-solving abilities and experience the consequences of mounting unresolved issues. As children, with or without additional mood and anxiety disorders, their ability to adapt to new situations is so impaired that they withdraw, avoid, or even become aggressive in new situations, such as school. When subject to residential instability, moving from family to family, as is frequently the case during foster and adoptive care, those affected show poor adjustment and manifest aggression, withdrawal, and insecure attachment. Anxiety, depression, and sleep difficulties are common reactions and create some of the early comorbid mental health symptoms that interface with FASD and mental disorder.

Aside from a few differences unique to those with ND-PAE/FASD, most features of its clinical manifestations are shared by many disorders. One significant feature of PAE and its outcomes involves deficits in executive function. Differentiating PAE deficits from similar deficits shared by 50%–75% of those diagnosed with ADHD is difficult. Social deficits that lead to social inhibition occur similarly in both autism spectrum disorder and in PAE and its consequences, although the latter manifest with a bit more disinhibition. In an effort to define the features of ND-PAE/FASD, manifesting symptoms were compared with several other disorders, especially in childhood. Disinhibition, poor social skills, impulsive behavior, perseveration, explosive anger, and sleep difficulties are a few brain-based features common in ND-PAE/FASD. These same features occur frequently in pervasive developmental disorders, mood disorders, disruptive behavior disorders, and intellectual disability disorders. In older subjects, lack of maturity, poor personal relations, poor understanding of personal boundaries, and becoming easily overwhelmed, which are characteristic of ND-PAE/FASD, can be true for a number of mental disorders. Patients manifesting a lack of maturity show wide variations in different areas of development. Patients with a well-developed expressive language will not necessarily have as good self-regulatory or memory abilities, for example. The consequences of these deficits and direct expression mimic antisocial personality behaviors, socially deficient negative symptoms, and borderline personality disorder.

Moving from a symptom-based conceptualization, ND-PAE/FASD has three domains of symptom clusters (self-regulatory, adaptive, and neurocognitive). These converge, and the spread of and correlation among their symptoms provide strong internal consistency. As such, the diagnostic criteria are highly reliable and well accepted, and their clinical utility is robust.

Clinically, PAE and comorbid conditions have a cumulative diagnostic relationship. Comorbid manifestations are more common in those with PAE, and a history of comorbid conditions increases the chances of an FASD diagnosis. Such was the case when the trajectories of 154 children were reassessed for an FASD diagnosis. Two years after initial assessment, impaired brain function, postnatal risk, and comorbidities predicted an FASD diagnosis in the one-third of subjects who were diagnosed on second assessment (Flannigan et al. 2019; Temple et al. 2019). Another finding in the relationship between FASD and ADHD has clinical utility: FASD with or without ADHD produced a poorer behavioral and cognitive profile in a study of 164 patients. The profile, along with externalizing behavior, hyperactivity, higher levels of atypicality, and aggression, differentiated ADHD from the impact of FASD, which can be a clinical indication for a comprehensive FASD assessment referral (Raldiris et al. 2018). Collateral information from teachers—high scores in learning problems, inattention, and poor adaptive skills—correlated strongly with an FASD diagnosis in 345 children with FASD (Taylor and Enns 2019). If replicated, this ability to differentiate ADHD and FASD symptoms could streamline diagnostic efficiency and encourage mental health professionals to participate in detection of PAE and FASD.

Conclusion

In completing an assessment of a person with PAE, noting that complaints may appear to be about something different than the PAE effects, mental health professionals should consider the nature of the whole-body disorder.

When the invisible nature of FASD is undetected and neglected, negative outcomes are more pronounced. The characteristic features of ND-PAE/FASD are shared with many disorders, but some symptoms and signs are pathognomonic for detecting PAE effects. Functional assessment is crucially important becasue it informs treatment even if the pathognomonic signs are present.

CLINICAL PRACTICAL APPLICATIONS

- The diagnostic process constitutes an essential therapeutic component of the patient's recovery.

- Physical examination of the features of PAE should consider ethnic variations of facial structures and measures.

- Clinicians interested in learning about the training and use of facial photographic software can access the FAS Diagnostic and Prevention Network website (https://depts.washington.edu/fasdpn/htmls/face-software.htm).

- Physical examination and laboratory investigations of patients should target indicia of thyroid, iron, and protein deficiency.

- Early research findings suggest that FASD alone produces a worse clinical picture than ADHD or a combination of ADHD and FASD.

- A PAE-lens perspective on the commonly occurring suicide attempt should target contributory factors of impulsivity, lack of attention to risk, cognitive inflexibility, childhood trauma, and sensory processing problems.

- Patients who reveal a previous history of assessment during which they were told there was "nothing wrong" with them should prompt the mental health professional to adopt a PAE perspective.

- A multidisciplinary method of diagnosis is preferred over other approaches.

References

Anderson T, Mela M, Rotter T, Poole N: qualitative investigation into barriers and enablers for the development of a clinical pathway for individuals living with fasd and mental disorder/addictions. Canadian Journal of Community Mental Health 38(3):43–60, 2020

Astley SJ: Diagnostic Guide for Fetal Alcohol Spectrum Disorders: The 4-Digit Diagnostic Code, 3rd Edition. Seattle, University of Washington Publication Services, 2004. Available at: http://depts.washington.edu/fasdpn/pdfs/guide04.pdf. Accessed October 2, 2020.

Astley SJ: Palpebral fissure length measurement: accuracy of the FAS facial photographic analysis software and inaccuracy of the ruler. J Popul Ther Clin Pharmacol 22(1):e9–e26, 2015

Astley SJ, Clarren SK: Diagnosing the full spectrum of fetal alcohol-exposed individuals: introducing the 4-digit diagnostic code. Alcohol Alcohol 35(4):400–410, 2000

Astley SJ, Clarren SK: Measuring the facial phenotype of individuals with prenatal alcohol exposure: correlations with brain dysfunction. Alcohol Alcohol 36(2):147–159, 2001

Astley SJ, Bailey D, Talbot C, Clarren SK: Fetal alcohol syndrome (FAS) primary prevention through fas diagnosis: II. A comprehensive profile of 80 birth mothers of children with FAS. Alcohol Alcohol 35(5):509–519, 2000

Baer JS, Sampson PD, Barr HM, et al: A 21-year longitudinal analysis of the effects of prenatal alcohol exposure on young adult drinking. Arch Gen Psychiatry 60(4):377–385, 2003

Barr HM, Bookstein FL, O'Malley KD, et al: Binge drinking during pregnancy as a predictor of psychiatric disorders on the Structured Clinical Interview for DSM IV in young adult offspring. Am J Psychiatry 163(6):1061–1065, 2006

Bell CC: Fetal alcohol exposure among African Americans. Psychiatr Serv 65(5):569, 2014

Bell CC: High rates of neurobehavioral disorder associated with prenatal exposure to alcohol among African Americans driven by the plethora of liquor stores in the community. J Fam Med Dis Prev 2(2):033, 2016

Bodnarchuk J, Patton D, Rieck T: Adolescence without Shelter: A Comprehensive Description of Issues Faced by Street Youth in Winnipeg. Winnipeg, MB, Addictions Foundation of Manitoba, 2006

Breen C, Burns L: Improving Services to Families Affected by FASD. Sydney, NSW, Australia, National Drug and Alcohol Research Centre, University of New South Wales, November 2012

Brintnell ES, Sawhney AS, Bailey PG, et al: Corrections and connection to the community: a diagnostic and service program for incarcerated adult men with FASD. Int J Law Psychiatry 64:8–17, 2019

Brown J, Mitten R, Carter MN, et al: Fetal Alcohol Spectrum Disorder and Sexually Inappropriate Behaviors: A Guide for Criminal Justice and Forensic Mental Health Professionals. Concordia St. Paul Blog & News Updates, October 2018

Brown NN, Burd L, Grant T, et al: Prenatal alcohol exposure: an assessment strategy for the legal context. Int J Law Psychiatry 42:144–148, 2015

Burd L: FASD and ADHD: Are they related and how? BMC psychiatry 16(1):325, 2016

Byrne C: The Criminalization of Fetal Alcohol Syndrome (FAS). 2002 Available at: http://www.americanbar.org/content/dam/aba/migrated/child/PublicDocuments/cfas.authcheckdam.pdf. Accessed February 23, 2019.

Chasnoff IJ, Wells AM, King L: Misdiagnosis and missed diagnoses in foster and adopted children with prenatal alcohol exposure. Pediatrics 135(2):264–270, 2015

Choate P, Badry D: Stigma as a dominant discourse in fetal alcohol spectrum disorder. Adv Dual Diagn 12:36–52, 2018

Clark E, Lutke J, Minnes PM, Ouellette-Kuntz H: Secondary disabilities among adults with fetal alcohol spectrum disorder in British Columbia. J FAS Int 2(e13):1–12, 2004

Clarren SK, Chudley AE, Wong L, et al: Normal distribution of palpebral fissure lengths in Canadian school age children. Can J Clin Pharmacol 17(1):e67–e78, 2010

Cook JL, Green CR, Lilley CM, et al: Fetal alcohol spectrum disorder: a guideline for diagnosis across the lifespan. CMAJ 188(3) 191–197, 2016

Dube SR, Anda RF, Felitti VJ, et al: Childhood abuse, household dysfunction, and the risk of attempted suicide throughout the life span: findings from the Adverse Childhood Experiences Study. JAMA 286(24):3089–3096, 2001

Fang S, McLaughlin J, Fang J, et al: Automated diagnosis of fetal alcohol syndrome using 3D facial image analysis. Orthod Craniofac Res 11(3):162–171, 2008

Fast DK, Conry J, Loock CA: Identifying fetal alcohol syndrome among youth in the criminal justice system. J Dev Behav Pediatr 20(5):370–372, 1999

Flannigan K, Pei J, Stewart M, Johnson A: Fetal alcohol spectrum disorder and the criminal justice system: a systematic literature review. Int J Law Psychiatry 57:42–52, 2018

Flannigan K, Gill K, Pei J, et al: Deferred diagnosis in children assessed for fetal alcohol spectrum disorder. Appl Neuropsychol Child 8(3):213–222, 2019

Grant TM, Brown NN, Graham JC, et al: Screening in treatment programs for fetal alcohol spectrum disorders that could affect therapeutic progress. Int J Alcohol Drug Res 2(3):37–49, 2013

Greenspan S, Driscoll JH: Why people with FASD fall for manipulative ploys: ethical limits of interrogators' use of lies, in Fetal Alcohol Spectrum Disorders in Adults: Ethical and Legal Perspectives: An Overview on FASD for Professionals (International Library of Ethics, Law, and the New Medicine, Vol. 63). Edited by Nelson M, Trussler M. Cham, Switzerland, Springer, 2016, pp 23–38

Gudjonsson GH, Clare ICH: The relationship between confabulation and intellectual ability, memory, interrogative suggestibility and acquiescence. Pers Individ Diff 19(3):333–338, 1995

Hagan JF Jr, Balachova T, Bertrand J, et al: Neurobehavioral disorder associated with prenatal alcohol exposure. Pediatrics 138(4):e20151553 2016

Huebert K, Raftis C: Fetal Alcohol Syndrome and Other Alcohol-Related Birth Defects, 2nd Edition. Edmonton, AB, Alberta Alcohol and Drug Abuse Commission, 1996

Kable JA, Coles CD: Evidence supporting the internal validity of the proposed ND-PAE disorder. Child Psychiatry Hum Dev 49(2):163–175, 2018

Kennedy SH, Lam RW, McIntyre RS, et al: Canadian Network for Mood and Anxiety Treatments (CANMAT) 2016 clinical guidelines for the management of adults with major depressive disorder: section 3: pharmacological treatments. Can J Psychiatry 61(9):540–560, 2016

Kodituwakku PW: Neurocognitive profile in children with fetal alcohol spectrum disorders. Dev Disabil Res Rev 15(3):218–224, 2009

LaDue RA, Streissguth AP, Randels SP: Clinical considerations pertaining to adolescents and adults with fetal alcohol syndrome, in Perinatal Substance Abuse: Research Findings and Clinical Implications. Edited by Sonderegger TB. Baltimore, MD, The Johns Hopkins University Press, 1992, pp 104–131

Lange S, Probst C, Gmel G, et al: Global prevalence of fetal alcohol spectrum disorder among children and youth: a systematic review and meta-analysis. JAMA Pediatr 171(10):948–956, 2017

Lebel CA, McMorris CA, Kar P, et al: Characterizing adverse prenatal and postnatal experiences in children. Birth Defects Res 111(12):848–858, 2019

Leibson T, Neuman G, Chudley AE, Koren G: The differential diagnosis of fetal alcohol spectrum disorder. J Popul Ther Clin Pharmacol 21(1):e1–e30, 2014

Lunsky Y: Suicidality in a clinical and community sample of adults with mental retardation. Res Dev Disabil 25(3):231–243, 2004

Mattson SN, Riley EP: Parent ratings of behavior in children with heavy prenatal alcohol exposure and IQ-matched controls. Alcohol Clin Exp Res 24(2):226–231, 2000

Mela M, Okpalauwaekwe U, Anderson T, et al: The utility of psychotropic drugs on patients with fetal alcohol spectrum disorder (FASD): a systematic review. Psychiatry and Clinical Psychopharmacology 28(4):436–445, 2018

Moore ES, Ward RE, Wetherill LF, et al: Unique facial features distinguish fetal alcohol syndrome patients and controls in diverse ethnic populations. Alcohol Clin Exp Res 31(10):1707–1713, 2007

Mutsvangwa TE, Meintjes EM, Viljoen DL, Douglas TS: Morphometric analysis and classification of the facial phenotype associated with fetal alcohol syndrome in 5-and 12-year-old children. Am J Med Genet Part A 152(1):32–41, 2010

O'Connor MJ, Shah B, Whaley S, et al: Psychiatric illness in a clinical sample of children with prenatal alcohol exposure. Am J Drug Alcohol Abuse 28(4):743–754, 2002

Popova S, Lange S, Shield K, et al: Comorbidity of fetal alcohol spectrum disorder: a systematic review and meta-analysis. Lancet 387(10022):978–987, 2016

Price A, Cook PA, Norgate S, Mukherjee R: Prenatal alcohol exposure and traumatic childhood experiences: a systematic review. Neurosci Biobehav Rev 80:89–98, 2017

Raldiris TL, Bowers TG, Towsey C: Comparisons of intelligence and behavior in children with fetal alcohol spectrum disorder and ADHD. J Atten Disord 22(10):959–970, 2018

Rangmar J, Sandberg AD, Aronson M, Fahlke C: Cognitive and executive functions, social cognition and sense of coherence in adults with fetal alcohol syndrome. Nord J Psychiatry 69(6):472–478, 2015

Rasmussen C, Andrew G, Zwaigenbaum L, Tough S: Neurobehavioural outcomes of children with fetal alcohol spectrum disorders: a Canadian perspective. Paediatr Child Health 13(3):185–191, 2008

Roebuck TM, Simmons RW, Richardson C, et al: Neuromuscular responses to disturbance of balance in children with prenatal exposure to alcohol. Alcohol Clin Exp Res 22(9):1992–1997, 1998

Safe B, Joosten A, Giglia R: Assessing motor skills to inform a fetal alcohol spectrum disorder diagnosis focusing on persons older than 12 years: a systematic review of the literature. J Popul Ther Clin Pharmacol 25(1):e25–e38, 2018

Sanders JL, Breen RE, Netelenbos N: Comparing diagnostic classification of neurobehavioral disorder associated with prenatal alcohol exposure with the Canadian fetal alcohol spectrum disorder guidelines: a cohort study. CMAJ Open 5(1):E178–E183, 2017

Shelton D, Reid N, Till H, et al: Responding to fetal alcohol spectrum disorder in Australia. J Paediatr Child Health 54(10):1121–1126, 2018

Singal D, Brownell M, Chateau D, et al: The psychiatric morbidity of women who give birth to children with fetal alcohol spectrum disorder (FASD): results of the Manitoba Mothers and FASD study. Can J Psychiatry 62(8):531–542, 2017

Streissguth AP, Barr HM, Kogan J, Bookstein FL: Understanding the Occurrence of Secondary Disabilities in Clients with Fetal Alcohol Syndrome (FAS) and Fetal Alcohol Effects (FAE), Final Report to the Centers for Disease Control and Prevention (CDC) (Tech Rep No 96-06). Seattle, University of Washington, Fetal Alcohol and Drug Unit, 1996

Streissguth AP, Bookstein FL, Barr HM, et al: Risk factors for adverse life outcomes in fetal alcohol syndrome and fetal alcohol effects. J Dev Behav Pediatr 25(4):228–238, 2004

Substance Abuse and Mental Health Services Administration: Addressing Fetal Alcohol Spectrum Disorders (FASD). Treatment Improvement Protocol (TIP) Series 58. HHS Publication No (SMA) 13-4803. Rockville, MD, Substance Abuse and Mental Health Services Administration, 2014

Taylor NM, Enns LN: Factors predictive of a fetal alcohol spectrum disorder diagnosis: parent and teacher ratings. Child Neuropsychol 25(4):507–526, 2019

Temple K, Cook VL, Unsworth J, et al: Mental health and affect regulation impairment in fetal alcohol spectrum disorder (FASD): results from the Canadian national FASD database. Alcohol Alcohol 54(5):545–550, 2019

Thanh NX, Jonsson E: Life expectancy of people with fetal alcohol syndrome. J Popul Ther Clin Pharmacol 23(1):e53–e59, 2016

Wattendorf DJ, Muenke M: Fetal alcohol spectrum disorders. Am Fam Physician 72(2):279–282, 285, 2005

Weyrauch D, Schwartz M, Hart B, et al: Comorbid mental disorders in fetal alcohol spectrum disorders: a systematic review. J Dev Behav Pediatr 38(4):283–291 2017

CHAPTER 7

Mental Disorder Manifestation of Fetal Alcohol Spectrum Disorder

WHAT TO KNOW

The clinical disadvantages ascribed to PAE include misdiagnosis (a different diagnosis apparently explains the presentation) and comorbidity (most patients with ND-PAE/FASD commonly have additional and often multiple other diagnoses).

The phrases "peas in a pod" and "hand in glove" are aphorisms that convey the complex, intricate, and reciprocal nature of the link between ND-PAE/FASD and mental disorder.

Adult diagnosis of ND-PAE/FASD is complicated by the mother's absence, unavailability of birth records, identification with a substitute diagnosis, and physical changes over the lifespan.

The intellectual deficit of individuals with PAE provides little contribution to understanding their neurodevelopmental disorders because only about a quarter of affected individuals have an IQ <70.

Training mental health professionals on identification and recognition of the consequences of PAE in various contexts is greatly needed because of the many affected patients in the mental health system.

Clinicians who treat patients with mental disorder aspire to the goal of recovery for their patients. Patients who are least able to achieve recovery experience more severe, long-standing, and treatment-resistant symptoms. They typically have a greater share and weight of negative prognostic factors. Having multiple disorders, *comorbidity*, is one of the most significant factors contributing to poor outcomes. Two or more disorders in the same person reduce access to the right treatment and limit the effectiveness of treatment, which is usually directed toward one disorder but not the others. Treatment focused on one disorder without attending to the other comorbid states or disorders is inadequate because the synergistic effect of interacting symptoms creates additive symptoms that contribute to outcomes. It has been observed that in addition to lack of awareness of the history of PAE, patients at the interface of coexisting ND-PAE/FASD and mental disorder experience chronic symptoms on account of the interactive effect at that interface. The mental health and addiction systems are also reported to be ill-informed about these interactions. When professionals train to recognize mental disorder manifestations in patients with PAE, more appropriate clinical care is directed toward the patient and outcomes are improved. Some of these mental disorder symptoms are unique, but some are common symptoms that are disguised or misinterpreted because of PAE-related neurocognitive deficits.

Professionals need to adjust their practice methods and recognize the multifactorial causes of clinical symptoms, so that they are considered and addressed in patients who present to mental health and addiction services. The need for such modifications is crucial in the care of patients with ND-PAE/FASD and mental disorder. This reorientation should ensure patient-centered decisions, high-quality care, effective treatment, and best clinical practices—principles that embody the highest standard in the delivery of care. For the adjustments to be relevant, the minor as well as monumental differences in presentation by people who share common clinical features and yet have different disorders must be understood. Features of mental disorder exist in patients with ND-PAE/FASD, and the occurrence of both disorders (known as comorbidity or dual diagnosis) complicates the expected manifestations in affected individuals.

Overrepresentation of mental disorder among patients with neurodevelopmental disorder due to PAE is well established in cross-sectional, case ascertainment, and cohort studies and is reported in many countries (Barr et al. 2006; O'Connor and Paley 2009). It is necessary to understand the obvious and the hidden relationships of mental manifestations when a person at the ND-PAE/FASD and mental disorder interface presents to any professional. Indices and diagnosis of different categories of mental disorder (e.g., substance use disorder, personality disorder, suicidal behavior, learning disorder) appear in greater prevalence in those with ND-PAE/FASD. This suggests that mental health professionals will regularly encounter those with PAE and should have a high index of suspicion for comorbidity. These professionals will be more effective if they know the specific mental disorders that are more prevalent in the types of patients they see. Children and adolescents, pregnant women with substance use disorder, and geriatric patients exposed to alcohol prenatally likely present with different rates of comorbidity. The manifestations and knowledge about their impact are helpful guides for ease of identification.

The relationship between mental disorder and ND-PAE/FASD is one that is intricately complex and reciprocally linked. Mental disorder compounds the cognitive and maladaptive behavioral difficulties associated with ND-PAE/FASD because the variability of the diagnosis depends on in utero exposure to alcohol and the interaction of alcohol with genetic and environmental factors. Compared with diagnosis in children and youth, adult diagnosis is complex. The diagnostic process is challenged by the unavailability of the mother to confirm PAE, absence of birth records, changes in weight and height over the lifespan, and indistinct facial features. These unique features can be distorted from injury to the face, body weight, and muscle mass changes to the face.

Frequency of Comorbidity

Individuals with PAE diagnosed with FASD manifest a high prevalence of psychiatric problems. In a follow-up of 415 patients diagnosed with FASD, 92% had at least one additional mental disorder diagnosis. Drug and alcohol use disorder, suicidal ideation and behaviors, sexual dysfunction, and maladaptive behaviors were identified as indicators of additional mental disorder (Astley 2010; Streissguth et al. 1996).

Early studies reported an overrepresentation of mental disorders in subjects with PAE. It was not immediately clear if this was a case of dual diagnosis (intellectual and mental disorders coexisting in the same person). The initial idea of the uniqueness of FASD from other neurodevelopmental disorders, especially intellectual disability, was studied among patients diagnosed with FASD who had an IQ higher than the cutoff score for intellectual disability (Famy et al. 1998). The study reported a high risk of psychopathological conditions in adults linked to PAE. This was separate from the effect of intellectual disability. Other unusual findings were noted in support of the uniqueness of FASD. Researchers reported an equal sex ratio for major depression in those with the risk factor of PAE and those not exposed to alcohol prenatally (Astley 2010; Dirks et al. 2019). In addition, the rate of psychosis was high in adults with PAE. The type of psychosis was not schizophrenia (the most enduring psychotic disorder) (Astley 2010; Famy et al. 1998).

Prevalence rates of mental disorder and clinical manifestations of patients with mental disorder have been reported in different populations, which has practical clinical implications for the mental health subspecialties (McGee and Riley 2007; Stringaris 2011). Most studies focus on the rates of diagnosable mental disorder among those with PAE and not on the rates of PAE in those already diagnosed with a mental disorder. Those different studies (Famy et al. 1998; Mela et al. 2013; O'Connor and Paley 2009), usually from an FASD diagnostic clinic or among patients diagnosed with FASD, agree on the over-representation of mental disorder (Weyrauch et al. 2017). However, they report slightly different rates when the studies are conducted in different groups: children, adults, forensic patients, inpatients, or community samples. This has led to study synthesis in the form of systematic reviews and meta-analysis to determine which mental disorders are more prevalent (Weyrauch et al. 2017).

Most outcome studies report an overrepresentation of ADHD, mood and anxiety disorders, and personality disorders (Mela et al. 2013) in people with FASD. The reported rates for substance use and psychotic disorders have been inconsistent, varying depending on the population studied. In a German specialized adult psychiatric clinic for FASD, for instance, the rates for comorbid mental disorders were low compared with rates reported among patients with FASD in whom the occurrence of mental disorder was determined at a later follow-up period (Landgraf et al. 2013). A potential factor affecting the consistency of rates is the mean age of the sample. This may be the reason samples with a younger age range are characterized by lower numbers of those with mental disorder associated with a shorter duration to follow-up. It is proposed that the longer the experience of the psychosocial burden of the developmental problems, the more likely mental disorders will emerge as a consequence. Support for this hypothesis is not available from current epidemiological studies. The developmental origins of disease and health and the stress-diathesis model explain emerging outcomes (Benz et al. 2009; Walthall et al. 2008). These outcomes arise because the brain impaired by neurocognitive deficits is more vulnerable to stress over time. Overburdened and overtasked, the exposed person's resources cannot respond adequately, thus setting up a later development of mental disorder. Substance use disorders, for example, frequently develop because a substance is used as a poor coping mechanism to manage psychosocial problems (McGee and Riley 2007).

Manifestation of Mental Health Symptoms

A broad range of effects and symptoms caused by PAE has been grouped under the term *fetal alcohol spectrum disorder* (Cook et al. 2016). Specific developmental damage affecting brain regions in control of behavior and function means that most people affected with consequences of PAE experience mental health symptoms across the lifespan. Evaluating patients with FASD reveals age-dependent manifestations. In children, for instance, symptom manifestations of PAE include undercontrolled, acting-out, and delinquent behaviors. These behaviors are expected because of the nature of the neurodevelopmental CNS impairment central to the effect of PAE. Clinicians should be aware that these behaviors engender differential diagnoses that should be systematically investigated. Clinically, they are recognized and identified when patients' aggression, anger, defiance, destruction of property, hostility, noncompliance, and violations of social rules are directed toward the external environment.

The rates of externalizing symptoms manifested by those with FASD were noted in a sample of children ages 6–18 years, using the Child Behavior Checklist. Seventy-five percent of the sample met the clinical cutoff for externalizing behaviors (Franklin et al. 2008). Other research has indicated that compared with IQ-matched peers without PAE, subjects diagnosed with FASD had elevated rates of externalizing behaviors (Mattson et al. 2011). The presence of these disruptive symptoms is enough to trigger a suspicion of ND-PAE/FASD. At the same time, the relevant mental disorders characterized by similar manifestations should be recognized. Externalizing behaviors, such as hyperactivity, impulsivity, and delinquency, are prominent in oppositional defiant disorder (ODD), conduct disorder, ADHD, and autism spectrum disorder.

Because these behaviors commonly occur across varied diagnostic criteria, clinicians need to elicit the differential diagnoses. Indeed, the different disorders can coexist as comorbid conditions. The astute clinician must attempt to disentangle the disorders that share common manifestations. One helpful step is for evaluators to seek out the teratological history for all children with any neurodevelopmental disorder (especially those manifesting externalizing disorders). When the contribution of PAE is isolated in patients, the quality of care is enhanced by apportioning the neurocognitive deficit part of the presentation to the correct diagnosis. The ultimate next step is directing appropriate support to address the impairing symptoms. By implication, health care providers must routinely consider PAE in the differential diagnosis of behavioral problems (Lange et al. 2017).

Clinical Vignette

During a team meeting, the social worker in charge of the care of a school-boy presents his case and requests your expert advice. As the school social worker, she visits the school to explain the meaning and ramifications of the diagnosis of ND-PAE/FASD to the teachers, parents, and staff. The social worker describes the young boy as being unsuccessful in multiple foster placements because of externalizing behaviors. The boy shows significant adaptive dysfunction, and teachers and parents are becoming exhausted. He has been diagnosed with ADHD and ODD. Recently, he was diagnosed with ND-PAE/FASD, and that is why the social worker became involved. The question has come up as how to differentiate the patient's behaviors in order to understand what is causing the repeated breakdown in residential placements. Parents report they are sure that when the patient misbehaves, it is done deliberately. He refuses to follow simple instructions, and, when challenged, parents say he "lies." He is doing poorly in school, and his place at the school is also threatened because he is suspected of twice throwing objects at the teacher.

In responding to questions, the clinician should adopt an educational role. The social worker's awareness of the cause of behavior will help her explain the behaviors to the teachers, who will then be better able to support the boy, which will in turn reduce frustration. This has the potential to positively influence the boy's trajectory. PAE is understood by the kind of brain damage associated with the timing of exposure. The outcome depends on many factors and the specific damage. In PAE-related neurocognitive damage, instructions do not register, so the boy's reactions may be oppositional. As shown in the table developed by Dan Dubovsky (see Table 7–1), a person with PAE is different from a person with ODD. The latter person registers, understands, and can recall the information but makes a deliberate choice to disobey, unlike someone with ADHD who gets distracted. Each person's behavior is best managed from the perspective of the specific damage. This knowledge is crucial for the mental health professional in order to provide support for the patient, his family, and teachers.

Clinical Application of the Findings

Studies have sought to explain the co-occurrence of mental disorder and ND-PAE/FASD among patients found to have both disorders. One study reported an abnormally high incidence of significant adverse life events and specific social determinants of health in the trajectory of subjects studied. Most of the social determinants reported were psychosocial determinants such as financial problems, low social support, impulsiveness, or a history of trauma (Pei et al. 2011). For the mental health professional, these are helpful clues when dealing with patients with mental disorder experiencing these life events. Although such psychosocial factors are also common in garden-variety mental disorders, they can serve as indicators of PAE. The determinants rise to the level of clinical red flags when they occur in patients whose mental disorder manifestations are related to chronic comorbid

TABLE 7–1. Differentiating the underlying behavior and responsive intervention in three mental conditions

	FASD	**ADHD**	**ODD**
Behavior	Does not complete tasks	Does not complete tasks	Does not complete tasks
Underlying cause of the behavior	May or may not take in the information	Takes in the information	Takes in the information
	Cannot recall the information when needed	Can recall the information when needed	Can recall the information when needed
	Cannot remember what to do	Gets distracted	Chooses not to do what they are told
Interventions for the behavior	Provide one direction at a time	Limit stimuli and provide cues	Provide positive sense of control, limits, and consequences

Note. ODD=oppositional defiant disorder.
Source. Developed by Dan Dubovsky, M.S.W., FASD Specialist and Consultant, Philadelphia, Pennsylvania, 2002. Used with permission.

symptoms and resistance to regular traditional treatment. Other features highly indicative of PAE in patients with mental disorder are based on the common neurocognitive deficits. Profiling those in patients is the subject of Chapter 8 ("Profile of Associated Mental Disorders").

Given the crossover of symptoms of FASD and mental disorder, it is likely that the reported overrepresentation of mental disorder was a result of misinterpretation of common symptoms. For the untrained clinician, features known to occur in the sequelae of PAE will be labeled as features of mental disorder. Antisocial personality disorder, conduct disorder, and ODD can easily be invoked in the context of a patient's adaptive dysfunction and poor impulse control. Emotional regulation problems are common and foundational in PAE and its sequelae; they may, however, be mislabeled as an anxiety or mood disorder.

There are likely risk and protective factors unique to those who do or do not develop additional disorders despite PAE. These factors have yet to be determined, but this area of inquiry calls for increased attention. For instance, in samples with sufficient support systems, patients do not manifest as much comorbid mental disorder as do those who are living or have lived in unstable and unsupported environments. These same settings are usually not conducive to even normal mental development. Support also facilitates access to early and appropriate interventions, including financial, health, and social assistance. Because of educational, health, housing, and financial support, a lower rate of negative outcomes was reported in a cohort of 79 patients with significant PAE (Rangmar et al. 2015). Other researchers also reported lower rates of secondary mental disorder in a special FASD outpatient clinic. The main reason was that each diagnosed patient was given the requisite support and supervision (Mukherjee et al. 2019). In addition to identifying people with PAE, mental health clinicians need training in how to provide appropriate intervention with components linked to positive outcomes. The apparent resistance to treatment and rather complicated diagnostic picture of patients with PAE are, after all, responsive to proven methods of instruction. Clinical care just needs to be modified once patients are identified as having PAE.

The most reported category of PAE-related symptoms manifesting as mental disorder involve behavioral and neurocognitive deficits. Externalizing features are ADHD-type manifestations of hyperactivity, impulsivity, and behavioral consequences of mood dysregulation. The consistency of these manifestations across the lifespan is being studied. However, to improve the diagnosis and care of a patient with comorbid conditions, the clinician should seek to clarify the contribution of the different determinants to these conditions. Deficits in neurocognitive functions manifest as intellectual disability. The manifestations vary by age. In the mental health setting, patients with similar symptoms (e.g., low mood, anxiety) are classified as either having a mental disorder or additional and related psychosocial stresses. Because these symptoms can be attributed to both ND-PAE/FASD and mental disorder, another perspective for the mental health clinician is to understand their interaction at the interface. These symptoms are related by causation, pathophysiology, clinical presentation, social background, and sometimes similar treatment approach.

Infants with PAE, for instance, present with irritability, jitteriness, low levels of arousal, and disturbed sleep pattern. Children with PAE were described as having poor attention, increased activity, increased emotional reactivity, and irritability similar to common features of other mental disorders. For instance, the emotional dysregulation observed in children with ADHD or behavioral difficulties in disruptive mood disorder are not different from these types of symptoms. Completed clinical assessments of those at the interface of PAE and mental disorder reveal significant similarities. Other researchers have suggested that because of this association, PAE is a major risk factor for different mental disorders. A large sample of individuals diagnosed with ND-PAE/FASD was followed up for one such disorder (somatoform disorder) (Barr et al. 2006). Even across age groups and diagnostic types, behavioral problems manifested among the patients were classified at clinical threshold levels. They were severe enough to require intensive care and multidisciplinary involvement. In reviewing the disturbed child–maternal interaction among the patients, attachment difficulties and disorders featured prominently. The patients also manifested a rapidly changing mood state, which contributed to irritable and aggressive behavior. Interpreting these manifestations is clinically important if appropriate interventions are to be applied. If wrongly interpreted, the less-effective approaches perpetuate the symptoms and contribute to poor prognosis because the deficits have a direct and continuous impact on activities of daily living.

Another factor of clinical relevance to the manifestations of mental disorder is related to fatal outcomes. Suicidal behavior in the form of ideation and attempts was reported to be between 23% and 40% in samples with PAE (Dirks et al. 2019). Explained as a product of mood disorder, poor impulse control, and the consequences of psychosocial stress, these behaviors were also noted as contributing to the unusual high mortality rate. Suicide and high-risk behavior were rated highly as contributing to a significantly lower life expectancy among those with PAE. Suicidal behavior in adolescents diagnosed with FASD was 19 times higher than the general population (O'Connor et al. 2019). The rates in adults was five times higher than the general population (Huggins et al. 2008). Given that mental health clinicians are tasked, rightly or wrongly, with identifying, managing, and preventing suicide, this rather unacceptable rate suggests many patients are falling between the cracks in the system. A fatal outcome in an exposed person at the interface appears more likely if mood, anxiety, and poor impulse control are ascribed to other non-PAE-related factors. The therapeutic efforts are then at odds with the PAE-informed approaches. Clinicians with a high suspicion of PAE and ready to apply their knowledge of alternative approaches are better placed to prevent suicidal behavior.

Cognitive and behavioral deficits that overlap in both mental disorder and FASD impact function and quality of life the most. Apart from the cumulative adverse consequences of the comorbid conditions, care is complicated by the environmental instability influenced by internalizing and externalizing behavior problems. This was the explanation proposed in a study of children with PAE in whom mood disorders were greater than in those without PAE (O'Connor and Paley 2009). Anxiety and attachment insecurity are characteristically found in children with PAE. Combined with the high rates of mood dysregulation, anxiety and attachment difficulties complicate each other; if the interaction of these conditions is unrecognized, treatment failure contributes to create conditions in which negative outcomes thrive.

Conclusion

Throughout the life cycle, the expertise of the psychiatrist is vital to the person who is born with, lives with, is negatively affected by, and ages with the diverse problems associated with the teratogenic effect of PAE. Knowledge of PAE is important for all mental health professionals, who possess the skills for differentiating the shared features of comorbid disorders, a necessary component in providing effective care for patients at the interface of PAE and mental disorder.

CLINICAL PRACTICAL APPLICATIONS

- For patients in the mental health and addiction systems, it is clinically astute to consider prenatal exposures as factors that contribute to treatment resistance, chronicity, and dysfunction, especially when recognized treatments seem to be ineffective.

- Obtaining comprehensive neurocognitive assessment (focused on deficits and strengths) of difficult-to-treat patients is a judicious requirement for optimizing care.

- Various manifestations of PAE cluster in particular patients, and well-informed clinicians should identify indices that support easier recognition of ND-PAE/FASD, as well as presentations that vary according to developmental trajectory.

- Other useful clues for the identification of PAE in patients in the mental health system include a history of trauma, financial problems, poor social support, and impulsiveness.

- Providing structure, supervision, and support proves to be protective against the internalizing and externalizing behavioral consequences of PAE.

References

Astley SJ: Profile of the first 1,400 patients receiving diagnostic evaluations for fetal alcohol spectrum disorder at the Washington State Fetal Alcohol Syndrome Diagnostic & Prevention Network. Can J Clin Pharmacol 17(1):e132–e164, 2010

Barr HM, Bookstein FL, O'Malley KD, et al: Binge drinking during pregnancy as a predictor of psychiatric disorders on the Structured Clinical Interview for DSM-IV in young adult offspring. Am J Psychiatry 163(6):1061–1065, 2006

Benz J, Rasmussen C, Andrew G: Diagnosing fetal alcohol spectrum disorder: history, challenges and future directions. Paediatr Child Health 14(4):231–237, 2009

Cook JL, Green CR, Lilley CM, et al: Fetal alcohol spectrum disorder: a guideline for diagnosis across the lifespan. CMAJ 188(3):191–197, 2016

Dirks H, Francke L, Würz V, et al: Substance use, comorbid psychiatric disorders and suicide attempts in adult FASD patients. Adv Dual Diag 12(1/2):6–13, 2019

Famy C, Streissguth AP, Unis AS: Mental illness in adults with fetal alcohol syndrome or fetal alcohol effects. Am J Psychiatry 155(4):552–554, 1998

Franklin L, Deitz J, Jirikowic T, Astley S: Children with fetal alcohol spectrum disorders: problem behaviors and sensory processing. Am J Occup Ther 62(3):265–273, 2008

Huggins JE, Grant T, O'Malley K, Streissguth AP: Suicide attempts among adults with fetal alcohol spectrum disorders: clinical considerations. Mental Health Aspects of Developmental Disabilities 11(2):33, 2008

Landgraf MN, Nothacker M, Heinen F: Diagnosis of fetal alcohol syndrome (FAS): German guideline version 2013. Eur J Paediatr Neurol 17(5):437–446, 2013

Lange S, Probst C, Gmel G, et al: Global prevalence of fetal alcohol spectrum disorder among children and youth: a systematic review and meta-analysis. JAMA Pediatr 171(10) 948–956, 2017

Mattson SN, Crocker N, Nguyen TT: Fetal alcohol spectrum disorders: neuropsychological and behavioral features. Neuropsychol Rev 21(2):81–101, 2011

McGee CL, Riley EP: Social and behavioral functioning in individuals with prenatal alcohol exposure. Int J Disabil Hum Dev 6(4):369–382, 2007

Mela M, McFarlane A, Sajobi TT, Rajani H: Clinical correlates of fetal alcohol spectrum disorder among diagnosed individuals in a rural diagnostic clinic. J Popul Ther Clin Pharmacol 20(3):e250–258, 2013

Mukherjee RAS, Cook PA, Norgate SH, Price AD: Neurodevelopmental outcomes in individuals with fetal alcohol spectrum disorder (FASD) with and without exposure to neglect: clinical cohort data from a national FASD diagnostic clinic. Alcohol 76:23–28, 2019

O'Connor MJ, Paley B: Psychiatric conditions associated with prenatal alcohol exposure. Dev Disabil Res Rev 15(3):225–234, 2009

O'Connor MJ, Portnoff LC, Lebsack-Coleman M, Dipple KM: Suicide risk in adolescents with fetal alcohol spectrum disorders. Birth Defects Research 111(12):822–828, 2019

Pei J, Denys K, Hughes J, Rasmussen C: Mental health issues in fetal alcohol spectrum disorder. J Ment Health 20(5):438–448, 2011

Rangmar J, Hjern A, Vinnerljung B, et al: Psychosocial outcomes of fetal alcohol syndrome in adulthood. Pediatrics 135(1):e52–58, 2015

Streissguth AP, Barr HM, Kogan J, Bookstein FL: Understanding the Occurrence of Secondary Disabilities in Clients with Fetal Alcohol Syndrome (FAS) and Fetal Alcohol Effects (FAE). Final Report to the Centers for Disease Control and Prevention (CDC), August 1996. Tech Rep No 96-06. Seattle, WA, University of Washington, Fetal Alcohol & Drug Unit, 1996. Available at: http://lib.adai.uw.edu/pubs/bk2698.pdf. Accessed October 2, 2020.

Stringaris A: Irritability in children and adolescents: a challenge for DSM-5. Eur Child Adolesc Psychiatry 20(2):61–66, 2011

Walthall J, O'Connor MJ, Paley B: A comparison of psychopathology in children with and without prenatal alcohol exposure. Mental Health Aspects of Developmental Disabilities 11(3):69–78, 2008

Weyrauch D, Schwartz M, Hart B, et al: Comorbid mental disorders in fetal alcohol spectrum disorders: a systematic review. J Dev Behav Pediatr 38(4):283–291, 2017

CHAPTER 8

Profile of Associated Mental Disorders

WHAT TO KNOW

The behavioral and cognitive manifestations of PAE are in keeping with the neurocognitive deficits, such as executive dysfunction, which contributes to an inability to learn from past mistakes.

Behaviors labeled treatment interference, such as self-harm, noncompliance, and missed appointments, may be construed differently using an FASD lens and thus better addressed by well-informed professionals.

Children with PAE have fifteen-fold, fivefold, threefold, and twofold odds for ADHD, oppositional defiant disorder, conduct disorder, and autism spectrum disorder, respectively.

Low IQ is detrimental as it significantly influences adaptive dysfunction across the neurocognitive deficits of language, attention, executive function, and memory.

ADHD-related manifestation of PAE is characterized by slow cognitive tempo and frontal dopamine D_1 dysfunction preferentially responsive to amphetamines.

The phenotypic presentation of nondysmorphic individuals with FASD is similar in many ways to the population of patients in the mental health system. Recognizing the neurobehavioral disorders and neurocognitive deficits of PAE is crucially important in differentiating those exposed from those not exposed. The differences are not always clinically obvious. As such, a longitudinal perspective on the variation of abilities and comprehensive functional assessment are important to identify patients with PAE. It is clear that PAE and the conditions that increase its risk together constitute significant risk of pathogenesis of mental disorder. The scatter of strengths and weaknesses associated with individual assessment, especially manifesting as inconsistent clinical and functional ability, support the neurodevelopmental outcome of PAE. These strengths and weaknesses can form different recognizable patterns. More circumscribed deficits suggest mental disorder, and when affected individuals respond to typical behavioral and psychological interventions, one can almost rule out PAE as the major risk factor. In this chapter, I describe the likely patterns that could assist clinicians in their ability to differentiate patients with PAE, even when comorbidity with other mental conditions exists.

Profile of Mental Disorders With FASD

One of the fundamental problems in those with FASD is their inability to cope with daily living because of their adaptive dysfunction. By the nature of the combined executive function and learning deficits, individuals struggle to solve daily problems and meet their hygiene, financial, and social needs. This means that dependent rather than independent living is the norm. Understanding the profile of those with FASD among the population of patients with mental disorder not only is important for recognition of those with FASD but also highly critical for intervention and prevention of adverse outcomes. When mental health patients show an inordinate frequency or pattern of responding impulsively and show repeated inability or reduced ability to learn from consequences, clinicians should consider the possibility of FASD. Patients who seem unable to understand simple instructions and who manifest a profile of impairments in planning, verbal reasoning, emotional regulation, memory, and learning are particularly likely to require a full FASD assessment.

Although gullibility and unawareness of risk seem to follow the pattern described in those with a similar, but non-PAE-related, portrait of adaptive dysfunction, these features are not always easy to identify clinically. Because the neurocognitive deficits align with a lack of strategic thinking ability, a longer period of observation is required to detect a profile. Clinicians will observe over a period of time that FASD is indicated in those struggling to assimilate and understand societal norms. Such patients seem not to avoid dangerous people and to gravitate toward negative influences in spite of suffering negative impacts. They are more at risk of exploitation if their social interactions are not monitored and scrutinized closely. These neuro-cognitive deficits also manifest in an inability to remember information such as appointment dates and times. Partial or lack of compliance with intervention may be the only identifiable link to neurocognitive deficits in those with FASD in the mental health system. Affected individuals display inability to cope with daily stresses and use extreme acts to draw attention to their needs. Self-harm and suicidal gestures are expressed regularly and are understood clinically in a large proportion of those with FASD as a means of communicating distress. Presenting as an emergency, patients with these profiles frequently are referred to mental health professionals. These cues must be attended with a view to establishing a fuller clinical picture. The process is usually supported by gathering examples of behaviors that indicate poor coping, which constitute a pattern.

A wide spectrum of cognitive disabilities in patients with FASD makes it difficult to pinpoint a valid and unified profile specific to FASD. Attempts to develop evidence-based useful portraits of FASD have yielded no unique pattern. Clinicians experienced with the population apply pattern recognition in dealing with patients presenting with deficits. It is hoped that such efforts will accord with research endeavors to generate a lasting profile. The clinical relevance of having such a profile is its usefulness in initiating appropriate interventions directed at the discovered deficits.

Profiles of those with FASD have been associated with characteristics that clinicians need to evaluate, such as involvement with the criminal justice system. Multiple disorders are common, which means that mental health professionals should view these co-occurring disorders and other negative life experiences as potential indicators of FASD (Table 8–1). These disorders co-occur in different age groups, and the person's age and specific disorder should direct the clinician to comprehensive evaluation with complete neurocognitive assessment.

Table 8–1 shows the most commonly diagnosed mental disorders in patients with FASD. Mental health clinicians were asked to identify these from a list of mental disorders (Brown and Harr 2019). Schizophrenia and sleep, mood, and anxiety disorders are also common. Bipolar disorder and borderline personality disorder may be confused with features of mood dysregulation, especially when patients with FASD manifest self-harm and destructive behaviors (Temple et al. 2019). Several studies identify high rates of mental disorders in individuals with FASD. A clinician may begin to formulate a profile for a patient with early onset of symptoms who presents atypically

TABLE 8–1.   Common diagnoses identified in those with ND-PAE/FASD

ADHD
Autism spectrum disorder
Oppositional defiant disorder
Conduct disorder
Reactive attachment disorder
Learning disorder
Intellectual disorder

and characterize that patient as noncompliant or resistant to treatment (Brown and Harr 2019; Grant et al. 2013). To understand the co-occurrence of multiple diagnoses, simple explanations are not helpful. Factors that mediate the risk of mental disorders considered in the context of multiple exposures have better clinical utility and should be put forward.

Risks Associated With Exposure to Illicit Substances

Longitudinal cohort studies have helped clarify the weight of several risk factors in outcomes of mental disorder. On follow-up, children exposed to several prenatal substances experience and manifest multiple internalizing and externalizing behavioral symptoms. Evidence came from evaluating the clinical presentations of school-age children exposed to multiple substances prenatally. Exposure to marijuana was associated with impulsivity, inattention, and increased hyperactivity as measured using the Swanson, Noland, and Pelham (SNAP) checklist (Goldschmidt et al. 2000). Symptoms of ADHD and autism spectrum disorder (ASD) are consistently reported not only for heavy substance exposure but also low and moderate exposures. Neurobehavioral and cognitive deficits were suggested as mediating the final outcome in schoolage children with exposure to cannabis and alcohol (Huizink and Mulder 2006). Therefore, inattention, hyperactivity, and impulsivity, individually and collectively, are a possible symptom profile that should arouse suspicion of PAE. When evaluating schoolage children, overrepresentation of these features is a red flag for exposure to multiple substances.

Specifically, a high rate of ASD and traits were noted in a cross-sectional study of children exposed to heavy alcohol use prenatally. Subsequent case-control studies were completed to understand the relationship (Mukherjee et al. 2011). In the first of these, alcohol-exposed children carefully matched with a reference group were assessed utilizing a scale to estimate the autistic score in study participants. Individuals with PAE were 17 times more likely to have a high score on the autism spectrum scale than those without PAE (Mukherjee et al. 2011). In the same special clinic sample of 99 individuals with prenatal exposure to alcohol and other substances, high rates of ASD and ADHD were reported (Mukherjee et al. 2019). These rates of disorders helped identify risk factors for negative outcomes. Factors present in those with mental disorders included neonatal abstinence syndrome, placement in nonbiological families, and placement before the age of 1 year (Gallagher et al. 2018). Additionally, having a low IQ, even without the risk of foster care placement, predicted mental disorder in the offspring. Neonatal abstinence syndrome was a specific predictor of inattention according to parent-reported SNAP-IV findings.

To explain the interaction between the different risk factors, it was noted that offspring may already be vulnerable and genetically predisposed. The nongenetic environment needed for acquisition of symptoms includes the social difficulties common in those who develop mental disorders. The factors of adverse childhood experience, psychological deprivation, and their interaction during critical periods of development affect brain development generally. Mediated through low IQ, parental inefficiency associated with high levels of substance use, and direct trauma to the offspring create the environment for many co-occurring presentations. Thus, a profile is noted in subjects with similar backgrounds. Externalizing behaviors are common and when they occur in environments of social disadvantage, this combination of factors supports the formulation of a mental disorder profile (Lange et al. 2018).

Psychological deprivation is associated with long-term neurocognitive and behavioral difficulties. Recognizing these factors is not conclusive because the biological, neural, and behavioral profiles associated with PAE have been reported to be unique and unaffected by neglect, a social disadvantage (Mukherjee et al. 2019; Nelson et al. 2019). It is therefore necessary to be cautious in screening for risk factors because they may apply in certain cases and not others.

Profile of Mental Disorder in Those With PAE

Externalizing behavior is the predominant manifestation of the consequences of PAE. Anger, hostility, destruction of property, defiance, and violation of rules typify externalizing behavior. Patients present with these challenging behaviors in the context of a variety of diagnoses. Children with hyperactive, impulsive, disruptive, or delinquent behaviors are characterized as having externalizing behavior. Instruments used to estimate the presence or absence of externalizing behavior have a clinical cutoff score that is computed using standardized scales. A significant proportion of individuals with PAE achieve clinically positive scores when assessed. In children with PAE, the odds of ADHD (15:1), ASD (2:1), oppositional defiant disorder (ODD) (5:1), and conduct disorder (3:1) were significantly higher than those without PAE (Lange et al. 2018). To be supportive of the neurocognitive deficits of their patients, mental health clinicians should evaluate and address the manifesting externalizing behaviors, especially those commonly associated with mental disorders in patients with PAE and exposure to other substances. A viable profile is available for a few of the common comorbid conditions. This should be useful in differentiating FASD from certain idiopathic neurodevelopmental disorders.

Autism Spectrum Disorder

Although initial cross-sectional studies and conceptual articles pointed to a high prevalence of ASD and autistic traits in individuals with PAE, this is not conclusive. Case-control research reports an association between heavy alcohol exposures in utero and ASD (Mukherjee et al. 2011). This association was refuted after a cohort study in children reported that the prevalence of ASD was not associated with light, moderate, or heavy alcohol use in a cohort of 12,000 participants (Gallagher et al. 2018). Separate, yet related, factors were associated with ASD. Identifying factors such as smoking in pregnancy, abnormal BMI, ethnicity, and income should form part of the assessment of risk factors contributing to the profile (Singer et al. 2017).

The profile of ASD in those with FASD is based on multiple retrospective and prospective studies. Risk factors for increased odds in specialized clinic patients may be overestimated, and clinical and environmental factors may represent differences in clinical presentation. A more severe form of externalizing behavior is associated with ASD and ND-PAE/FASD. This is associated with additive effects of the contributory factors of both conditions. Research also implicates the effect of poor parent–child interaction, poor attachment, and disrupted residential placement in increasing vulnerability in those with PAE. PAE combined with these forms of postnatal adversity therefore produces externalizing behavior of clinical significance. These factors are helpful in clinically categorizing the patients. Patients are also viewed from a developmental perspective, so much so that their functioning appears inconsistent. This is because patients may exhibit weakness in some functions but excel in others.

Clinical Vignette

A 23-year-old man is described as a "frequent flyer" at the emergency room (ER) of a city hospital. His attendance is, on average, every other day; on severe days, he appears in the ER two or three times. He usually presents with fear of having a heart attack, threatens to harm or kill himself, reports hearing voices, and requests admission. He regularly refers to his symptoms as "my anxiety is flaring up." The repeated psychiatric opinions are similar on most occasions when he is referred by ER doctors. He is diagnosed with panic disorder, mild alcohol use disorder, and borderline personality disorder. He lost his group home placement because he threatened to set fire to the home if the group home operator refused to take him to the ER; the operator had declined because the home had a signed contract with the hospital restricting his attendance. The patient is usually partially compliant with his medication regimen (paroxetine 20 mg and quetiapine 75 mg hs).

What are the red flags in this vignette? This young patient shows a pattern of dependent living and an inability to cope with distressing situations. Requesting hospitalization and repeated presentations conveys a lack of understanding of guidelines and social norms. Repeated self-harming and suicidal behaviors, threats of arson, partial compliance with treatment, and inability to maintain a stable residence insinuate impulsivity and lack of awareness of risk. These are suggestive of an absence of strategic thinking, which may or may not be PAE related.

What should change in the management of this patient? Repeated visits to the ER and unsuccessful interventions call for a change of approach and a modified strategy. The behaviors manifested by this young man may or may not suggest PAE in the overall understanding. Given the protracted and challenging nature of the clinical conundrum he presents, some assumptions may include the possibility of PAE and its consequences. If the possibility of PAE is acknowledged, review of the case using an FASD lens will search for additional and collateral information about prenatal and postnatal experiences. With sufficient indicators, a request for neurocognitive assessment may help clarify several of the resistant symptoms. The nature and expression of the anxiety, characterized by verbal and nonverbal expressions, could be atypical compared with those in the general population. Individuals with PAE who have difficulties with reading and comprehension may complete self-report questionnaires incorrectly. The labels used in regular questionnaires may be inadequate for eliciting an accurate response. When administering an assessment tool, someone who knows the patient should use concrete examples for the questions related to anxiety. Clinicians who identify physical symptoms and signs stand a better chance of detecting the types of symptoms that bring this patient to the ER.

The following questions could be asked directly during an assessment: What do you feel in your gut? Describe how your breathing has changed. When did that happen? Do you get scared? What happens after you sleep? What happens after you eat food? These open-ended questions using words familiar to the cognitively impaired person provide a more accurate estimation of anxiety and may also, incidentally, provide an indication of interoceptive awareness.

If the neurocognitive features of FASD were previously unrecognized, a modified approach is to request a comprehensive functional and neurocognitive assessment focused on eliciting the patient's strengths and weaknesses. A relevant and well-accepted communication strategy is using the same words the patient uses and ensuring the patient understands words and phrases used during a clinical assessment. It is also known that patients with slow speed of information processing provide better responses if they are allowed time to think before answering. Any sense that they are being rushed will lead to inexact responses. Clinicians who adopt less sophisticated language in keeping with the patient's level of comprehension connect better with those patients. This approach is associated with better understanding, which could clarify sources of distress and enhance compliance with the current treatment.

The overall treatment plan should be based on the neurocognitive deficits guiding specific modifications. Before the patient can be placed in a new group home, the patient's lack of risk perception necessitates the assignment of a mentor. The best possible mentor is one who is experienced with the expression and amelioration of distress in FASD. There is usually a surprising recognition of previously undetected intellectual disorder, which can open up new funding opportunities for support related to intellectual disability services. These services are usually dependent on the level of impairment; in the vignette, the young man's illness is severe enough to warrant support. Support could fund help with the activities of daily living through the new group home, extra leisure activities with the mentor, and supported employment placement for the patient.

Current evidence indicates that people with PAE appreciate a balanced level of occupation. Such a balance involves providing structure to the day, supervision by a job coach or recreation specialist, and access to an expert in managing anxiety. These are important steps for managing distress. Patients who feel supported and who engage in an occupation report better self-esteem. A team with an interest in the patient's overall neurocognitive function based on identified strengths places more emphasis on the zone of proximal development (Pavlov et al. 1999). This allows the team to assign tasks that are easily completed by the patient with or without assistance.

With regard to pharmacotherapy, evidence has shown that most patients affected by PAE will respond to ligand-specific medications, but others may not (Mela et al. 2018). An algorithmic approach to the pharmacological treatment of impulsiveness and anxiety from hyperarousal or affect dysregulation may call for consideration and choice of an α-adrenergic agonist (clonidine or guanfacine) over other antianxiety medications. Use of a selective serotonin reuptake inhibitor (e.g., fluoxetine) initiated at a low dose conforms to management principles for neurodevelopmental disorder (Ji and Findling 2016); slowly increasing that dose has the potential for success (Doig et al. 2008). A functional behavioral analysis should be used to monitor progress. To continue to minimize the "flaring" of anxiety, promoting positive behavior activation, such as games, exercises, and interactions, and social engagement in fun activities acceptable to the patient should be pursued (Petrenko 2015).

Attention-Deficit/Hyperactivity Disorder

ADHD remains the most prevalent mental disorder among people with PAE (Fryer et al. 2007; Weyrauch et al. 2017). PAE is a relevant factor to consider in the pathogenesis of psychiatric disorders, especially disorders of childhood development. The initial clinical presentation comprises the core symptoms of ADHD, which has led to several efforts to disentangle the causes, pathophysiology, and treatment of the two disorders (Mukherjee 2016). In clinical settings, the ability to tell PAE from ADHD may depend on the clinician's orientation. The relative risk of ADHD in those with PAE is very high. The profile included provides guidance for recognizing shared as well as distinguishing features.

ADHD was shown in a systematic review to be the most prevalent mental disorder in those with PAE (Weyrauch et al. 2017); the rates for having full-syndrome ADHD or most of its clinical features range from one-third to almost 100% (Astley 2010). The relationship between FASD and ADHD has many facets. Clinically, some differences have been described. Predominantly, impaired attention, inattention, higher executive dysfunction, and impulsivity are featured in patients with PAE outcomes and diagnosed with FASD. The executive dysfunction in individuals with PAE (without ADHD) manifests as significant deficits in planning, set-shifting, working memory, and fluency compared with those with ADHD (without PAE) (Kingdon et al. 2016). Attention deficits and distraction seem to be the core findings in many clinical studies of patients with PAE.

Etiologically, the relationship between FASD and ADHD may be purely coincidental, based on shared neurological factors, or genetic. Mothers with ADHD act impulsively and are said to more readily drink alcohol, and thus,

TABLE 8–2.   Some of the clinical and psychological findings potentially differentiating ADHD with and without PAE

ADHD WITH PAE	ADHD WITHOUT PAE
Worse behavioral and cognitive deficits, full-scale IQ (verbal and performance), perceptual reasoning, verbal comprehension, and working memory	More externalizing behavior, hyperactivity, higher levels of atypicality and aggression More impulsivity
Weaker verbal comprehension	Increased focus and sustained attention
Visual attention deficits	
Slower reaction test	Increased risk of psychiatric diagnoses
Deficiency in shifting attention (planning, fluency, and set-shifting)	Synergistic effect on conduct disorder
Deficits in cognitive flexibility, response inhibition, planning, and concept formation	Synergistic effect on externalizing behavior
High rates of sluggish cognitive tempo	
Preference for dexamphetamine use	

they may share the required genetic predisposition with their offspring (Graham et al. 2012). In addition, the neurological deficits identified in animal PAE studies were similar to deficits found in ADHD (Petrelli et al. 2018). Individuals with PAE were found to have elevated scores on a behavioral phenotype measured as sluggish cognitive tempo (Table 8–2). High sluggish cognitive tempo scores were positively associated with both internalizing and externalizing behaviors in this and other studies recognizing cognitive factors in patients with ADHD and were specifically related to PAE (Fryer et al. 2007; Kodituwakku and Kodituwakku 2014).

Explanations about etiology, underlying brain function, and phenomenological outcomes remain unclear because of the types of samples used to study the relationship between ADHD and the consequences of PAE (Burd 2016). Initial results suggesting they are clinically different were based on case series and a few clinical control studies. Cohort studies are needed to estimate the contribution of PAE to the rates of ADHD and ND-PAE/FASD. Treatment of individuals with ADHD and PAE has provided a potential explanation for this relationship. Specific dopamine receptors in the prefrontal and frontal brain areas were found to be more responsive to dexamphetamine supplements than to methylphenidate. These receptors were also identified as more effective in improving deficits in attention, which are more prominent in PAE. Treatment of ADHD based on decision tree considerations was effective and resulted in positive outcomes (Pliszka et al. 2006). Approaching treatment using a decision tree that follows a step-by-step choice of medication can improve outcomes and may be applicable to PAE and its consequences. However, there is limited information on effective strategies. The goals of treatment should be to reduce polypharmacy and improve the patient's functioning as well as the clinician's confidence in managing comorbidity.

A consensus panel of experts recognized the relationship between FASD and ADHD (Young et al. 2016). They proposed certain clinical red flags to identify those with ADHD who are likely to require special attention on account of a history of PAE. These red flags are new and have not yet been studied. According to the panel's recommendations, PAE can be confirmed if the patient shows a predominance of inattentive symptoms combined with impulsive behaviors. Having an IQ < 50, poor response to the first-line medication methylphenidate, lack of response to typical behavioral interventions, and any features suggestive of maternal risks of PAE support an FASD diagnosis. These features, the panel argued, will cue the clinician to adopt new strategies, including the use of nonpharmacological approaches (Young et al. 2016).

Anxiety and Mood Disorders in FASD

The hypothalamic-pituitary-adrenal axis is credited with the shared expression of anxiety and mood dysregulation in individuals with PAE. The pattern is similar to what occurs in patients with diagnosed anxiety, mood, and personality disorders. Stress is mediated by complex pathways, including the hypothalamic-pituitary-adrenal axis associated with mental disorders. Neurodevelopmental and mental disorders associated with anxiety and mood closely correlate with the manifestations of early childhood trauma (Hellemans et al. 2010). Deprivation, abuse, social isolation, and neglect have been shown to increase disordered development and thus contribute to psychiatric conditions (Nelson et al. 2019). Stresses in childhood also contribute to common behavioral disorders such as ODD (Oberlander et al. 2010; Pei et al. 2011). Manifestations of anxiety begin early in patients with PAE, and the rates are higher than in those without PAE (Astley 2010; Famy et al. 1998; O'Connor et al. 2002). The confluence of environmental, genetic, and neurobehavioral factors contributes to the long-standing adult manifestations of symptoms of anxiety and mood disorders. People with PAE who demonstrate a repertoire of risky behaviors do so because of their poor coping methods, demonstrating poor decision-making abilities and judgment. That is likely why suicidal behaviors are accentuated in ND-PAE/FASD, especially when anxiety and depression are frequent and rampant.

Other Disorders

Although the clinician requires a long-standing relationship to identify individuals with atypical presentation, research continues to identify clinical and treatment variations between patients with PAE and those without. A group of disorders (PTSD, sleep disorders, psychosis in adults, personality disorders, and substance use disorders) are highly prevalent in people with PAE (Wengel et al. 2011). This knowledge should encourage clinicians to continue assessing for perinatal insults and to identify failed interventions with the goal of introducing more effective strategies to their patients. The many manifestations of mental disorder among those with PAE should be recognized, and interventions should be tailored to improve function.

Conclusion

Clinicians need to align symptoms and signs to particular disorders. PAE creates a challenge in that multiple diagnoses are commonly found in patients. Specifically, the preponderance of clinical syndromes such as ADHD, ASD, and mood and anxiety disorders raises questions of etiology, clinical presentation, differential diagnosis, and management. A few recognized differences can help distinguish patients with PAE. This is a valuable step in understanding the profiles of people with PAE who have additional mental disorder.

CLINICAL PRACTICAL APPLICATIONS

- There are times when clinicians should protect patients who show a lack of strategic thinking, gullible behavior, risk unawareness, and ease of exploitation caused by neurocognitive deficits.

- To enhance communication with patients who have slow processing ability, they should be allowed plenty of time to consider a question before responding or answering.

- Clinicians should tailor language to account for identified deficits and pitch conversation at a level that facilitates understanding.

- Deficits in sustained attention, impulse control, and higher executive function, manifested by disturbed set-shifting, working memory, planning, and fluency, affect individuals with combined ADHD and PAE more severely than those with ADHD without PAE.

- Clinicians should be conversant with the common disorders and profiles of patients who have PAE and comorbid mental disorder.

References

Astley SJ: Profile of the first 1,400 patients receiving diagnostic evaluations for fetal alcohol spectrum disorder at the Washington State Fetal Alcohol Syndrome Diagnostic & Prevention Network. Can J Clin Pharmacol 17(1):e132–e164, 2010

Brown J, Harr D: Perceptions of fetal alcohol spectrum disorder (FASD) at a mental health outpatient treatment provider in Minnesota. Int J Environ Res Public Health 16(1):E16, 2019

Burd L: FASD and ADHD: are they related and how? BMC Psychiatry 16(1):325, 2016

Doig J, McLennan JD, Gibbard WB: Medication effects on symptoms of attention-deficit/hyperactivity disorder in children with fetal alcohol spectrum disorder. J Child Adolesc Psychopharmacol 18(4):365–371, 2008

Famy C, Streissguth AP, Unis AS: Mental illness in adults with fetal alcohol syndrome or fetal alcohol effects. Am J Psychiatry 155(4):552–554, 1998

Fryer SL, McGee CL, Matt GE, et al: Evaluation of psychopathological conditions in children with heavy prenatal alcohol exposure. Pediatrics 119(3):e733–e741, 2007

Gallagher C, McCarthy FP, Ryan RM, Khashan AS: Maternal alcohol consumption during pregnancy and the risk of autism spectrum disorders in offspring: a retrospective analysis of the Millennium Cohort Study. J Autism Dev Disord 48(11):3773–3782, 2018

Goldschmidt L, Day NL, Richardson GA: Effects of prenatal marijuana exposure on child behavior problems at age 10. Neurotoxicol Teratol 22(3):325–336, 2000

Graham DM, Crocker N, Deweese BN, et al: Prenatal alcohol exposure, attention-deficit/hyperactivity disorder, and sluggish cognitive tempo. Alcohol Clin Exp Res 37(suppl 1):E338–E346, 2012

Grant TM, Brown NN, Graham JC, et al: Screening in treatment programs for fetal alcohol spectrum disorders that could affect therapeutic progress. Int J Alcohol Drug Res 2(3):37–49, 2013

Hellemans KG, Sliwowska JH, Verma P, Weinberg J: Prenatal alcohol exposure: fetal programming and later life vulnerability to stress, depression and anxiety disorders. Neurosci Biobehav Rev 34(6):791–807, 2010

Huizink AC, Mulder EJ: Maternal smoking, drinking or cannabis use during pregnancy and neurobehavioral and cognitive functioning in human offspring. Neurosci Biobehav Rev 30(1):24–41, 2006

Ji NY, Findling RL: Pharmacotherapy for mental health problems in people with intellectual disability. Curr Opin Psychiatr 29(2):103–125, 2016

Kingdon D, Cardoso C, McGrath JJ: Research review: executive function deficits in fetal alcohol spectrum disorders and attention-deficit/hyperactivity disorder—a meta-analysis. J Child Psychol Psychiatry 57(2):116–131, 2016

Kodituwakku P, Kodituwakku E: Cognitive and behavioral profiles of children with fetal alcohol spectrum disorders. Current Developmental Disorders Reports 1(3):149–160, 2014

Lange S, Rehm J, Anagnostou E, Popova S: Prevalence of externalizing disorders and autism spectrum disorders among children with fetal alcohol spectrum disorder: systematic review and meta-analysis. Biochem Cell Biol 96(2):241–251, 2018

Mela M, Okpalauwaekwe U, Anderson T, et al: The utility of psychotropic drugs on patients with fetal alcohol spectrum disorder (FASD): a systematic review. Psychiatry Clin Psychopharmacol 28(4):436–445, 2018

Mukherjee R: The relationship between ADHD and FASD. Thrombus 8:4–7, 2016

Mukherjee R, Layton M, Yacoub E, Turk J: Autism and autistic traits in people exposed to heavy prenatal alcohol: data from a clinical series of 21 individuals and a nested case control study. Advances in Mental Health and Intellectual Disability 5(1):42–49, 2011

Mukherjee RAS, Cook PA, Norgate SH, Price AD: Neurodevelopmental outcomes in individuals with fetal alcohol spectrum disorder (FASD) with and without exposure to neglect: clinical cohort data from a national FASD diagnostic clinic. Alcohol 76:23–28, 2019

Nelson CA 3rd, Zeanah CH, Fox NA: How early experience shapes human development: the case of psychosocial deprivation. Neural Plast 2019:1676285, 2019

Oberlander TF, Jacobson SW, Weinberg J, et al: Prenatal alcohol exposure alters biobehavioral reactivity to pain in newborns. Alcohol Clin Exp Res 34(4):681–692, 2010

O'Connor MJ, Shah B, Whaley S, et al: Psychiatric illness in a clinical sample of children with prenatal alcohol exposure. Am J Drug Alcohol Abuse 28(4):743–754, 2002

Pavlov I, Watson J, Skinner BF, et al: What Is the Zone of Proximal Development? 1999

Pei J, Denys K, Hughes J, Rasmussen C: Mental health issues in fetal alcohol spectrum disorder. J Ment Health 20(5):473–483, 2011

Petrelli B, Weinberg J, Hicks GG: Effects of prenatal alcohol exposure (PAE): insights into FASD using mouse models of PAE. Biochem Cell Biol 96(2):131–147, 2018

Petrenko CL: Positive behavioral interventions and family support for fetal alcohol spectrum disorders. Curr Dev Disord Rep 2(3):199–209, 2015

Pliszka SR, Crismon ML, Hughes CW, et al: The Texas Children's Medication Algorithm Project: revision of the algorithm for pharmacotherapy of attention-deficit/hyperactivity disorder. J Am Acad Child Adolesc Psychiatry 45(6):642–657, 2006

Singer AB, Aylsworth AS, Cordero C, et al: Prenatal alcohol exposure in relation to autism spectrum disorder: findings from the Study to Explore Early Development (SEED). Paediatr Perinatal Epidemiol 31(6):573–582, 2017

Temple VK, Cook JL, Unsworth K, et al: Mental health and affect regulation impairment in fetal alcohol spectrum disorder (FASD): Results from the Canadian national FASD database. Alcohol Alcohol 54(5):545–550, 2019

Wengel T, Hanlon-Dearman AC, Fjeldsted B: Sleep and sensory characteristics in young children with fetal alcohol spectrum disorder. J Dev Behav Pediatr 32(5):384–392, 2011

Weyrauch D, Schwartz M, Hart B, et al: Comorbid mental disorders in fetal alcohol spectrum disorders: a systematic review. J Dev Behav Pediatr 38(4):283–291, 2017

Young S, Absoud M, Blackburn C, et al: Guidelines for identification and treatment of individuals with attention deficit/hyperactivity disorder and associated fetal alcohol spectrum disorders based upon expert consensus. BMC Psychiatry 16(1):324, 2016

PART IV

Assessment and Diagnosis

CHAPTER 9

Neuroimaging

WHAT TO KNOW

Neuroimaging is heralded as a potential diagnostic tool even though findings from studies of individuals with PAE are not yet consistent enough to elevate its use in clinical practice.

Specific findings (cortical thinness, abnormalities of the corpus callosum, and white matter changes) have been linked to PAE.

Interesting findings on diffusion tensor imaging of lower fractional anisotropy and high mean diffusivity align with neurobehavioral consequences of PAE-related deficits and may be considered for future biomarkers.

The corpus callosum, cerebellum, and frontotemporal parietal areas of the brain are the most studied for changes related to PAE.

Most mental health professionals are knowledgeable about the regional and illness-specific brain changes associated with findings on neuroimaging. Unlike neurological injury that depends on such techniques as structural and functional MRI (fMRI), positron emission tomography (PET), single-photon emission computed tomography (SPECT), and optical imaging for diagnosis, this is not yet the case for mental disorders. It is hoped that in a not too distant future, psychoradiology may guide diagnosis and treatment. The scope of this chapter is limited to information about interesting findings of neuroimaging techniques when patients with PAE are studied. Most information now relies on comparative studies with nonclinical subjects.

There is no current test to diagnose ND-PAE/FASD or the presence of PAE in especially nondysmorphic cases. Ancillary neurophysiological investigations, including saccadic eye movement, are paving the way for future diagnostic utility. Noninvasive imaging, structural and functional, illuminates the deficits of PAE, complements the existent neuropsychological and clinical phenotype, and may contribute to monitoring changes in treatment outcomes. The first reported images of the brain of those affected with PAE were dramatically abnormal because they represented severe cases arising from heavy PAE. However, there are more subtle PAE cases involving minor brain changes that neuroimaging cannot easily detect. Still, impaired brain connectivity was demonstrated for language, memory, and processing speed deficits, which manifested as an inability for information sharing from one side of the brain to the other. The major techniques used to study the effect of PAE include MRI, fMRI, magnetic resonance spectroscopy (MRS), PET, and diffusion tensor imaging (DTI).

Reduced brain volume and cortical thinness and thickness are the more consistent neuroimaging findings in individuals with PAE. The location of the volumetric and architectural damage on the cerebrum and cerebellum informs clinical neurocognitive findings, but findings are not yet consistent. Some findings relate to frontotemporal areas; other findings suggest that the parietal lobe and all brain regions are sensitive to insult from PAE (O'Hare et al. 2005; Sowell et al. 2002).

Clinical Vignette

A radiologist contacted an expert in ND-PAE/FASD after discovering corpus callosum agenesis in a 35-month-old child. After consulting with a geneticist, a formal disorder could not be confirmed. The radiologist wants to know if the child could have ND-PAE/FASD, given that his mother died at birth. The discussion with the radiologist provides an opportunity for the geneticist to describe the existing standard for diagnosis: a multidisciplinary functional assessment, in which neuroimaging is considered research evidence. Being aware that specific findings and the emerging use of deep machine learning could begin to offer refinement to diagnostic approaches, the clinician who specializes in ND-PAE/FASD sets up a meeting with the radiologist, who offers to participate in a literature review of the current research findings on neuroimaging.

The findings likely to be obtained remain at the level of research, with the hope of specific clinical indications. In the past decade, findings from clinical presentations of those with ND-PAE/FASD stimulated research in identifying a profile of neurocognitive deficits that could reliably diagnose patients (Table 9–1) (Kodituwakku 2009). This in turn led to research in neuroimaging to characterize and profile the neural circuit deficits associated with PAE (Barrett et al. 2019; Spadoni et al. 2007). It is worth noting that advancement in the field is rapidly turning emerging evidence into clinical practice in cases with high indication for neuroimaging. It is expected that in the near future, these techniques will predominate in the diagnostic assessment of patients with PAE.

Examining the White Matter

Postmortem findings of hypoplasia and agenesis of the corpus callosum were confirmed using neuroimaging techniques. Midline defects especially of white matter have been associated with PAE. DTI now depicts global white matter changes indicative of microstructural problems. The changes detected also align with deficits of working memory and speed of information processing. DTI is credited with the advancement of the in vivo characterization of neural macrostructure and microstructure, especially of the white matter (Ghazi Sherbaf et al. 2019). Compared with control subjects, researchers identified subjects with FASD as having lower fractional anisotropy. Explained at first as a result of the teratogenesis of alcohol, the finding was later said to be related to neurobehavioral sequelae of executive dysfunction and visual processing deficits (Fryer et al. 2009).

The technical aspects of DTI are beyond the scope of this book, but it is worth noting that white matter abnormalities are detected by measuring water movement in brain organelles. The direction of movement is indirectly measured by fractional anisotropy (FA). FA serves as a biomarker of the integrity of white matter. Thus, lower FA indicates disruption and damage of white matter. On the other hand, mean diffusivity reflects the total amount of water in the voxel, irrespective of the direction (Ghazi Sherbaf et al. 2019). Other autopsy-based findings of white matter abnormalities have been supported by DTI studies (Wozniak et al. 2006). In a systematic review of 23 studies, lower FA and higher mean diffusivity and radial diffusivity were reported more consistently in the corpus callosum, cerebellar peduncles, cingulum, and longitudinal fasciculi connecting frontal and temporoparietal regions (Ghazi Sherbaf et al. 2019). Figure 9–1 depicts how white matter fibers are represented in DTI studies. Although it is still early for clinical use, comprehensive understanding of the heterogeneity of PAE through neuroimaging was recommended as an essential step in the future diagnosis and treatment of ND-PAE/FASD (Ghazi Sherbaf et al. 2019).

TABLE 9–1. Summary of findings in the past decade on PAE and neuroimaging (2010–2020)

NEUROIMAGING TECHNIQUE	NEUROIMAGING FINDINGS	POTENTIAL CLINICAL IMPLICATIONS
Structural (MRI, CT)	Thicker cortices in frontal, parietal, and temporal regions (Yang et al. 2012)	Widespread deficits that require individual treatment planning
	Larger cortical thickness in those with FASD than in those with ADHD (Fernández-Jaén et al. 2011)	
	Widespread cortical thinning (Zhou et al. 2011)	
	Reductions in global and regional cortical thickness, while the pattern and degree of cortical thickness asymmetry were preserved (Zhou et al. 2018)	
Functional (fMRI)	Compared with control subjects, those with FASD use subnetwork of cerebellar regions and parietal cortex for verbal working memory tasks (Diwadkar et al. 2013)	Parietal networks may be impaired; deficits in spatial working memory
	Those with FASD use additional parietal networks to perform proximal judgment and tasks of addition (Meintjes et al. 2010)	
	Altered network connectivity in those with FASD (Wozniak et al. 2013)	
Metabolic (PET, SPECT)	Diminished tracer activity in bilateral thalami, basal ganglia, and temporal lobes (Codreanu et al. 2012)	Important for affect and memory issues
Other (DTI, NRI)	Significant reduction in the superior long fasciculus, and superior and inferior fronto-occipital fasciculus	Reduced PFC activity but increased oxygen consumption without sufficient oxygen replacement
	Reduced prefrontal cortex HBO and increased HBR in the inhibitory condition	

Note. CT=computed tomography; DTI=diffusion tensor imaging; HBO= oxyhemoglobin; HBR=deoxyhemoglobin; NRI=near-infrared spectroscopy; PFC=prefrontal cortex; SPECT=single-photon emission computed tomography.

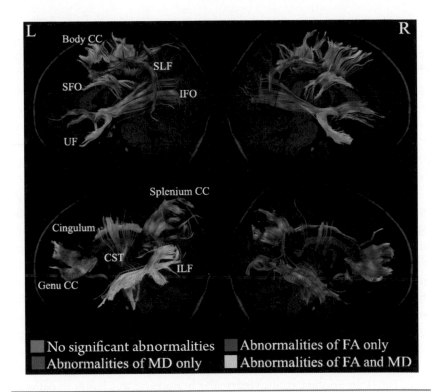

FIGURE 9-1. White matter mapping using diffusion tensor imaging showing the presence or absence of abnormalities in those with fetal alcohol spectrum disorder. (See Plate 1 to view this figure in color.)

CC=corpus callosum; CST=corticospinal tract; FA=fractional anisotropy; IFO=inferior fronto-occipital fasciculus; ILF=inferior longitudinal fasciculus; L=left; MD=mean diffusivity; R=right; SFO=subfornical organ; SLF=superior longitudinal fasciculus; UF= uncinate fasciculus. Both FA and MD are measures of white matter microstructure.

Source. From Lebel C, Rasmussen C, Wyper K, et al.: "Brain Diffusion Abnormalities in Children With Fetal Alcohol Spectrum Disorder." *Alcoholism: Clinical and Experimental Research* 32(10):1732–1740, 2008. Copyright ©2008 John Wiley and Sons. Used with permission.

Examining the Grey Matter

MRI was used to detect volumetric changes of the hippocampi, which were smaller in those with FASD (Norman et al. 2009). The finding was used to verify histopathology results of hippocampal damage in animal models. This is the basis for defects of laying down new memories, which is associated with learning difficulty. MRI findings also identified smoothness and reduced elevation of the brain cortex gyri. This was correlated with low intelligence.

Brain damage as foundational to PAE was supported when a study using neuroimaging with three subgroups of exposed subjects and a group of control subjects found high correlations of damage in those with PAE (Astley et al. 2009). This study used comprehensive assessments and neuroimaging techniques—MRI, MRS, and fMRI—and identified alterations in neurochemistry, neurostructure, and neurometabolism consistent with brain damage. Confirming such damage via the use of these sensitive neuroimaging techniques may be of future clinical utility (Astley et al. 2009). The incidental finding of abnormalities among control subjects compared with subjects with FASD was not significantly different. A recent study in more than 300 participants suggested that clinical MRI is not diagnostic in subjects with FASD (Treit et al. 2020). This suggests a need for advanced imaging.

When MRI was used to study the effect of PAE on the brain, changes in brain size and volume were detected using quantitative structural analysis. Applied to group differences, significant findings were reported in certain brain areas among subjects with PAE and diagnosed with FAS compared with the control group. Like neuroanatomical studies of brain structure in mental illness, the more sensitive indices used to detect abnormalities are the ratio of total brain volume to intracerebral volume and the ventricular brain ratio. In schizophrenia, for example, such volumetric changes were reported on these indices. In bipolar disorder, right-sided ventricular enlargement was detected using MRI. This was the only significant finding in a systematic review that comprised 28 studies with 404 patients (McDonald et al. 2004). In another study, ventricular brain ratio was larger in patients with bipolar disorder and schizophrenia but not in patients with schizoaffective disorder compared with control subjects who did not have these disorders (Reite et al. 2010).

Still, clinical utility of neuroimaging in the diagnosis of ND-PAE/ FASD must wait for more evidence. Available research findings need to be collated, for example, through meta-analysis, to detect the best evidence of the benefit of neuroimaging. This more rigorous approach helps refine inconclusive brain-related MRI findings, as carried out for other mental disorders. Uncertainties still exist surrounding findings from those disorders, even with a longer period of research evidence. After many years of neuroimaging studies in schizophrenia, no specific significant finding was recommended for clinical use (Woolley and McGuire 2005). Decreased cortical and hippocampal volumes and increased ventricular volumes have been the more consistently reported in cross-sectional studies of schizophrenia. The inadequacy of using cross-sectional samples led to a cohort study over a duration of 13 years. In patients with schizophrenia, a 3% reduction in brain volume was detected, but this was not significant (Reite et al. 2010). Further studies clarified the reported brain reductions. The progressive reductions, compared with control subjects, were located in the frontal and temporal lobes (Guo et al. 2014).

There are still lessons to learn from those areas of mental disorder attempting to improve the diagnostic value of MRI. Even before clinical use is pronounced, findings help align or explain certain brain-based clinical presentations. In a cohort of 33 patients with schizophrenia, compared with 71 control subjects, decline in social and occupational functioning was associated with right supramarginal gyrus reduction (Guo et al. 2015). The same reduction was credited for mediating progressive brain volume changes. It is expected that in both the field of mental disorder and the study of the consequences of PAE, the advancement of neuroimaging combined with clinical neurophysiological findings holds promise for reliable and valid diagnosis (Suttie et al. 2018) and may also be used in monitoring treatment progress.

In PAE, the timing of alcohol exposure is important but is not the only factor in determining the damage to the temporal, inferior parietal, and frontal lobes. Therefore, initial reports of the regional reductions in volume and tissue density are being clarified. Research has shown specific reduction in cranial vault, brain size, and parietal lobes of those with PAE. Additional abnormalities detected in parietal and temporal lobes affected the perisylvian cortices, which showed relative increases in grey matter and decreases in white matter (Sowell et al. 2001b).

The effect of PAE in altering sensorimotor structure and function has been implied when resting state fMRI found increased functional connectivity between the sensorimotor brain network and the striatum and brain stem (Donald et al. 2016). PAE subjects had increased functional connectivity between sensorimotor regions to the default mode network and salience network, which control motor function, cognitive function, emotions, and consciousness. Alterations in sensorimotor connectivity were related to the extent of facial dysmorphology (Long et al. 2018). Compared with control subjects, those with PAE were shown to have significantly smaller brain volume.

The future benefit of this type of research finding is to link detected brain changes with neuropsychological abnormalities that are relevant to clinical features. For instance, response inhibition, behavioral control, and executive functions in children with PAE are related to difficulties of frontal-lobe neurocognition. These in turn mirror findings of reduced brain growth in the ventral portions of the frontal lobes and narrowing at sites with increased grey matter density, albeit this is not reported in all studies. Longitudinal studies demonstrated cortical thinning in control subjects in the medial and lateral surfaces of the cerebral hemispheres as depicted in Figure 9–2.

Changes related to cerebellar volume reduction were significant in both FAS and nondysmorphic FASD. They were more localized at the anterior

Control subjects

FASD

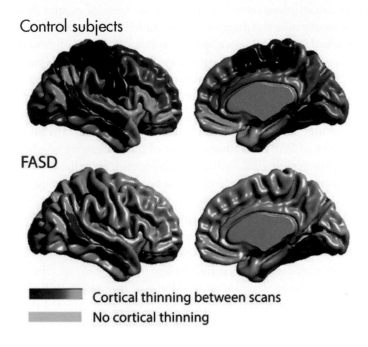

■■■■ Cortical thinning between scans
■■■■ No cortical thinning

FIGURE 9–2.   Medial and lateral surface of the right hemisphere showing more longitudinal cortical thinning in control subjects than children with FASD. (See Plate 2 to view this figure in color.)

Source.   Courtesy Sarah Treit, Ph.D., Department of Biomedical Engineering, University of Alberta.

vermis than the posterior. MRI was used to detect agenesis and alterations in the size and shape of the corpus callosum. These findings are among the most replicated. Evidence that links neuroimaging findings with established neuropathology has been accumulating. This evidence is specific to the cerebellum (anterior vermis), cerebrum (frontal-temporal-parietal area), basal ganglia, and corpus callosum. More anterior displacement of the corpus callosum correlated with impairment in verbal learning tasks in those with FASD (Sowell et al. 2001a). The subcortical group of neurons are sensitive to PAE and function in the control of movements by connecting the thalamus with the cortex. The basal ganglia volume, especially of the caudate nucleus, was reduced in those with FASD compared with control subjects.

   The reasons these discoveries have yet to trigger clinical use of neuroimaging rest on inconsistent findings and the difficulty of isolating the profound environmental effect of brain plasticity in response to experience (Kolb and Whishaw 1998). Some study subjects are not comparable with those who take medications because some medications can affect brain volume. Publishing only significant studies, differences in the resolutions used, and small numbers of subjects studied contribute to the inconsistencies.

In a sizable number of subjects with dysmorphic and nondysmorphic outcomes of PAE, similar findings on DTI were identified. Specific regions were mapped along the DTI indices. These included the left inferior longitudinal fasciculus, splenium, and isthmus. Further analysis indicated that the impairment in white matter mediated the adverse effects of PAE on information processing speed and eye-blink conditioning (Fan et al. 2016). In a larger sample of children with PAE who underwent brain MRI and participated in eye movement tasks and psychometric tests, FA was decreased in specific white matter tracts compared with control subjects. There was a sex difference in that females in the PAE group had lower FA than female control subjects for certain tracts. Measures of eye movements were suggested as possible biomarkers of PAE because there was no correlation between eye movement and DTI in the PAE group although a correlation was found in control subjects (Paolozza et al. 2017).

Conclusion

These are exciting times for the field of study involving the differentiation of patients exposed to PAE and manifesting clinical symptoms of mental disorder. Although neuroimaging approaches are not yet ready to play a definitive diagnostic role in the clinical setting, advances in technology make possible new and innovative research findings with various combinations of neuroimaging. With artificial intelligence and deep machine learning on the horizon, diagnosis and treatment should not be as complicated and uncertain as previously. Neuroimaging findings on white and grey matter are laying the foundation for establishment of biomarkers, although these are likely to be derived from a combination of clinical, psychological, and neuroimaging domains. Similar innovations are occurring in the mental health fields, and these should be complementary to the goal of improved diagnosis and treatment of individuals affected by PAE.

CLINICAL PRACTICAL APPLICATIONS

- MRI findings of smaller hippocampi in individuals with PAE support the clinical and neurocognitive indices of memory challenges mental health professionals will encounter in patients with PAE.
- Diffusion tensor imaging, MRI, magnetic resonance spectroscopy, and functional MRI have so far been the most promising in the emerging techniques for studying the brain function and structure of PAE-affected individuals.

- Clinicians can now refine diagnosis and treatment of patients by combining findings from neuroimaging studies with their clinical impression and their knowledge of the neuropsychological abnormalities associated with ND-PAE/FASD.

- When using neuroimaging, the distinction between dysmorphic and nondysmorphic PAE is blurred; thus, neuroimaging may hold promise for universal clinical use.

References

Astley SJ, Aylward EH, Olson HC, et al: Magnetic resonance imaging outcomes from a comprehensive magnetic resonance study of children with fetal alcohol spectrum disorders. Alcohol Clin Exp Res 33(10):1671–1689, 2009

Barrett CE, Kable JA, Madsen TE, et al: The use of functional near-infrared spectroscopy to differentiate alcohol-related neurodevelopmental impairment. Dev Neuropsychol 44(2):203–219, 2019

Codreanu I, Yang J, Zhuang H: Brain single-photon emission computed tomography in fetal alcohol syndrome: a case report and study implications. J Child Neurol 27(12):1580–1584, 2012

Diwadkar VA, Meintjes EM, Goradia D, et al: Differences in cortico-striatal-cerebellar activation during working memory in syndromal and nonsyndromal children with prenatal alcohol exposure. Hum Brain Mapp 34(8):1931–1945, 2013

Donald KA, Ipser JC, Howells FM, et al: Interhemispheric functional brain connectivity in neonates with prenatal alcohol exposure: preliminary findings. Alcohol Clin Exp Res 40(1):113–121, 2016

Fan J, Jacobson SW, Taylor PA, et al: White matter deficits mediate effects of prenatal alcohol exposure on cognitive development in childhood. Hum Brain Mapp 37(8):2943–2958, 2016

Fernández-Jaén A, Fernández-Mayoralas DM, Quiñones Tapia D, et al: Cortical thickness in fetal alcohol syndrome and attention deficit disorder. Pediatr Neurol 45(6):387–391, 2011

Fryer SL, Schweinsburg BC, Bjorkquist OA, et al: Characterization of white matter microstructure in fetal alcohol spectrum disorders. Alcohol Clin Exp Res 33(3):514–521, 2009

Ghazi Sherbaf F, Aarabi MH, Hosein Yazdi M, Haghshomar M: White matter microstructure in fetal alcohol spectrum disorders: a systematic review of diffusion tensor imaging studies. Hum Brain Mapp 40(3):1017–1036, 2019

Guo JY, Huhtaniska S, Miettunen J, et al: Longitudinal regional brain volume loss in schizophrenia: relationship to antipsychotic medication and change in social function. Schizophr Res 168(1-2):297–304, 2015

Guo X, Li J, Wang J, et al: Hippocampal and orbital inferior frontal gray matter volume abnormalities and cognitive deficit in treatment-naive, first-episode patients with schizophrenia. Schizophr Res 152(2-3):339–343, 2014

Kodituwakku PW: Neurocognitive profile in children with fetal alcohol spectrum disorders. Dev Disabil Res Rev 15(3):218–224, 2009

Kolb B, Whishaw IQ: Brain plasticity and behavior. Annu Rev Psychol 49:43–64, 1998

Long X, Little G, Beaulieu C, Lebel C: Sensorimotor network alterations in children and youth with prenatal alcohol exposure. Hum Brain Mapp 39(5):2258–2268, 2018

McDonald C, Zanelli J, Rabe-Hesketh S, et al: Meta-analysis of magnetic resonance imaging brain morphometry studies in bipolar disorder. Biol Psychiatry 56(6):411–417, 2004

Meintjes EM, Jacobson JL, Molteno CD, et al: An FMRI study of number processing in children with fetal alcohol syndrome. Alcohol Clin Exp Res 34(8):1450–1464, 2010

Norman AL, Crocker N, Mattson SN, Riley EP: Neuroimaging and fetal alcohol spectrum disorders. Dev Disabil Res Rev 15(3):209–217, 2009

O'Hare ED, Kan E, Yoshii J, et al: Mapping cerebellar vermal morphology and cognitive correlates in prenatal alcohol exposure. Neuroreport 16(12):1285–1290, 2005

Paolozza A, Treit S, Beaulieu C, Reynolds JN: Diffusion tensor imaging of white matter and correlates to eye movement control and psychometric testing in children with prenatal alcohol exposure. Hum Brain Mapp 38(1):444–456, 2017

Reite M, Reite E, Collins D, et al: Brain size and brain/intracranial volume ratio in major mental illness. BMC Psychiatry 10:79, 2010

Sowell ER, Mattson SN, Thompson PM, et al: Mapping callosal morphology and cognitive correlates: effects of heavy prenatal alcohol exposure. Neurology 57(2):235–244, 2001a

Sowell ER, Thompson PM, Mattson SN, et al: Voxel-based morphometric analyses of the brain in children and adolescents prenatally exposed to alcohol. Neuroreport 12(3):515–523, 2001b

Sowell ER, Thompson PM, Peterson BS, et al: Mapping cortical gray matter asymmetry patterns in adolescents with heavy prenatal alcohol exposure. Neuroimage 17(4):1807–1819, 2002

Spadoni AD, McGee CL, Fryer SL, Riley EP: Neuroimaging and fetal alcohol spectrum disorders. Neurosci Biobehav Rev 31(2):239–245, 2007

Suttie M, Wozniak JR, Parnell SE, et al: Combined face-brain morphology and associated neurocognitive correlates in fetal alcohol spectrum disorders. Alcohol Clin Exp Res 42(9):1769–1782, 2018

Treit S, Jeffery D, Beaulieu C, Emery D: Radiological findings on structural magnetic resonance imaging in fetal alcohol spectrum disorders and healthy controls. Alcohol Clin Exp Res 44(2):455–462, 2020

Woolley J, McGuire P: Neuroimaging in schizophrenia: what does it tell the clinician? Advances in Psychiatric Treatment 11(3):195–202, 2005

Wozniak JR, Mueller BA, Chang PN, et al: Diffusion tensor imaging in children with fetal alcohol spectrum disorders. Alcohol Clin Exp Res 30(10):1799–1806, 2006

Wozniak JR, Mueller BA, Bell CJ, et al: Global functional connectivity abnormalities in children with fetal alcohol spectrum disorders. Alcohol Clin Exp Res 37(5):748–756, 2013

Yang Y, Roussotte F, Kan E, et al: Abnormal cortical thickness alterations in fetal alcohol spectrum disorders and their relationships with facial dysmorphology. Cereb Cortex 22(5):1170–1179, 2012

Zhou D, Lebel C, Lepage C, et al: Developmental cortical thinning in fetal alcohol spectrum disorders. Neuroimage 58(1):16–25, 2011

Zhou D, Rasmussen C, Pei J, et al: Preserved cortical asymmetry despite thinner cortex in children and adolescents with prenatal alcohol exposure and associated conditions. Hum Brain Mapp 39(1):72–88, 2018

CHAPTER 10

Psychological Testing

WHAT TO KNOW

Although promising, the search for a specific profile based on psychological test results has not yet yielded the desired diagnostic characterization of ND-PAE/FASD.

DSM-5 recognizes the domains of neurocognitive functioning, behavior regulation, and adaptive functioning to be central in diagnosing ND-PAE/FASD.

Notwithstanding the term *spectrum*, and with most diagnostic guidelines requiring three impaired psychological brain domains, patients with ND-PAE/FASD are significantly impaired.

Irrespective of IQ scores, other neurocognitive findings, executive function especially, have influential effects on patients.

Examples of domains to be assessed for ND-PAE/FASD diagnosis include attention, language, motor skills, memory, executive function, affect regulation, neurophysiological variables, cognition, academic achievement, and adaptive functions.

Experts are attempting to develop a streamlined list of specific domain testing tools and instruments.

Until more specifically refined and valid tests become available and clinically useful, psychological assessment remains the gold standard for identifying deficits in those with PAE, with or without specific mental disorders. Detecting functional and behavioral difficulties is achieved by interpreting information gathered from the patient and reliable collateral sources. Profiles (behavioral, motor, diagnostic, and treatment) of clinical subtypes based on PAE-induced neurocognitive deficits and neurodevelopmental disorder are needed to reliably identify and treat patients. Organizing the abundance of clinical features into manageable categories currently requires multiprofessional team involvement with each patient. A variety of clinical features assessed by different specialists can be pulled together to provide relevant information for creating a treatment plan. The effectiveness of this plan rests on correctly maximizing strengths and correcting the PAE-induced weaknesses recognized in the patient. Because psychiatric classification systems are only beginning to recognize the role of PAE in diagnosis, it will be a while before aspects of its categories become applicable in clinical settings. This means seeking information about presentations and patterns with clinical usefulness, especially to reorient the mental health system to the obvious needs of patients with PAE.

In this chapter, I review the development of psychological tests in the field of ND-PAE/FASD treatment and report attempts to create profiles and consensus on tests for neurocognitive deficits. The clinical utility and future implications of tests and their limitations are covered as well.

Development of Psychological Profiles in ND-PAE/FASD

Clinical phenotypes are helpful in clinical management. They are developed when identified clinical features and standard test scores are combined to create an accurate patient profile. When the features are valid and reliable, subjects with similar profiles are conceptualized as a group and managed consistently. There have been several clinical and research attempts to characterize symptoms of those with PAE in order to create unique subtypes. Research targeting a unique clinical profile for the consequences of PAE have so far yielded few useful results. However, progress is being made, and mental health professionals currently have a set of behavioral neurocognitive phenotypes to continue the search for one, or a few, predictive profiles. The hope for a blueprint for treatment interventions may rest firmly on the discovery of such patterns.

After reviewing multiple studies and clinical cases, some indicators were acknowledged as useful in forming a profile for detecting PAE in patients.

Deficits related to adaptive functioning, which regularly included dependent living and behaviors that compromised patient safety, were noted as significantly challenging for these patients. Variations in learning and inconsistent language abilities were also thought to be part of the profile. Multiple deficits associated with reasoning and lower intelligence, especially verbal, were found to predominate in standardized test results (Clarren et al. 2015; Kodituwakku 2007). A high percentage of individuals with PAE demonstrated deficits in attention, memory, and specific math ability, which, with other decision-making problems, were linked to executive function deficits. Socially, patients displayed impaired relationships and experienced poor sensory integration of multiple stimuli. Using standard psychological tests to generate patterns of various combinations of deficits, screening tools were proposed. It was later thought that the test results could yield different profiles that could be grouped as clinical cases and subgroups within these clinical cases. The search for unique and specific profiles is ongoing (Fast and Conry 2009; Mattson and Riley 2011). Other researchers have focused on the most predictive standard test deficits as representative of the majority of those with PAE. A number of systematic reviews have attempted this type of profile research, but none has yet reached a level of significance to become part of the diagnosis of ND-PAE/ FASD (Kodituwakku 2007; Koren et al. 2014; Mattson and Riley 2011). A consensus process among researchers determined three similar behavioral patterns and deficits that form diagnostic profiles. These were defined as PAE-influenced superdomains (i.e., neurocognitive functioning, behavior regulation, and adaptive functioning) (Sanders et al. 2017) and were recommended for the DSM-5 diagnosis of ND-PAE (American Psychiatric Association 2013).

The clinical utility of this profile stems, first, from the similarities found in the criteria for ND-PAE and nondysmorphic consequences of PAE. Even when populations of both dysmorphic and nondysmorphic FASD were compared along the diagnostic criteria of ND-PAE, those superdomains identified specific profiles. Recent approaches include focusing on profiles of subtests and combined standardized psychological tests among patients diagnosed with FASD and subjects prenatally exposed to alcohol but not diagnosed. At times, indices and subindices of the tests are combined to identify any profiles, and at other times, the study population will be restricted by age or comorbid condition. In a large sample of patients, the deficits detected by some psychological tests were found to be effective in correctly identifying those with a diagnosis of FASD. Psychological tests of intelligence, academic achievement, memory, and executive functioning accurately identified up to three-quarters of those with a diagnosis (Enns and Taylor 2018). Enns and Taylor suggested that subindices of these tests produce the best classification rate, thus potentially positioning a profile to enhance efficiency in diagnosis by reducing the number of tests. Perhaps, psychological tests in the future will not only identify the most effective tests through an algorithm but also hold the promise of easy and accurate profiles for identifying clinical subjects. The efficacy of combining psychological test results with clinical features and neuroimaging findings to predict a diagnostic profile is still being explored (Suttie et al. 2018).

Clinical Vignette

A 39-year-old woman refers herself to a multidisciplinary diagnostic team for neurodevelopmental disorders. The patient is living with her adoptive mother and is struggling with her 5-year-old son, who is displaying severe temper tantrums. Her mother was recently diagnosed with anxiety and depression in the context of caregiver burnout. Because the care of her three children has now been transferred to her, the patient is seeking help with how to manage. She forgets to take her daughter to her dance classes, cannot keep the house clean, and is feeling overwhelmed by the noise in the house. She has been prescribed some medications, but she cannot remember their names.

The patient was adopted at birth, struggled in school, and only completed ninth grade through a modified program. When she found a job, she was assigned to the cash register in a fast food restaurant. Despite coaching, she made so many mistakes that she was let go after 2 weeks. Her records show that the patient had an IQ test when she was in the third grade. Her full-scale IQ score was 85. At the time, a more comprehensive assessment was not required. Prompted by her son's doctor asking if she drank alcohol during pregnancy, she decided to ask her adoptive mother about her own behavior as a 5-year-old. Her mother describes similar temper tantrums when the patient was about her son's age. Her birth records provide scant information.

To obtain a clearer picture of the seeming forgetfulness, lack of ability to plan, past history of school difficulties, employment failure, and temper tantrums, the team seeks to examine as many brain domains as will elicit a comprehensive picture of the patient's case. These findings are necessary if an adequate treatment plan is to be put into effect. The psychologist on the team and the occupational therapist help in completing the tests (see test examples in Table 10–1) to determine any brain domain deficits. The test score assumes clinical relevance when the person scores 1.5–2.0 standard deviations below the normed population mean, after the raw score has been converted and compared with the population mean. Another criteria used is when scores of the different subscales show marked variance between them. Each neurocognitive domain is evaluated against this criteria, and a diagnosis of ND-PAE/FASD is made when at least three brain domains meet the test criteria. The domains are functionally assessed by age-specific tests.

TABLE 10–1. Test examples

NEUROCOGNITIVE DOMAIN	TEST (AGE SPECIFIC)*
Motor skills	Abnormal Involuntary Movement Scale
	Finger-tapping test
Neurophysiology/ Neuroanatomy	Measurement of head circumference to detect microcephaly, electroencephalogram (EEG), MRI
Cognition	Wechsler Adult Intelligence Scale (WAIS)
	Wechsler Intelligence Scale for Children (WISC)
	Bayley Scales of Infant and Toddler Development—Third Edition (Bayley-III)
Language	Peabody Picture Vocabulary Test (PPVT)
	Expressive Vocabulary Test (EVT)
Academic achievement	Woodcock–Johnson Tests of Achievement
	Wechsler Individual Achievement Test (WIAT)
Memory	A Developmental NEuroPSYchological Assessment—Second Edition (NEPSY-II)
	Wechsler Memory Scale (WMS)
Attention	Conners' Continuous Performance Test (CPT)
	Child Behavior Checklist (CBCL)
Executive function	Wisconsin Card Sorting Test (WCST)
	Behavior Rating Inventory of Executive Function (BRIEF)
Affect regulation	Clinical interview and anxiety and mood questionnaires
Adaptive behavior, social skills, OR social communication	Vineland Adaptive Behavior Scales (VABS) Adaptive Behavior Assessment System (ABAS)

*Tests vary with age, normed data, and the tester's preference and experience (see Coons-Harding et al. 2019).

Arrangements should be made to complete the assessment of the patient. These tests last more than 4 hours, and so frequent breaks and support after the tests are essential for the patient's stamina and self-esteem. An IQ of 85 may fluctuate, depending on factors such as alcohol use, medications, trauma, and head injury since the last assessment. Because of the diffuse nature of the damage in PAE, IQ results do not determine the level of deficits in other areas—executive function, memory, and language—which could be severely impaired and could explain the poor coping the subject of the vignette expresses.

Clinical Utility of Psychological Tests

Identifying a neuropsychological profile of the person with FASD provides several advantages, especially diagnostic accuracy and ease of classification. These two objectives have remained elusive given the multiple domains assessed and ascribed to PAE. Current evidence for the diagnostic value of neuropsychological tests is lacking; yet, tests of planning, set-shifting, fluency, and working memory may be instrumental in precisely defining the clinical phenotype of FASD. The "red flag" is a concept that is clinically useful. Referral for a comprehensive assessment is indicated when patients demonstrate numerous critical features of a given disorder. To be effective, clinicians should be acutely aware of factors responsible for variations in the neurocognitive profile of their patients. Neurocognitive impairments, ascertained from test results across the lifespan, affect independent functioning and become more pronounced with increasing age. Knowledge about the factors precipitating neurocognitive variations and how neurocognitive deficits manifest over time permits clinical features to be used to develop a profile and helps to determine which team members are invited to contribute their assessment skills in identifying the neuropsychological deficits.

Scope of Psychological Testing

Neurocognitive and neuropsychological testing are used interchangeably even though the extent of their application may have glaring or subtle differences. *Neurocognitive* testing employs noninvasive means of measuring the normal function of the brain, such as cognition, memory, language, and attention. *Neuropsychological* testing is inferred when processes and tests attempt to link brain parts with the impairment in function. The structure and pathways of the brain produce specific test patterns, which can be clinically identified, tested, and measured. These measurements compare the patient's scores with normative data to determine if and how extensive the function varies from the expected norm. Evaluations of this form are well known in the mental health system. They are indicated when evaluating the impairment arising from the disease process of severe and persistent mental illness, such as schizophrenia, bipolar disorder, schizoaffective disorder, and major depressive disorder. The request for neurocognitive evaluation is also essential to the process used to diagnose major and minor neurocognitive disorders, such as dementia; sequelae of traumatic brain injury; and neurodevelopmental disorders, such as autism spectrum disorder.

Neurocognitive and neurodevelopmental evaluation is an integral part of the diagnostic assessment of ND-PAE/FASD. It establishes maladaptation related to brain dysfunction and is foundational to treatment planning. Comprehensive treatment planning involves multidisciplinary team members with roles catering to specific individual deficits. Treatment has to respond to the deficits identified in a habilitation or rehabilitation mode of care (serving to train, retrain, or help acquire and improve functional skills).

Treatment planning is limited by inadequate domain assessment and absence of a list of psychosocial strengths. This occurs in areas with few psychological services and where psychologists are under pressure to diagnose a target number of patients. They therefore strategize the administration of the tests to maximize time by sequentially detecting the minimum required domains. Stopping at that point rather than completing the full battery of tests is a service-specific challenge. These time-saving solutions present ethical issues about comprehensibility and efficiency (Coons-Harding et al. 2019).

Differentiating the Neuropsychological Profile of ADHD

The relationship between ND-PAE/FASD and ADHD continues to be the subject of research and much interpretation. The shared variables between the two entities have prompted explanations for developing profiles with diagnostic capabilities. PAE produces a poorer behavioral and cognitive profile than ADHD. Studies comparing the consequences of PAE use different outcomes (Raldiris et al. 2018). In patients with the combination of ND-PAE/FASD and ADHD, certain features combine to act as warning signs and should trigger a request for more comprehensive assessment. Subjects with ND-PAE/FASD alone showed worse deficits in full-scale IQ, perceptual reasoning, verbal comprehension, and working memory compared with those with ADHD alone (Raldiris et al. 2018; Taylor and Enns 2018). Differences in externalizing behavior and hyperactivity and higher levels of atypicality and aggression were ADHD related. Weaker verbal comprehension was uniquely associated with those with PAE combined with ADHD.

Many patients with FASD qualify for an ADHD diagnosis. Deficits in visual attention were found to be more representative of alcohol exposure, whereas impulsivity was prevalent in children with ADHD who were not exposed to alcohol. Reaction time, a cognitive measure of processing speed, was slower in alcohol-exposed children. This was particularly related to a higher demand in the choice reaction time, which tests general alertness and motor speed by providing the test taker with two possible stimuli and two possible responses.. Findings of abnormalities in visuospatial processing and memory in alcohol-exposed children invoke difficulties in shifting attention, which is likely related to the reduced cerebellar vermis. Reduction in frontal lobes and basal ganglia and their distorted connection was put forward as an explanation for the perseveration noted in alcohol-exposed children. Also, children with FASD showed significant impairment in cognitive flexibility, response inhibition, planning, concept formation, and reasoning domains of executive functioning. Verbal and nonverbal fluency are equally impaired, and those impairments are suspected as arising from deficits related to the reduction and thinning of the frontal lobes and reduction in the basal ganglia, which are connected through the frontal-subcortical circuit. These deficits may also be related to deficits in spatial memory, perseverative tendencies, and attentional problems (Raldiris et al. 2018; Riley and McGee 2005).

Profiling Without Psychological Tests

Without psychological tests, for the most part those affected by PAE are detected coincidentally and sometimes accidentally or in unusual circumstances. Individuals are currently diagnosed most often in a research sample during the research project. The failure to diagnose patients outside of the case ascertainment setting reveals the difficulty of identification in clinical settings. To improve on the current anecdotal discovery, psychological tests offer a more systematic approach. This is why elaborate and resource-dependent psychological testing is needed. Depending on the resources and types of services accessible to mental health professionals, obtaining psychological tests may feel overwhelming and discouraging. Although the gold standard of psychological assessment involves evaluating the scores of multiple neurocognitive domains to determine adaptive dysfunction, other reported attempts at profiling those with PAE and its outcomes may be instructive to the professional. Teachers, more than parents, were reported as accurately identifying those with ND-PAE/FASD using teacher-reported observation questionnaires with students (Taylor and Enns 2018). Correctional officers were asked to refer a group of individuals in their facility for a comprehensive neurodevelopmental assessment. More than 95% of those referred were ultimately diagnosed with ND-PAE/FASD. No training was offered for the referring correctional officers (Brintnell et al. 2019). These nonclinicians seem to be able to recognize those who fall within the continuum of ND-PAE/FASD. Thus, it is likely that even without a commonly accepted profile for those with PAE and its outcomes, training will improve recognition. Features that identify people with PAE in nonclinical settings, such as a classroom and correctional setting, seem to adequately differentiate them from unaffected nonclinical cases.

To select the correct predictive tests in nonclinical settings, teacher ratings were also compared with parent ratings and found to be superior to parent ratings in 345 child and adolescent cases. This study was instructive in identifying FASD diagnosis using specific ratings associated with adaptive and executive dysfunction (Enns and Taylor 2018). Those features, rated by nonclinicians, were compared with a retrospective diagnosis of subjects. Worse ratings on learning issues, attention, and adaptive skills were associated with a 1.5- to 2.0-fold increase in diagnosis of FASD among an alcohol-exposed group. If replicated, the use of collateral information from teachers could carry reasonable weight in increasing the reliability of diagnosis. Depending on the rating scale used, the profiles of the impairment are different, so diagnostic outcomes will vary as well. In a comparative study examining the clinical utility of executive function tests and subtests, ratings by caregivers were compared with the clinical scores of patients. A Behavior Rating Inventory of Executive Function (BRIEF) was completed by caregivers of those with FASD, and the Delis-Kaplan Executive Function System (D-KEFS) was completed by clinicians. Three executive function domains in the BRIEF showed clinically significant elevations, but the two scales bore little resemblance (Mohamed et al. 2019; Mukherjee et al. 2019). The useful BRIEF scale is recommended by various guidelines for assessment and diagnosis of ND-PAE/FASD (Cook et al. 2016; Sanders et al. 2017).

The importance of a profile applies when differentiating clinical populations. The diagnosis of ND-PAE/FASD should be made separately from diagnosis of those with other mental disorders (e.g., depression, anxiety, PTSD, conduct disorder) but without ND-PAE/FASD. The ability to separate these categories is limited, and perpetuated, by current explanatory models of the sequelae of PAE, for example, viewing PAE's damage as nonspecific and, at best, characterized as diffuse brain dysfunction (Clarren 1986; Mattson and Riley 1996). Given that comorbidity with multiple mental disorders is the norm, the disorders are complicated further because they share similar pathophysiology and neuroimaging features (Johnson et al. 2018; Mattson et al. 2011). Shared features did not stop clinicians in a study from apportioning differing weights to the role of PAE in the mechanism of disorders. Study subjects identified PAE as the significant factor in ND-

PAE/FASD but did not give quite enough weight to PAE in other conditions comorbid with PAE. Using vignettes and their experience with those patients at the interface, clinicians listed adaptive and executive function impairments and deficits as features that separate ND-PAE/FASD from other clinical entities (Chudley 2018; Doyle and Mattson 2015). Screening tests can be developed using the features identified and determined by similar experienced clinicians as significantly related to PAE. A substantial number of diagnostic clinics insist on confirming PAE in referred cases, which delays access to diagnosis. Using a consensus approach, patterns can be developed from the selected impairments and then rigorously tested. Reassuringly, application of this approach aligns with the finding that referral services that do not insist on PAE still receive a large proportion of those diagnosed with ND-PAE/FASD. In a study of the reasons for referral, behavioral and adaptive function problems were relatively stable reasons; this validates the findings of the comprehensive psychological tests (Chudley 2018).

Specific maladaptive functions have been selected to improve screening of those with ND-PAE/FASD. As indicated in Chapter 6 ("Clinical Presentation"), these lists require formal validation, but they are useful for mental health professionals who do not have access to resources for obtaining psychological testing. Patients identified as manifesting those dysfunctions should be referred to be formally and comprehensively assessed. Other strategies that require validation include those suggesting improved recognition by nonclinical professionals. Some easy-to-identify factors endorsed by caregivers include level of parenting stress, scales that measure infant behaviors as early as the first year of life, which are helpful for recognition when clinical services are extremely limited. These may point to individuals exposed to alcohol during gestation. In the study by Enns and Taylor (2018), neurobehavioral outcomes were useful in separating individuals exposed to heavy alcohol use from those without heavy alcohol exposure.

Executive dysfunction was thought to selectively identify alcohol-exposed children because it occurred frequently in ND-PAE/FASD, but poor executive functioning also occurs frequent in other disorders, such as ADHD (Nguyen et al. 2014). Parent ratings using the BRIEF compared with neuropsychological testing using D-KEFS were noted earlier (Mukherjee et al. 2019; Taylor and Enns 2018). Results from studies comparing the two measures found the main effects to be indicative of a neurobehavioral pattern capable of separating subjects with PAE from those without. In search of a psychological profile, psychological tests cannot be avoided. That is why a comprehensive approach involves multiple tests (Coons-Harding et al. 2019). Consequently, implicit memory was found to be no different between the alcohol-exposed group and the control group of non-exposed children. Deficits in memorizing information were ascribed to a deficiency in acquisition rather than inability to remember (Riley and McGee 2005). FASD patients were significantly impaired in word comprehension and naming components of language.

Comparing various diagnostic guidelines, it was recommended that 10 brain domains be comprehensively assessed for diagnosis (Cook et al. 2016). Arguably, these features can be monitored during intervention. The same domains have been proposed for the more readily used diagnostic guidelines in multiple countries—Australia, Scotland, and New Zealand. Those who administer the different tests were given options to select the more valid tests. Preferences and experience with certain tests will affect compliance with the recommended lists (Coons-Harding et al. 2019). It is time to evaluate the clinical utility of existing psychological test instruments specific to the consequences of PAE. Most of the tests were conceptualized in different contexts, and their cutoff criteria may be arbitrary. Some mental health professionals determine impairment at 1.5 standard deviations from the mean; others use 2.0. Trained psychologists are the major professional group that tests subjects. Occupational therapists, language and speech pathologists, behavior therapists, and rehabilitation consultants have various aspects that they can contribute to the assessment. The goal of psychological testing is to identify significant impairments and areas or domains of strength. Researchers indicate that parent-report measures are clinically useful in predicting alcohol exposure regardless of other disorders such as ADHD. Whether one domain or a combination of domains can form a profile to identify those with PAE remains to be confirmed.

Occupational therapists are important members of diagnostic teams, especially with children. They are a clinical resource for mental health clinicians by providing alternate assessments, especially in the absence of psychological tests. Fine-motor speed and coordination are impaired in those with FASD, who appear to rely more on somatosensory input. These patients are reported as being at high risk for problem behaviors that can interfere with their participation in home, school, and social environments. Impairments in social skills are explained by arrested development. Hence, for patients younger than 12, assessment can be requested for fine-motor skills, visual-motor integration, and balance skills. These areas are the purview of occupational therapists, and test result deficits in motor features were found to persist in patients with PAE (Safe et al. 2018). In subjects with historical or neurological evidence of motor skills deficit, occupational therapy assessments confirming these provide additional diagnostic and possibly therapeutic information (Mattson et al. 2011). In patients suspected of having ND-PAE/FASD, occupational therapy assessments for executive function and other cognitive deficits should be sought during mental health assessments, especially when PAE indicators are suspected.

Profile of Neuropsychological Assessments

The search for a characteristic neurocognitive profile in ND-PAE/FASD is based on CNS abnormalities. Exact profiles are not yet available for clinical use. Current profiles use the most frequently impaired brain domain functions noted in neurodevelopmental psychological assessments. When a pattern of these deficits is identified as prevalent in those ultimately diagnosed with ND-PAE/FASD, a profile is suggested (Bakhireva et al. 2018). Stand-alone and combination profiles have been studied, with the goal of improving validity and reliability of identification. Current research findings recommend combining wide-ranging CNS damage, such as microcephaly, with other features (facial dysmorphia, neuroimaging, and other face-brain images) to identify predictive models (Peadon et al. 2008; Pei and Rinaldi 2004; Suttie et al. 2018).

Predictive profiles using databases of psychological tests completed in FASD diagnostic clinics are being examined. These allow maternal factors, results of neuroimaging studies, clinical information, and psychological tests to be linked (Astley 2010; Singal et al. 2016; Wozniak et al. 2019). The beauty of this research is the large numbers of diagnosed patients with multiple points of data that can aid in the creation of profiles. For instance, outcomes of psychological tests of dysfunction in social communication, executive function, and adaptive function in more than 3,000 patients are now analyzable (Astley 2010). In a retrospective comparison data analysis of those with PAE, psychological predictors can be identified using logistic regression. Analyzing subindices of neuropsychological tests in a large number of patients has the potential to improve classification of individuals with PAE. Research goals include refining the number of such indices so that, in combination, they can potentially enhance efficiency in diagnosis. Parsimoniously, using an algorithm allows a reduced number of tests (test battery) and still facilitates effective assessment, and that should inform more effective intervention (Enns and Taylor 2018).

Practical Evolution and Future of Psychological Testing

In a survey of multidisciplinary diagnostic clinics, specialized training was reported in virtually all of them, and psychological testing took the longest allotted time (Peadon et al. 2008). Most clinics run for about 1–2 days, and in-person psychological testing lasts an average of 6 hours. Processes have evolved, and most clinics have developed processes and procedures to effectively diagnose and make recommendations about those they assess. Completed psychological testing forms a major part of the documentation, which allows recommendations to be neurocognitive specific (Astley 2004; Pei and Rinaldi 2004).

Synthesizing neurocognitive and brain–face abnormality testing results holds promise for diagnostic validity, efficiency, and reliability. Research used dense surface models of facial features and the surface shape of specific neuroanatomical landmarks in relationship with neurocognitive correlates of ND-PAE/FASD. Analysis of high-resolution three-dimensional facial images with MRI images of cortical structures known to be damaged by PAE was completed. Caudate nucleus asymmetry was reduced in FAS among those heavily exposed to prenatal alcohol compared with control subjects. Caudate nucleus asymmetry is strongly associated with general cognitive ability, verbal learning, and recall (Suttie et al. 2018). Combined with neurocognitive correlates, this area of exploration could potentially revolutionize FASD diagnosis.

People perform and react differently to the process of psychological testing. Clinical sensitivity to the effects of patients' effort, motivation, and persistence is necessary. Those who have PAE already experience problems with self-esteem, organization, and comprehension, which exert differential restrictions on the conduct and interpretation of test results. Results are also varied, and PAE-induced neuropsychological deficits are contextualized to the person. For instance, results of assessment of IQ were reported to range widely from 20 to 120. About one-quarter of most patients with FASD score in the IQ range of mental retardation (Riley and McGee 2005). Although most test results are variable, research studies overall report lower scores in the dysmorphic FASD group (Doyle and Mattson 2015). The variation and atypicality of test results place ND-PAE/FASD among the most challenging and yet clinically fulfilling encounters when the right approach is applied. With computerized scales and games, the future application and implications of psychological tests are promising to facilitate understanding and interventions not previously imagined or studied.

Clinicians were surveyed to determine the consistency of psychological tests used for neurobehavioral and cognitive assessments. Similar to what was obtained in other settings, the results from a single jurisdiction made up of 23 clinicians showed an overlap of the measures used. Although still using a variety of tests, combining direct and indirect measures, the clinicians made useful recommendations in line with supporting patients assessed by those tests (Coons-Harding et al. 2019). The study found commonalities between tests and strong convergence of direct and indirect measures to assess brain function. Training, keeping up with current best practices, and using comprehensive and reliable psychological tests were recommended as the essential practices to ensure the diagnostic accuracy of the assessment. The surveyed clinicians recognized the importance of identifying challenges as well as strengths as a way to improve functional abilities in all those tested (Coons-Harding et al. 2019). This completes the loop of recognizing cognitive deficits and then assessing individuals using noninvasive psychological tests to attempt to ameliorate the deficits clinically.

Conclusion

The value of psychological tests and results in the case formulation of patients with ND-PAE/FASD and similar complex presentations cannot be overestimated. Research indicates that no single profile has been identified to represent individuals with PAE. Strategies to obtain full assessments include referral to experts in the field, access to psychologists as team members, use of other professionals with testing abilities (e.g., occupational therapists), and employing nonclinical sources (teachers and parents). The goals are to target the independence and adaptive functioning level of the patient and to streamline testing through the use of algorithmic steps. The results are unique to each patient and should inform interventions and outcomes. It is likely that more than one profile exists for the consequences of PAE. It is more efficient to conceptualize valid profiles by combining test results and other clinical and neuroimaging indices to form a robust gestalt of identification.

CLINICAL PRACTICAL APPLICATIONS

- There is sufficient evidence to allow clinicians conversant with diagnosing ND-PAE according to DSM to be confident that their diagnostic process and outcomes generally aligns with other diagnostic schemes.

- If a clinician's resources allow a limited amount of tests, at the very least, intelligence, academic achievement, memory, and executive functioning should be assessed in order to provide as robust an understanding of the patient as possible.

- Access should be improved for clinicians to request the assessment of normal brain function (neurocognitive) or impaired brain function (neuropsychological); these assessments should be an accepted clinical standard of care in managing complex cases.

- Effective treatment planning should recognize strategies that correct the deficits identified through psychological testing.

- In addition to a psychological test result, differentiating ADHD from PAE-induced ADHD requires a stepwise sorting of collated referral, clinical, collateral, and treatment features.

- In the absence of psychological testing, proxy psychological measures like Behavior Rating Inventory of Executive Function and parent and teacher rating scales may be clinically useful because worse scores on these measures correlate with PAE.

References

American Psychiatric Association: Diagnostic and Statistical Manual of Mental Disorders, 5th Edition. Arlington, VA, American Psychiatric Association, 2013

Astley SJ: Diagnostic Guide for Fetal Alcohol Spectrum Disorders: The 4-Digit Diagnostic Code, 3rd Edition. Seattle, WA, University of Washington, 2004

Astley SJ: Profile of the first 1,400 patients receiving diagnostic evaluations for fetal alcohol spectrum disorder at the Washington State Fetal Alcohol Syndrome Diagnostic & Prevention Network. Can J Ther Clin Pharmacol 17(1):e132–e164, 2010

Bakhireva LN, Lowe J, Garrison LM, et al: Role of caregiver-reported outcomes in identification of children with prenatal alcohol exposure during the first year of life. Pediatr Res 84(3):362–370, 2018

Brintnell ES, Sawhney AS, Bailey PG, et al: Corrections and connection to the community: a diagnostic and service program for incarcerated adult men with FASD. Int J Law Psychiatry 64:8–17, 2019

Chudley AE: Diagnosis of fetal alcohol spectrum disorder: current practices and future considerations. Biochem Cell Biol 96(2) 231–236, 2018

Clarren SK: Neuropathology in fetal alcohol syndrome, in Alcohol and Brain Development. Edited by West JR. New York, Oxford University Press, 1986, pp 158–166

Clarren S, Halliwell CI, Werk CM, et al: Using a common form for consistent collection and reporting of FASD data from across Canada: a feasibility study. J Popul Ther Clin Pharmacol 22(3):e211–e28, 2015

Cook JL, Green CR, Lilley CM, et al: Fetal alcohol spectrum disorder: a guideline for diagnosis across the lifespan. CMAJ 188(3):191–197, 2016

Coons-Harding KD, Flannigan K, Burns C, et al: Assessing for fetal alcohol spectrum disorder. J Popul Ther Clin Pharmacol 26(1):e39–e55, 2019

Doyle LR, Mattson SN: Neurobehavioral disorder associated with prenatal alcohol exposure (ND-PAE): review of evidence and guidelines for assessment. Curr Dev Disord Rep 2(3):175–188, 2015

Enns LN, Taylor NM: Factors predictive of a fetal alcohol spectrum disorder: neuropsychological assessment. Child Neuropsychol 24(2):203–225, 2018

Fast DK, Conry J: Fetal alcohol spectrum disorders and the criminal justice system. Dev Disabil Res Rev 15(3):250–257, 2009

Johnson S, Moyer CL, Klug MG, Burd L: Comparison of alcohol-related neurodevelopmental disorders and neurodevelopmental disorders associated with prenatal alcohol exposure diagnostic criteria. J Dev Behav Pediatr 39(2):163–167, 2018

Kodituwakku PW: Defining the behavioral phenotype in children with fetal alcohol spectrum disorders: a review. Neurosci Biobehav Rev 31(2):192–201, 2007

Koren G, Zelner I, Nash K, Koren G: Foetal alcohol spectrum disorder: identifying the neurobehavioural phenotype and effective interventions. Curr Opin Psychiatry 27(2):98–104, 2014

Mattson SN, Riley EP: Brain anomalies in fetal alcohol syndrome, in Fetal Alcohol Syndrome: From Mechanism to Prevention. Edited by Abel EL. Boca Raton, FL, CRC Press, 1996, pp 51–68

Mattson SN, Riley EP: The quest for a behavioral profile of heavy prenatal alcohol exposure. Alcohol Res Health 34(1):51–55, 2011

Mattson SN, Crocker N, Nguyen TT: Fetal alcohol spectrum disorders: neuropsychological and behavioral features. Neuropsychol Rev 21(2):81–101, 2011

Mohamed Z, Carlisle ACS, Livesey AC, Mukherjee RAS: Comparisons of the BRIEF parental report and neuropsychological clinical tests of executive function in fetal alcohol spectrum disorders: data from the UK national specialist clinic. Child Neuropsychol 25(5):648–663, 2019

Mukherjee RA, Cook PA, Norgate SH, Price AD: Neurodevelopmental outcomes in individuals with fetal alcohol spectrum disorder (FASD) with and without exposure to neglect: clinical cohort data from a national FASD diagnostic clinic. Alcohol 76:23–28, 2019

Nguyen TT, Glass L, Coles CD, et al: The clinical utility and specificity of parent report of executive function among children with prenatal alcohol exposure. J Int Neuropsychol Soc 20(7):704–716, 2014

Peadon E, Fremantle E, Bower C, Elliott EJ: International survey of diagnostic services for children with fetal alcohol spectrum disorders. BMC Pediatr 8:12, 2008

Pei J, Rinaldi C: A review of the evolution of diagnostic practices for fetal alcohol spectrum disorder. Developmental Disabilities Bulletin 32(2):125–139, 2004

Raldiris TL, Bowers TG, Towsey C: Comparisons of intelligence and behavior in children with fetal alcohol spectrum disorder and ADHD. J Atten Disord 22(10):959–970, 2018

Riley EP, McGee CL: Fetal alcohol spectrum disorders: an overview with emphasis on changes in brain and behavior. Exp Biol Med (Maywood) 230(6):357–365, 2005

Safe B, Joosten A, Giglia R: Assessing motor skills to inform a fetal alcohol spectrum disorder diagnosis focusing on persons older than 12 years: a systematic review of the literature. J Popul Ther Clin Pharmacol 25(1):e25–e38, 2018

Sanders JL, Breen RE, Netelenbos N: Comparing diagnostic classification of neurobehavioral disorder associated with prenatal alcohol exposure with the Canadian fetal alcohol spectrum disorder guidelines: a cohort study. CMAJ Open 5(1):E178–E183, 2017

Singal D, Brownell M, Hanlon-Dearman A, et al: Manitoba mothers and fetal alcohol spectrum disorders study (MBMomsFASD): protocol for a population-based cohort study using linked administrative data. BMJ Open 6(9):e013330, 2016

Suttie M, Wozniak JR, Parnell SE, et al: Combined face-brain morphology and associated neurocognitive correlates in fetal alcohol spectrum disorders. Alcohol Clin Exp Res 42(9):1769–1782, 2018

Taylor NM, Enns LN: Factors predictive of a fetal alcohol spectrum disorder diagnosis: parent and teacher ratings. Child Neuropsychol 25(4):507–527, 2018

Wozniak JR, Riley EP, Charness ME: Clinical presentation, diagnosis, and management of fetal alcohol spectrum disorder. Lancet Neurol 18(8):760–770, 2019

CHAPTER 11

Laboratory Testing

WHAT TO KNOW

PAE affects all organs and should prompt an active search for medical conditions through rational laboratory investigations.

Thyroid, iron, and immune deficiency are subtle abnormalities well detected by blood tests.

Reliable laboratory tests should be considered because the patient may not be forthcoming with relevant clinical information.

Metabolic syndrome arising from medications should be diagnosable from physical examination and confirmed with laboratory indices.

Genetic testing and neuroimaging are combined for more specific diagnostic investigation in ND-PAE/FASD.

There is no laboratory test for diagnosing ND-PAE/FASD. Purposes for ordering tests in patients diagnosed with ND-PAE/FASD include general screening, diagnostic confirmation, and monitoring and risk management. Mental health professionals should be aware that where laboratory investigations are required, patients should be supported through the arrangement and completion of testing. This is particularly important because of neurocognitive deficits in memory, planning, impulse control, and sensory processing. These can interfere with management. Being hyper- or hypo-sensitive to different sensory stimuli could manifest in some patients as avoiding venipuncture, for instance. A patient with memory deficits is at an increased risk of failing to recall clinical information from past encounters. Patients may fail to disclose information necessary to rule out other relevant medications used or medical conditions. Knowing the level of concentration of medications, maintaining the therapeutic window of potentially toxic medications, and determining blood levels of electrolytes become dependent on laboratory testing.

Although there is no clinical consensus on what tests constitute the requisite general screening panel, some should be considered essential. Tests classified as baseline in patients help to establish current states, and changes in their levels can be monitored. Repeated over time, changes in test results are helpful indicators for various interventions and their consequences. For example, iron deficiency occurs in a significant proportion of patients with PAE. A baseline test confirming the level of iron deficiency should be followed with repeated tests to establish if levels have normalized.

Baseline Screening Tests

During the comprehensive assessments for individuals suspected of having PAE, indicators for specific laboratory tests and assays should be inquired about and sought. The consequences of PAE adversely affect virtually all organs of the body, a condition known as whole-body disorder (Shelton et al. 2018). This suggests that patients should be asked about current and past symptoms of bodily and organ-specific dysfunction, which is best achieved through a review of symptoms during history taking and a complete physical examination. Because of neurocognitive deficits, only a proactive search is likely to reveal any important symptoms and signs because patients may not report any symptoms or past episodes of many illnesses. PAE disrupts immune function in offspring through direct and indirect mechanisms, such as zinc depletion. The resulting immune deficiency predisposes those with PAE to significant inflammation, and some individuals also develop infections (Gano et al. 2017). Hyposensitivity to pain in a patient could cause unawareness of the pain from such infections. This, and many other pathways in which disease states are common in ND-PAE/FASD, calls for baseline tests. A complete blood count should be ordered to detect raised levels of white cell count, and an actual neutrophil count may uncover current infection. Abnormal levels of these indices of inflammation are helpful in guiding the choice of special tests to be requested. Serum levels of urea, electrolytes, and creatinine are usually ordered not only to establish a baseline but also to monitor the renal consequences of disease and medications. There are reported cases of renal complications from herbal preparations consumed by patients. Monitoring may indicate the effect of medications that are toxic to the kidneys, such as lithium prescribed for mood stabilization. Tests may also help to identify medical conditions such as anemia, diabetes mellitus, and immune deficiency. Immune deficiency can occur as a result of the natural depletion of interleukins, which has been noted in subjects with FASD.

Investigators attribute patients' poor judgment to executive dysfunction, which can increase high-risk behaviors. Common features associated with PAE explain how individuals with substance use disorder, impulsive acting-out behavior, poor awareness of boundaries, and sexual indiscretions interact to increase the risk of sexually transmitted diseases, including HIV/AIDS. Medical conditions are more prevalent in subjects with neurocognitive sequelae of PAE (Gauthier 2015). Baseline results of tests still must be repeated even when they are initially normal. Repeated tests detect changeable medication effects, future disease state, and new emerging illnesses. For clinicians who are seeking to obtain a full understanding of their patient's biochemical, hematological, and genetic status, a picture of the human body serves as a cue to include important tests. Figure 11–1 shows the location of the organs adversely affected by PAE and lists special tests for the person affected.

Special PAE-Related Tests

Special tests are indicated when baseline test results are abnormal or are associated with more PAE-specific indicators. Highly specific tests in ND-PAE/FASD include those for thyroid function beyond thyroid-stimulating hormone level, interleukin levels, and immunoglobulins. Iron and ferritin levels noted to be abnormal should be followed with tests for total iron-binding capacity.

If alcohol use during the last 6 months of pregnancy is suspected, at the time of delivery an assay of fatty acid ethyl esters can confirm if PAE occurred during the last half of the pregnancy. A sample of meconium is needed to estimate the level of fatty acid ethyl esters; >2 nmol/g is a strong biomarker of PAE (Riley et al. 2011). Clinicians should be aware of the ethical controversies associated with the test, for example, in situations in which the mother adamantly denies drinking alcohol, even though reliable sources report otherwise. The stigma associated with confirming alcohol use and being made to look deceitful may have unintended consequences (Bryanton et al. 2014). Mothers may blame themselves, which does not sup-

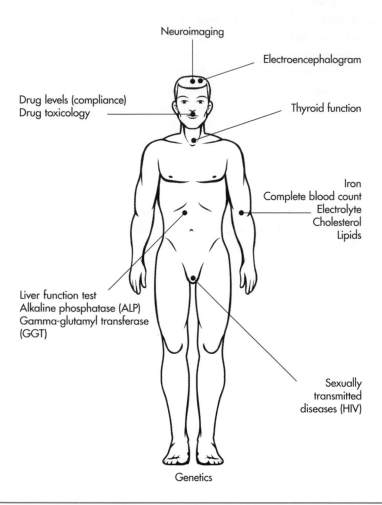

FIGURE 11–1. Recommended laboratory tests linked to various organs affected by PAE and useful in monitoring interventions and providing cues to clinicians.

port a patient-centered approach. To perform the test, fully informed consent from the mother is essential.

Tests for Diagnostic Confirmation

Currently, the diagnosis of ND-PAE/FASD is based on clinical information collated from multiple sources. Because multiple comorbid conditions are associated with ND-PAE/FASD, identifying those conditions requires highly specialized laboratory tests beyond the simple or baseline. The tests discussed here are also not specific for detecting conditions related to PAE.

They are mostly ordered for the assistance they provide in confirming or ruling out particular medical and mental diagnoses. Herein lies the value of a test when information is limited because the patient cannot remember or may be embarrassed to make a disclosure. A history of substance use, especially when there is a legal prohibition, falls within this category. Urine toxicology for illicit substances, blood alcohol levels, and liver function tests are important to detect substance use or confirm diagnosis. Alanine transaminase and aspartate transaminase are the hepatic enzymes released into the bloodstream as markers of liver injury. Higher than normal levels of alkaline phosphatase indicate liver injury, but a blockade of bile duct drainage is the significant contributor. Similarly, γ-glutamyltransferase is increased, but it is more sensitive to liver damage from alcohol use and other disorders including cancers, hepatitis, and nonhepatic acute coronary syndrome (see Figure 11–1). The blood levels of enzymes are helpful but not confirmatory in cases of patients who abuse alcohol. A biomarker that provides information for recent use is a *state marker*, and a few are highly specific. A test for carbohydrate-deficient transferrin, a protein that has received attention in recent years, can be requested. Another marker, N-acetyl-β-hexosaminidase, if available, can be helpful as a state marker. Clinical use includes identifying heavy use and chronic use of alcohol, which are common in ND-PAE/ FASD even when the information is not revealed (Chabenne et al. 2014; Lange et al. 2018).

If a laboratory test could be used in prevention, it would be important in deterring adverse consequences of alcohol use in offspring predisposed to severe injury. Other genetic markers support the identification of patients at an increased risk. That risk may be averted if it is known that the genetic trait is present. A cell membrane protein, adenylyl cyclase, uniquely identifies genetic risk and is sensitive to alcohol use and consumption of cannabis and other drugs (Peterson 2004–2005). Not all laboratories are equipped to measure this enzyme. Access to these diagnostic tests is important in the absence of clinical information, which is typical in ND-PAE/FASD.

Detecting medical conditions among those with ND-PAE/FASD calls for specific testing for Hb1C, hepatitis C, and HIV, for example. Measuring mean corpuscular volume is helpful for diagnosing types of anemia and alcohol use disorder. In females, pregnancy tests should be ordered because dates marking the last menstrual period may be inaccurate due to poor concentration, executive function, and memory.

In addition to blood tests, electrophysiological measures are important for assessing for comorbid conditions. Seizures and congenital cardiovascular disorders are common in patients with ND-PAE/FASD. An electroencephalogram and electrocardiogram (ECG) should be ordered as indicated. Although some eye movement tests associated with neurocognitive deficits are beginning to distinguish people with PAE, implementing clinical use will take some time.

Clinical Vignette

A patient presents in the emergency room with anxiety, fear of having a heart attack, sweating, and listlessness. She saw her family doctor a week earlier complaining of depression. Her diagnosis of complex partial seizures is managed using lamotrigine. Physical examination shows a maculopapular rash all over her back and other parts of her body. She complains of memory problems and has forgotten the schedule of the dosage increase of lamotrigine. Her past medical record confirms an electroencephalogram finding of the seizures and indicates that she has been referred to a multidisciplinary team to undergo functional assessment to determine if her memory problems are associated with thyroid deficiency or the effect of PAE.

Given that no pathognomonic tests are indicated for ND-PAE/FASD, it is wise to support this patient in various ways. The offending medication should be discontinued; any reintroduction or medication scheduling should use visual aids and pharmacist-led support, which could include more frequent contact to ensure appropriate use. The effect of PAE on various organs means that in addition to obtaining a complete blood count and eosinophil levels, other relevant tests based on the clinical picture should be ordered. Iron, folate, and thyroid levels are the immediate tests necessary to ascertain if they are associated with listlessness, anxiety, past suspicion of thyroid problems or PAE, and memory deficits. Table 11–1 shows some of the tests with relevant indications for use with patients diagnosed with ND-PAE/FASD.

Monitoring and Risk Management

Certain deficiencies in hormonal or metabolic syndromes are corrected by replacement substances prescribed for the patient. Treatment of these deficiencies, such as iron, requires supplementation. When repeated blood tests reveal that levels have normalized, it can then be deduced that the deficiency has been corrected. This is supportive evidence that the patient has complied with treatment. Memory and planning problems may indicate neurocognitive deficits, which may combine negatively with social problems such as financial constraints and poor social support. This may result in unintentional noncompliance. Therefore, monitoring laboratory test results ensures compliance and becomes a strategy to reduce risk of noncompliance. Levels of hormones are easy to monitor in that way. The necessary frequency of blood tests will vary, determined by the factors influencing

TABLE 11–1. Recommended laboratory tests and rationale for those with ND-PAE/FASD

TYPE OF TEST CATEGORY	EXAMPLES	RANGES	NOTE
Baseline screen	CSC Actual neutrophil count Electrolyte test Glucose test Urinalysis	Locally established normed levels	
PAE specific	Iron test Thyroid test Fatty acid ethyl esters in meconium	Being determined for those with PAE	Measure of oxidative stress
Comorbid detection	Baseline screen Liver function test Renal function test Interleukin 6 test Chest X-ray	Normed ranges	
Medication compliance	Lithium level Tricyclic antidepressant level Atypical neuroleptic level	Normed range	Provide written instruction and support adherence
Risk management tests	Metabolic panel Urine toxicology	Detection at cutoff level	
Soon to have clinical use	MicroRNA levels Neuroimaging	Dependent on normed sample See "Neuroimaging Investigations" section	State and trait biomarkers of substance use

Note. Tests of electrophysiology—electrocardiogram and electroencephalogram—are excluded.

compliance. Blood iron levels, medication blood levels, and proxy measures of compliance are examples of monitoring blood tests.

Blood tests should be ordered to manage the risk of side effects of medications prescribed for patients with ND-PAE/FASD. Where there are manifestations of mental health symptoms suggesting cognitive disadvantage from taking multiple medications, laboratory tests of medication levels can be lifesaving. There is no recognized indicator for these cognitive deficits, and patients who present with complicated features may be prescribed combinations of medications that have adverse effects. Carbamazepine may be prescribed and orally administered to patients with PAE who also manifest features of affect dysregulation, mood swings, seizures, aggression, and bipolar disorder. Lithium can be effective for treating bipolar disorder in a patient with ND-PAE/FASD and resistant depression. Some of the adverse effects from these medications, especially in combination, include agranulocytosis, aplastic anemia, Stevens-Johnson syndrome, and neurotoxicity. Patients may not be able to recall side effects when asked. A baseline blood test and repeated monitoring of laboratory levels can prevent or minimize these side effects. It may be expecting too much for the patient with neurocognitive deficits to monitor and identify indicators of these adverse effects; this may be better accomplished with blood tests. Such tests are really important because they can detect the changes in levels before the side effects occur. Side effects can be fatal in some situations, and patients should be monitored with laboratory tests, especially when because of sensory processing deficits, those with ND-PAE/FASD do not perceive accurately the sensations associated with side effects (pain from swellings, numbness, tingling, and variation in temperature). These abnormal sensations are clinically confusing, and thus objective laboratory tests may reduce the risk associated with medication.

Monitoring medication levels is also indicated for clozapine and atypical antipsychotics. These are regularly prescribed for multiple reasons, especially behavioral disturbance (Frankel et al. 2006; Mela et al. 2018; Ozsarfati and Koren 2015). Moreover, the role of clozapine in reducing the high prevalence of suicidal behavior in FASD is worth exploring. Both lithium and clozapine are reported to be antisuicide medications, but no direct association of this effect has been established with ND-PAE/FASD. Monitoring a patient's regularly occurring side effects is crucial. Antipsychotic medications contribute significantly to the emergence of metabolic syndrome. Lipid panels should be ordered to determine triglyceride levels in patients prescribed clozapine and lithium.

Considering the role of brain domains and the cognitive faculties necessary to understand instructions about medications, clinician monitoring of blood levels of medications is indicated to prevent negative outcomes. Adherence to a medication regimen requires patients to understand the instructions, organize, and sequence and execute actions. Because these faculties are adversely affected by PAE, patients on the FAS spectrum may be susceptible to unintended mistakes in following directions regarding their medications. They are more likely to use drugs of abuse. Body fluid monitoring via laboratory testing therefore becomes important in the evaluation, management, and monitoring of patients taking medications.

Patient safety is the priority for testing of those medications that are amenable to monitoring. Some medications administered incorrectly can become dangerous, and the concept of a therapeutic window underlies the use of monitoring to ensure safe levels. Blood tests can disclose whether a safe therapeutic level is being maintained. Lithium and nortriptyline, for example, which are used in mood disorders, both have narrow therapeutic windows. Only through drug monitoring can the levels be maintained in the therapeutic nontoxic range. Monitoring will help detect overdose or dangerous use.

Pregnancy can be adversely affected if certain medications are prescribed. Because neurocognitive deficits associated with PAE potentially disrupt sequencing and memory, clinicians should promptly ask about the date of the last menstrual period and follow up that inquiry on a regular basis to assess whether a laboratory pregnancy test needs to be ordered. This will help facilitate appropriate care during the pregnancy, if present, and serve as a PAE-preventive strategy. The conversation with the patient should also support her abstinence from alcohol and explain the value of the prescribed medications. Although vitamins, folate, and ferrous sulfate are not harmful per se, their ready availability should prompt caution. The disturbed pregnant patient with ND-PAE/FASD could mistakenly, and sometimes intentionally, take an overdose of these medications. Monitoring blood levels is therefore clinically indicated. Information on medications with teratogenic outcomes (e.g., carbamazepine, valproate) should be requested by the responsible medical professional and steps taken to confirm or rule them out using laboratory tests.

Monitoring Stimulant Medications

Stimulants are the most commonly prescribed psychotropic medications among children and adolescents with ND-PAE/FASD. The response rates of these patients to stimulants vary from those of patients with other disorders with indications for stimulant medication. The recommended strategies and procedures to safely prescribe and monitor stimulants have been established by the American Academy of Pediatrics (Subcommittee on Attention-Deficit/Hyperactivity Disorder et al. 2011). Prior to prescribing stimulants, a factor that should be carefully considered is the higher incidence of cardiovascular abnormalities in those with ND-PAE/FASD. High rates of alcohol and substance use disorders, impulsive tendencies, and memory problems also must be factored in; involving significant others in supporting adherence to a medication regimen should be considered. Educational and counseling support given to caregivers about the administration and dangers of stimulants and other medications is the most reliable approach to limiting diversion and misuse of medications by patients with neurocognitive deficits. Patients exhibit poor medication adherence for many reasons, for example, gullibility and high susceptibility to manipulation, desire to be accepted driven by low self-esteem, and general unawareness of risk; these are all common in patients with ND-PAE/FASD. In addition to initially recording baseline vital signs such as pulse rate and blood pressure and subsequent monitoring after a period of taking the medications and when dosages change, especially for stimulants, other investigations are desirable. Further reasonable baseline tests to administer are an ECG and a serum electrolyte level analysis. These measures should be ordered before and after stimulants are prescribed to detect any changes.

Other medications (antipsychotics, antidepressants, and adrenergic agonists) are frequently prescribed for older patients. Recommended guidelines and laboratory measurements should be followed. In the frequently used risperidone, clinicians should monitor the patient's weight, lipids, cholesterol, electrolytes, and serum levels of risperidone using the same guidelines used for adults without PAE. The inclusion of adults with PAE and without PAE recognizes that even without the neurocognitive deficits of PAE, patients prescribed medications, especially stimulants, have reported misuse and diversion (Lensing et al. 2013). In a number of reviews, the problems of nonmedical use of stimulants were outlined (Plant et al. 2011; Popova et al. 2013). Equally important is the link between the regionally specific dopamine increase in the brain that accounts for the efficacy of the medication and the root of the neural correlates of misuse (Clemow and Walker 2014). It is important in treating ND-PAE/FASD that efforts are made to protect the patient and not deny medication because of those mishaps (diversion and misuse).

One approach to fostering patient acceptance of medication adherence proposed by some clinicians and researchers is to establish a set of conditions listed in a formal treatment agreement and to obtain the patient's commitment to this agreement. Knowing about a patient's neurocognitive deficits affords the clinician the advantage of planning to protect the patient and adopting a problem-solving approach when the patient "breaks" the treatment agreement. The agreement incorporates urine monitoring, compliance checks, and ongoing psychoeducation. In a population of patients taking stimulants in a primary care setting, for instance, such an agreement produced improved adherence and reduced medication diversion (Downey et al. 2017). Most of the 2,500 patients in that study signed the agreement. The act of commitment through a signed agreement contributed to positive outcomes. In a general way, clinicians can modify this approach. Clinicians should explain the reasons for such an agreement. Stimulants are long-term, Schedule II medications. The risks of ingestion, diversion, and misuse are regularly balanced against the benefits of symptomatic and functional improvement. Strategies to support medication adherence using the agreement may involve other team members. Pharmacists play an active role in patient education; they may witness administration and may direct safer dispensing to minimize risk. Pharmacists may employ daily dispensing, use bubble packs, and communicate with the patient by text and phone messaging to enhance closer monitoring. Depending on their estimation of risk, pharmacists and technicians may recommend laboratory tests and clinical surveillance. An increased frequency of heart rate and blood pressure measurement and ECG are essential to minimize the risk of overdose or diversion. Electrolyte monitoring is part of the safety plan included in treatment agreements.

Neuroimaging Investigations

Although fractures from injuries that are common manifestations of PAE will be confirmed with X-ray, the place of neuroimaging in ND-PAE/FASD is more specific to detecting the biological correlates of PAE. The field of imaging (CT, MRI, and functional magnetic spectroscopy) is advancing and uncovering specific identifiable deficits. Unfortunately, there is yet to be discovered a clinically relevant profile with unique relations to ND-PAE/FASD that can be recommended for clinical use. Observing white matter abnormalities kindled a lot of interest. Diffuse tensor imaging studies show abnormalities in cortical white matter, which mediates the effect of PAE on information processing and eye blink conditioning (Fan et al. 2016). Clinicians may find reason to order these tests to exclude other brain-occupying lesions or to rule out other causes of neurocognitive deficits. Head trauma and degenerative disorders of the brain are commonly comorbid and need to be identified when they complicate the neurocognitive deficits associated with PAE. Still, correlating and interpreting significant clinical features and the findings of neuroimaging abnormalities are in line to support clinical application in the future (Suttie et al. 2018).

Genetic Testing

DNA methylation utilizing microarray has been proposed as a valuable tool ifor identifying those in whom PAE has altered epigenetic processes (Balaraman et al. 2016; Boyadjieva and Varadinova 2015). It is not yet clear how the tests can be interpreted and applied from a research context to the clinical environment. The weight of the environmental factors varies widely, and advanced analytical methods using large data sets are required to clarify the relationship of nature and nurture. It is likely that in the next one or two decades these types of testing will provide weighted measures of heritability, which will sufficiently apportion different weights to the several factors known to contribute to the development of ND-PAE/FASD, especially as they regularly coexist.

Microarray analysis falls into the realm of efforts to develop biomarkers for detecting those with PAE. Circulating microRNA levels are an example of such biomarkers (Balaraman et al. 2016; Chabenne et al. 2014) (see Figure 11–1). Others are being developed but are not yet ready for clinical use. Some biomarkers can be detected in maternal blood, whereas others are directly estimated in the offspring diagnosed with ND-PAE/FASD.

Conclusion

Laboratory tests are adjuncts to the clinical diagnosis and management of patients suspected of or confirmed to have been prenatally exposed to alcohol. The tests identify damaged organs and set the baseline for comparison when treatment is initiated. How comprehensive or focused those tests are depends on why they are ordered. Advances in technology and medical knowledge are contributing to the improved sensitivity and specificity of laboratory tests and to their usefulness in informing relevant interventions.

CLINICAL PRACTICAL APPLICATIONS

- Clinical staff should be aware that the neurocognitive deficits associated with PAE, such as memory deficits and sensory processing difficulties, may result in missed appointments and avoidance of procedures, respectively; these deficits create an added layer of significance for the consideration and use of laboratory investigations.

- Saccadic eye movements differentiate the neurocognitive deficits of PAE from other disorders and are diagnostically important.

- Pregnancy testing and monitoring of alcohol use during pregnancy are important preventive steps, but they should be conducted ethically.

- Monitoring blood levels of medications, prescribed or accidentally consumed, can be lifesaving in light of the poor memory and impulsivity that characterize patients with ND-PAE/FASD.

- ADHD practice guidelines for initiating and maintaining stimulant medications, including electrophysiological monitoring, should be followed.

References

Balaraman S, Schafer JJ, Tseng AM, et al: Plasma miRNA profiles in pregnant women predict infant outcomes following prenatal alcohol exposure. PLoS One 11(11):e0165081, 2016

Boyadjieva N, Varadinova M: Role of fetal alcohol exposure on molecular and epigenetic mechanisms of autism. Recent Advances in Autism 1–10, 2015

Bryanton J, Gareri J, Bosweall D, et al: Incidence of prenatal alcohol exposure in Prince Edward Island: a population-based descriptive study. CMAJ Open 2(2):E121–E126, 2014

Chabenne A, Moon C, Ojo C, et al: Biomarkers in fetal alcohol syndrome. Biomarkers and Genomic Medicine 6:12–22, 2014

Clemow DB, Walker DJ: The potential for misuse and abuse of medications in ADHD: a review. Postgrad Med 126(5):64–81, 2014

Downey E, Pan W, Harrison J, et al: Implementation of a Schedule II patient agreement for opioids and stimulants in an adult primary care practice. J Fam Med Prim Care 6(1):52–57, 2017

Fan J, Jacobson SW, Taylor PA, et al: White matter deficits mediate effects of prenatal alcohol exposure on cognitive development in childhood. Hum Brain Mapp 37(8):2943–2958, 2016

Frankel F, Paley B, Marquardt R, O'Connor M: Stimulants, neuroleptics, and children's friendship training for children with fetal alcohol spectrum disorders. J Child Adolesc Psychopharmacol 16(6):777–789, 2006

Gano A, Pautassi RM, Doremus-Fitzwater TL, Deak T: Conditioned effects of ethanol on the immune system. Exp Biol Med (Maywood) 242(7):718–730, 2017

Gauthier TW: Prenatal alcohol exposure and the developing immune system. Alcohol Res 37(2):279–285, 2015

Lange S, Rehm J, Popova S: Implications of higher than expected prevalence of fetal alcohol spectrum disorders. JAMA 319(5):448–449, 2018

Lensing MB, Zeiner P, Sandvik L, Opjordsmoen S: Adults with ADHD: use and misuse of stimulant medication as reported by patients and their primary care physicians. Atten Defic Hyperact Disord 5(4):369–376, 2013

Mela M, Okpalauwaekwe U, Anderson T, et al: The utility of psychotropic drugs on patients with fetal alcohol spectrum disorder (FASD): a systematic review. Psychiatry and Clinical Psychopharmacology 28(4):436–445, 2018

Ozsarfati J, Koren G: Medications used in the treatment of disruptive behavior in children with FASD: a guide. J Popul Ther Clin Pharmacol 22(1):e59–e67, 2015

Peterson K: Biomarkers for alcohol use and abuse—a summary. Alcohol Res Health 28(1):30–37, 2004–2005

Plant A, McDermott E, Chester V, Alexander RT: Substance misuse among offenders in a forensic intellectual disability service. Journal of Learning Disabilities and Offending Behaviour 2(3):127–135, 2011

Popova S, Lange S, Burd L, et al: Cost of specialized addiction treatment of clients with fetal alcohol spectrum disorder in Canada. BMC Public Health 13(1):570, 2013

Riley EP, Infante MA, Warren KR: Fetal alcohol spectrum disorders: an overview. Neuropsychol Rev 21(2):73–80, 2011

Shelton D, Reid N, Till H, et al: Responding to fetal alcohol spectrum disorder in Australia. J Paediatr Child Health 54(10):1121–1126, 2018

Subcommittee on Attention-Deficit/Hyperactivity Disorder; Steering Committee on Quality Improvement and Management, Wolraich M, et al: ADHD: clinical practice guideline for the diagnosis, evaluation, and treatment of attention-deficit/hyperactivity disorder in children and adolescents. Pediatrics 128(5):1007–1022, 2011

Suttie M, Wozniak JR, Parnell SE, et al: Combined face-brain morphology and associated neurocognitive correlates in fetal alcohol spectrum disorders. Alcohol Clin Exp Res 42(9):1769–1782, 2018

CHAPTER 12

Diagnostic Nosology

WHAT TO KNOW

Diagnostic classification serves many purposes, including enhancing communication, improving statistics for public health planning, supporting financial assistance for the diagnosed person, and informing treatment interventions.

PAE outcomes depend on combinations of maternal, genetic, environmental, and alcohol-related factors.

DSM-5 includes the current classification of ND-PAE with conditions for further study.

There are current research efforts to standardize diagnosis of the consequences of PAE.

Diagnosis is the important process necessary to understand, support, and intervene with individuals experiencing the multiple consequences of PAE. Two questions are important in addressing the classification of complex disorders such as PAE, with its multiple outcomes. First, are diagnostic terms based on etiological, phenotypical, or clinical description? Second, what is the public health perspective in understanding the etiology of FASD? In this chapter, I review the history of classification and diagnostic labels in the field of mental health as influenced by advances in the labels used to describe individuals affected by PAE. The various labels relating to PAE across the world are juxtaposed with the single system that categorizes psychiatric disorders. Internationally and in all jurisdictions, a universally accepted labeling method would be welcome, but the field is not yet at that level of agreement.

Why Is Diagnostic Nosology Important?

Until recently, the interface between mental disorders and the diagnostic outcomes of PAE were subject to two entirely different classification systems. Children were easily diagnosed with the various outcomes of PAE. As children with PAE became adults, they were shown to manifest unusually high rates of mental disorders (O'Connor 2014). The evolving mental disorders as long-term complications of PAE attracted researchers, who considered and explored the interface of the diagnostic relationship between mental disorders and PAE outcomes. To make sense of this endeavor, the purposes of diagnostic nosology should be understood.

As a communication tool, the system of diagnoses allows the use of ordinary language for the exchange of information about diagnostic outcomes. This exchange involves researchers, clinicians, international collaborators, policymakers, and families. Ultimately, people diagnosed with the consequences of PAE benefit from knowledge about their symptoms that forms a diagnostic entity. Similar to the role of classification in mental disorders, the nosological reference system provides a source of statistical records that are valuable for public health and preventive interests. Each diagnosis must be valid, reliable, and practical to be clinically useful. Clinical utility rests on an identified pattern that leads to consistency in group-based diagnoses, with specific treatments and prognoses at the interface of mental disorders and diagnostic outcomes of PAE. To refine the diagnoses within that interface, ideas and practices from both fields are integrated. Diagnostic systems are declared relevant and exact when their criteria have verifiable norms and verifiable variance from those norms. Criteria that have etiological and pathogenic explanations are understood as superior to those without those norms. The DSM classification of mental disorders is regarded as atheoretical and pragmatic (American Psychiatric Association 2013).

The need to combine approaches becomes even more important to understand the philosophical reasoning about psychopathogenic explanations. Classifications follow understanding of the theory about the disorders. Currently, mental disorders best align with the cluster system. Compared with the system based on etiology, the current system was socially constructed to support financial compensation. The classification also provides a practical explanatory model of mental disorders. DSM-5 criteria for ND-PAE recognize the causative role of PAE but also include the descriptive and practical aspects of the neurocognitive deficits (American Psychiatric Association 2013). Diagnosticians who use the classification understand the value of combined explanatory models, which, for practical purposes, show how the neurocognitive and behavioral symptoms manifest in an affected person. Additional benefit is obtained by the more inclusive disability and functional abnormality approach over a reductionist one.

Nosology is limited by the diversity and impact of the factors that influence the outcomes of PAE. A specific unifying etiological basis for diagnosis is lacking. Timing, quantity, and duration of alcohol use during pregnancy, as well as specific maternal and offspring factors (e.g., genetics, nutrition, psychosocial factors), determine the expression of the phenotype. With epigenetic studies, even the genotype is recognized as depending on various factors (e.g., DNA methylation, migration, proliferation of neurons).

How Classification of PAE Outcomes Applies to Mental Disorders

For wider application across the lifespan, diagnostic criteria should have clinical utility and be relevant for communication, research, and epidemiology. Epidemiological outcomes specific to PAE and the resulting mental disorders are different from outcomes with clinical relevance. The former arise from the finding that PAE is significantly associated with neurodevelopmental disorder. In epidemiological terms, PAE was dubbed the most common preventable cause of intellectual disability in developed countries (Tough et al. 2005). This is less certain considering the many associated risk factors, with none yet proven to specifically occupy a prime explanatory position. Other prominent maternal risk factors such as malnutrition, exposure to domestic violence, mental disorders, and prenatal use of other psychoactive substances contribute to the mechanisms that make negative outcomes in offspring more likely.

Researchers have shown that misdiagnosis of individuals with FASD in health and social systems is associated with the emergence and maintenance of negative outcomes (Chasnoff et al. 2015). It is paramount that classification systems that provide clinical guidelines be based on current evidence. Furthermore, any proposed changes should depend on additional evidence. Advances in knowledge should be reflected in updated diagnostic classifications. In turn, the ready availability of DSM-5 codes for clinicians should lead to wider recognition, improved access to care, and better-informed care for patients. The recent changes introduced in mental health and psychiatry with the DSM-5 classification are part of this scientific advancement. New knowledge clarifies and guides the processes and decisions related to current psychiatric terminology. There are benefits to modernizing diagnostic labels. It has been suggested that the stigma associated with mood disorder and externalizing disorders such as ADHD was reduced when the diagnostic criteria and their labels were updated (Kendler 2008). Terms such as *mental retardation* previously were associated with the diminution of a person's potential; for that reason, DSM-5 adopted the term *intellectual disability* in its place. Nowhere are such balancing acts more nearly essential, required, and useful than in the classification of FASD to ameliorate stigma.

Mental disorders and FASD are diagnostic terms applied when symptoms and signs meet the threshold criteria predetermined by some convention. In turn, classification of the diagnosis allows for clinical identification of the patient. From the clinical presentation, the clinician organizes treatment and constructs a prognostic formulation. Usually, the same outcome is shared by members of a subgroup of the whole population. Individuation is therefore lost when signs and symptoms are patterned and grouped to aid clinical reasoning. Symptoms vary in significance as the starting points of these clinical entities. They are important to patients because they exert an overall adverse effect, have negative impact, and have a unique meaning. To physicians, symptoms represent the pieces of the puzzle that illuminate understanding of patterns in the patients' suffering and the need for intervention. Unfortunately, patients' and physicians' meanings are sometimes at variance, but appreciating each other's position or emphasis allows for better doctor–patient collaboration. Nowhere is this collaboration more important than at the misunderstood interface of mental disorders and ND-PAE/FASD (diagnostic outcomes of PAE). Mental health professionals have a crucial role to play in diagnosis. Psychiatrists should have the competence to address and ameliorate the deficits associated with PAE (see Figure 12–1) throughout the patient's life span.

Diagnostic terms can refer to the underlying pathology or etiology of a clinical entity. It is desirable in medicine that etiological classification be achieved in order to support interventions. Examples of etiology-based diagnoses in mental health include PTSD and mood disorder associated with hypothyroidism. Generally, most mental disorders are labeled without reference to such etiological basis because causation is unknown. Unlike FASD, classification of mental disorders depends on patterns of clinical presentation and recognition of biopsychosocial factors that contribute to the various diagnoses. PAE is assumed to be the major contributing etiological factor in FASD. The consequences of PAE include identifiable neurocognitive deficits similar to the recognized deficits in some mental disorders. Mental disorders and the diagnostic outcomes of PAE appear to be like "peas in a pod." In spite of these similarities, DSM classification only adopted the diagnostic

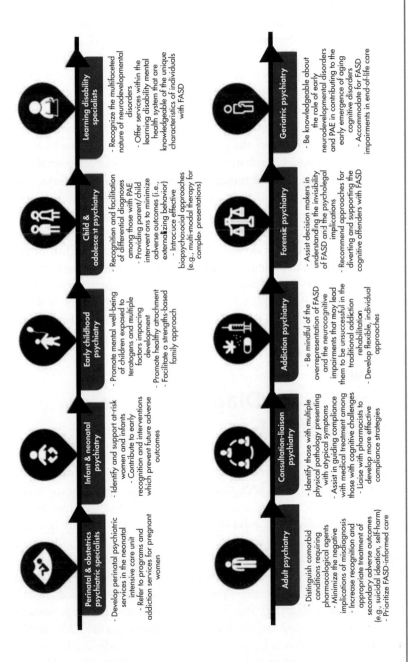

FIGURE 12–1. Role of psychiatry in treating patients with FASD across the lifespan.

Source. Reprinted from Mela M, Coons-Harding KD, Anderson T: "Recent Advances in Fetal Alcohol Spectrum Disorder for Mental Health Professionals." *Current Opinion in Psychiatry* 43(4):328–335, 2019. Copyright © 2019 Wolters Kluwer Health. Used with permission.

outcomes of PAE quite late in its evolution (after about 60 years) (American Psychiatric Association 2013).

The easily identifiable diagnostic outcomes of PAE (FASD) are anchored in four characteristic components: congenital physical anomalies, growth deficiency, neurocognitive abnormalities, and confirmed PAE. These components occur in varying degrees. PAE contributes to physical, mental, behavioral, and learning disabilities in affected offspring. The degree of disability and the factors that contribute to the disability help define the threshold for the symptoms adopted by the classification systems. These systems are based on more than five decades of studying PAE and its consequences. *Fetal alcohol syndrome* (FAS) was the prototypical diagnosis reserved for patients with the full dysmorphic characteristics criteria. These congenital features included sentinel facial features and specific growth, cognitive, and behavioral deficits. In contrast, *fetal alcohol effects* (FAE) was the term reserved for other manifestations of PAE that did not fulfill the same dysmorphic criteria. Symptoms of mental disorders featured prominently in the FAE category. *Alcohol-related neurodevelopmental disorder* (ARND), introduced in the Institute of Medicine criteria, represented the closest category of mental disorder to FAE. Owing to the indiscriminate application of FAE to all consequences of PAE, especially minor effects, it fell out of use. ARND referred to patients with CNS deficits or a complex pattern of behavioral or cognitive abnormalities. People diagnosed with ARND do not have the dysmorphic features.

Nosology in the Diagnostic Outcomes of PAE

Most mental health professionals may be unaware of the development of nosology as it related to PAE. FAS, the first clinical description of the medical consequences of PAE, was insufficient to explain the multiple-organ outcomes of PAE. Individuals were diagnosed with FAS not only because they possessed CNS dysfunction and growth deficiency but also because they manifested characteristic and specific craniofacial abnormalities (dysmorphia). Only about one-tenth of patients prenatally exposed to alcohol and inheriting characteristic features manifest those specific physical or sentinel features (May et al. 2010). When some of the dysmorphia was missing in the presence of the majority of diagnostic features, partial FAS (pFAS) was invoked. Nevertheless, a large number of exposed individuals without the characteristic facial features were noted to be adversely affected by the neurocognitive consequences of PAE. This led to the initial and amorphous term FAE to account for all other presentations outside of FAS and pFAS (Clarren and Smith 1978). As FAE fell out of use due to its nonspecificity, ARND was introduced. This was applied to patients with PAE outcomes who did not display physical and facial abnormalities but were affected by PAE-induced CNS dysfunction. FASD was the umbrella term for all of these groups of disorders. ND-PAE was introduced into the psychiatric nosology to identify the many people whose PAE caused the expression of the constellation of behavioral and cognitive manifestations. This is where the two classification systems meet to represent the many patients who navigate the systems, especially as adolescents and adults.

Although there are notable differences in the criteria and diagnostic processes, the overarching criteria in the existing clinical guidelines for diagnosing FASD overlap considerably (e.g., Astley 2004; Chudley et al. 2005; Hoyme et al. 2016; Landgraf et al. 2013; Watkins et al. 2013). Researchers compared the various diagnostic systems and found them superficially different but inherently similar. Clinical guidelines have arisen in different countries and systems in order to fill service gaps and facilitate classification of the diagnostic outcomes of PAE. Most guidelines incorporate the same items for diagnostic threshold: medical description of the genetic disorders, examination of facial dysmorphology, and growth indices. The combination of these elements furnishes the best estimate of significant PAE. Neuropsychological deficits are assessed through diagnostic processes to categorize the deficits consequent to PAE. The differences in criteria for a specific neurocognitive deficit include threshold levels for deviation from the norm in neurocognitive testing. Some systems adopt a 1.5 or 2.0 standard deviation from the normed mean for the population. Additionally, some systems require significant impairment in two or three neurocognitive domains; however, others have different lists of the specific domains invoked in PAE damage. A global effort is being made by researchers and clinicians to standardize the diagnoses arising from PAE.

The diagnostic guidelines seek to improve diagnostic validity and reliability, as well as clinical, policy, communication, and research utility. Given the dynamic climate of the mental health field, and judging from the regular updates and scientifically based improvements, a global unified diagnostic scheme may be developed. This is possible given that the foundational elements of diagnosis (i.e., PAE, dysmorphology, growth deficiencies, neurological/neuropsychological dysfunction) are widely accepted and have been referenced in previous and currently updated guidelines (Cook et al. 2016; Johnson et al. 2018). Mental health professionals should benefit from the historical origins and developmental improvements of the guidelines, most especially with the inclusion of ND-PAE in DSM-5, the diagnostic manual used by mental health professionals.

Existing Diagnostic Schemes

Characterizing the multiple outcomes of PAE required various schemes and approaches to guide diagnostic processes. These schemes originated from a collaboration of experts from pediatrics, genetics, and developmental neonatology. Experts recommended the use of multidisciplinary teams to evaluate components of the criteria and apply specific clinical skills by bringing together objective measurements (e.g., weight, facial measurements), clinical judgment (determination of nonbiased history of maternal alcohol use during pregnancy), and consensus (ascribing a specific diagnosis in place of an alternative differential diagnosis based on a predetermined threshold consistent with previously set criteria by consensus). Until recently, the only involvement of mental health professionals was providing objective measures with standardized instruments. The role of affect and self-regulation has now been made a significant component of diagnosis. Thus, the skills of mental health professionals are required in the range of activities necessary to arrive at a diagnosis. These professionals use their abilities to generate differential diagnoses. Table 12–1 depicts the various schemes and guidelines and is provided to help mental health professionals recognize their role in the formal FASD diagnostic processes. It is hoped that such knowledge will prompt mental health professionals to put forward their skills in screening, diagnosing, and supporting patients in their clinical population who may have been undiagnosed or misdiagnosed. It is hoped that understanding the steps to diagnosis outlined in the information in Table 12–1 will greatly increase the contribution of mental health professionals for patients at the interface of diagnosed mental disorder and outcomes of PAE.

Summary of the Diagnostic Systems of FASD

The first recommendation for diagnosing FASD was based on a case series. After examining medical outcomes in patients exposed to alcohol prenatally, Jones and Smith (1973) developed a set of clinical criteria to be used to diagnose those malformations caused by PAE. The cardinal features included microcephaly and other abnormal organogenesis. Although not a diagnostic guideline, this was the first clinical description, and it provided the essential criteria to identify clinical cases.

The Institute of Medicine initiated the development of criteria for FASD to facilitate communication and improve the reliability of diagnoses. The criteria were developed following a study by an expert committee that identified four different diagnoses (Stratton et al. 1996).

TABLE 12–1. Past to current diagnostic systems employed to diagnose FASD

DIAGNOSTIC SCHEME/GUIDELINE	REFERENCE	PRACTICE	COMMENTS
FAS diagnosis	Jones et al. 1973	Provided pure medical diagnosis	Clinical criteria developed, 1973
Fetal Alcohol Syndrome: Diagnosis, Epidemiology, Prevention, and Treatment	Stratton et al. 1996	Improved reliability and communication	Multiple diagnostic titles recommended as established diagnostic categories delineating the spectrums
Four-digit diagnostic code	Astley and Clarren 2000	Used in large samples of patients with validation studies	Multiple diagnoses created
Practical clinical approach to diagnosis	Hoyme et al. 2005	Used multinational data to operationalize diagnoses	FASD diagnoses standardized in clinical setting
DSM-5	American Psychiatric Association 2013	Used currently and for further studies, potentially leading to greater access to diagnosis	Specific criteria cutoff levels still needed and role of multidisciplinary teams uncertain
Australian diagnostic guidelines	Watkins et al. 2013	Combined four-digit diagnostic code and the Canadian guidelines for FASD diagnosis	Population-wide screening discouraged
"Updated Clinical Guidelines for Diagnosing Fetal Alcohol Spectrum Disorders"	Hoyme et al. 2016	Provided literature review and expert consensus	
First Canadian diagnostic guidelines	Chudley et al. 2005	Generated interest	Database of diagnosed children and adults created

TABLE 12–1. Past to current diagnostic systems employed to diagnose FASD *(continued)*

DIAGNOSTIC SCHEME/GUIDELINE	REFERENCE	PRACTICE	COMMENTS
Updated Canadian diagnostic guidelines	Cook et al. 2016	Provided reproducible systematic literature review, extensive clinic data and consensus	Existing evidence used to rename categories, specific sections for adults
"Diagnosis of Fetal Alcohol Syndrome (FAS): German Guideline Version 2013"	Landgraf et al. 2013	Provided rigorous scientific evidence	Confirmation of PAE not considered a prerequisite for diagnosis
Scottish guidelines	Wise 2019	Adopted previous guidelines, from Canada especially	Treatment emphasized

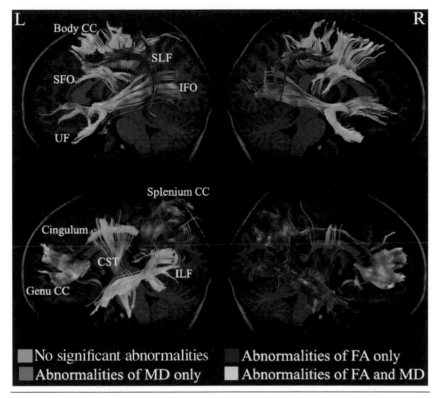

PLATE 1. White matter mapping using diffusion tensor imaging showing the presence or absence of abnormalities in those with fetal alcohol spectrum disorder.

CC=corpus callosum; CST=corticospinal tract; FA=fractional anisotropy; IFO= inferior fronto-occipital fasciculus; ILF=inferior longitudinal fasciculus; L=left; MD=mean diffusivity; R=right; SFO=subfornical organ; SLF=superior longitudinal fasciculus; UF= uncinate fasciculus. Both FA and MD are measures of white matter microstructure.

Source. From Lebel C, Rasmussen C, Wyper K, et al.: "Brain Diffusion Abnormalities in Children With Fetal Alcohol Spectrum Disorder." *Alcoholism: Clinical and Experimental Research* 32(10):1732–1740, 2008. Copyright ©2008 John Wiley and Sons. Used with permission.

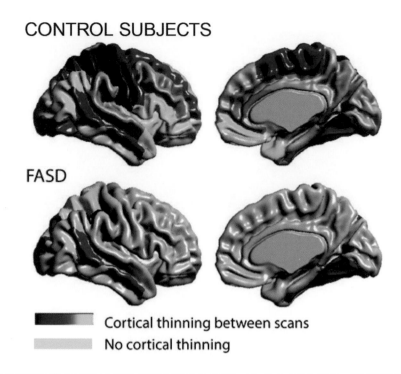

CONTROL SUBJECTS

FASD

Cortical thinning between scans
No cortical thinning

PLATE 2.   Medial and lateral surface of the right hemisphere showing more longitudinal cortical thinning in control subjects than children with FASD.

Source.   Courtesy Sarah Treit, Ph.D., Department of Biomedical Engineering, University of Alberta.

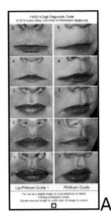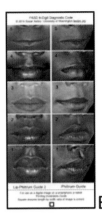

PLATE 3. Lip-philtrum guides 1 (**A**) and 2 (**B**) are used to rank upper lip thinness and philtrum smoothness.

The philtrum is the vertical groove between the nose and upper lip. Guide A is used for Caucasians and all other races with lips like Caucasians. Guide B is used for African Americans and all other races with similarly full lips. The guides reflect the full range of lip thickness and philtrum depth, with Rank 3 representing the population mean. Ranks 4 and 5 reflect the thin lip and smooth philtrum that characterize the FAS facial phenotype.

Source. Copyright © 2020, Susan (Astley) Hemingway, Ph.D., University of Washington. Used with permission. Free digital images of these guides for use on smartphones and tablets can be obtained from astley@uw.edu.

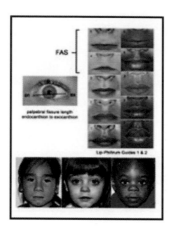

PLATE 4. The three diagnostic facial features of FAS include 1) short palpebral fissure lengths, 2) a smooth philtrum (Rank 4 or 5 on the Lip-Philtrum Guide), and 3) a thin upper lip (Rank 4 or 5 on the Lip-Philtrum Guide).

Lip-Philtrum Guides 1 and 2 are used to rank upper lip thinness and philtrum smoothness. The University of Washington guides reflect the full range of lip and philtrum shapes, with Rank 3 representing the population mean. Ranks 4 and 5 reflect the thin lip and smooth philtrum that characterize the FAS facial phenotype. Examples of the FAS facial phenotype are shown across three races: Native American, Caucasian, and African American.

Source. Copyright © 2020, Susan (Astley) Hemingway Ph.D., University of Washington. Used with permission.

The Washington State FAS Diagnostic and Prevention Network initiated a project to create a representative system for inclusion of individuals with PAE. This was arranged according to four diagnostic criteria (growth, face, brain, and alcohol exposure) scored on a Likert scale. With the third edition in 2004, supported by a number of studies validating its criteria, several modifications helped establish this system as a standard for many diagnostic clinics (Astley 2004; Clarren and Astley 1997). These efforts led to the development of standardized approaches for establishing and measuring deficits, especially facial dysmorphology (Figures 12–2 and 12–3).

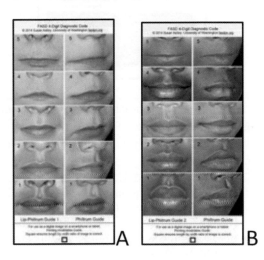

FIGURE 12–2. Lip-philtrum guides 1 (**A**) and 2 (**B**) are used to rank upper lip thinness and philtrum smoothness. (See Plate 3 to view this figure in color.)

The philtrum is the vertical groove between the nose and upper lip. Guide A is used for Caucasians and all other races with lips like Caucasians. Guide B is used for African Americans and all other races with similarly full lips. The guides reflect the full range of lip thickness and philtrum depth, with Rank 3 representing the population mean. Ranks 4 and 5 reflect the thin lip and smooth philtrum that characterize the FAS facial phenotype.

Source. Copyright © 2020, Susan (Astley) Hemingway, Ph.D., University of Washington. Used with permission. Free digital images of these guides for use on smartphones and tablets can be obtained from astley@uw.edu.

Using a multinational case ascertainment data set, the previously adopted Institute of Medicine criteria of 1996 were revised and updated for use with individuals 21 years or younger (Hoyme et al. 2005). These criteria were developed with practical application in mind; they clarified and operationalized the definitions for the different diagnoses and suggested a behavioral phenotype.

The Canadian Guidelines for Diagnosis of FASD were published by a committee of the Public Health Agency of Canada with widely based con-

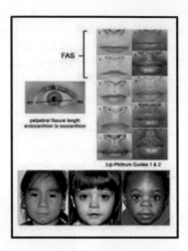

FIGURE 12–3. The three diagnostic facial features of FAS include 1) short palpebral fissure lengths, 2) a smooth philtrum (Rank 4 or 5 on the Lip-Philtrum Guide), and 3) a thin upper lip (Rank 4 or 5 on the Lip-Philtrum Guide). (See Plate 4 to view this figure in color.)

Lip-Philtrum Guides 1 and 2 are used to rank upper lip thinness and philtrum smoothness. The University of Washington guides reflect the full range of lip and philtrum shapes, with Rank 3 representing the population mean. Ranks 4 and 5 reflect the thin lip and smooth philtrum that characterize the FAS facial phenotype. Examples of the FAS facial phenotype are shown across three races: Native American, Caucasian, and African American.

Source.   Copyright © 2020, Susan (Astley) Hemingway, Ph.D., University of Washington. Used with permission.

sultation with experts in the field (Chudley et al. 2005). After a decade of use, the data emanating from clinics using the 2005 guidelines were reviewed by a select group of experts. Revised guidelines were produced by incorporating a comprehensive systematic literature review on diagnosis with expert consensus. These updated guidelines recommended, among other things, adult diagnosis, new affect regulation criteria, and new thresholds for establishing significant PAE (Chudley et al. 2005; Cook et al. 2016).

Identification of dysmorphology and heavy PAE based on standardized procedures were incorporated for diagnostic purposes by the Collaborative Initiative on Fetal Alcohol Spectrum Disorder (Mattson et al. 2010). After a strong recommendation from the DSM expert committee, DSM-5 recognized the sequelae of PAE in both the main diagnostic section and in the section for further study (American Psychiatric Association 2013).

Various countries observed their unique challenges with PAE and adopted region-specific guidelines. In Australia, a panel of 13 professionals collaborated to produce the consensus adaptation of elements from both the University of Washington four-digit diagnostic code and the Canadian guidelines for FASD diagnosis. This process produced the Australian diagnostic guidelines (Bower et al. 2017; Watkins et al. 2013). The German diagnostic guidelines specifically did not make PAE a prerequisite for diagnosis. Guidelines developed in Scotland were intended to improve accurate diagnosis and treatment and adopted the majority of the Canadian guidelines and the processes proposed in the German guidelines (Landgraf et al. 2013; Wise 2019).

Psychiatric Nosology of PAE Outcomes

Recognition of PAE in contributing to identifiable mental disorders dates back to DSM-III (American Psychiatric Association 1980). The *International Classification of Diseases* (ICD) recognized the diagnostic outcomes of PAE and used the label *noxious influences affecting the fetus or newborn* (code 760.7). The subcategory 760.71 refers to FAS. The first two editions of DSM were theoretical in their approach to psychoanalytic understanding (American Psychiatric Association 1952, 1968). Once the atheoretical underpinnings of the classification system of mental disorders were introduced in 1980, DSM recognized the influences of PAE in mental disorder nosology. This was short-lived, however; DSM-III-R (American Psychiatric Association 1987) excised the criteria that recognized FAS as a cause of mental retardation. Two subsequent versions, DSM-IV and DSM-IV-TR (American Psychiatric Association 1994, 2000), did not include PAE as part of psychiatric nosology (Mela 2006).

Currently, DSM-5 includes PAE as a significant risk factor, a predictor of diagnostic category, a diagnostic subgroup of neurodevelopmental disorders, and a condition for further study (ND-PAE). The section on intellectual disability paved the path for PAE when the diagnostic influence of IQ was indirectly reduced by ascribing equal weight to intellectual and adaptive deficits in the diagnostic criteria. This acknowledged that IQ alone cannot determine the level of deficiency in function, a view that aligns with the findings of the diffuse brain injury invoked in PAE. Specifiers now adopt cognitive, social, and practical deficits in determining the severity of the intellectual or adaptive deficits.

DSM-5 and the Consequences of PAE

FAS is recognized as a specifier in patients diagnosed with autism spectrum disorder, as are other medical and genetic disorders (e.g., Rett syndrome, fragile X syndrome). The environmental risk and prognostic factors associated with a diagnosis of ADHD in DSM-5 include PAE. PAE is recognized as occurring in a number of individuals who also report a history of child abuse, neglect, multiple foster placements, neurotoxin exposure (e.g., lead), and infections (e.g., encephalitis). The level of causality in this relationship is yet to be determined. DSM-5 recognition is seen as legitimizing a previously stigmatized and excluded risk factor. Prenatal smoking was strongly identified as a risk factor for ADHD diagnosis. PAE is also recognized as a risk factor for developmental coordination disorder, which manifests as motor coordination challenges. People affected face difficulties daily with motor coordination involving dressing, writing, and small muscle movements. Commonly, visual motor integration difficulties can be identified, and some aspects of clumsiness and dyspraxia serve as red flags when assessing patients with the consequences of PAE. Impaired academic achievement and poor physical fitness are affected by developmental coordination disorder. The corresponding intersection between DSM-5 and PAE is also seen in those with developmental coordination disorder. The relevant domains of motor abilities and academic achievements (evaluated in the comprehensive neurocognitive assessment of PAE) are the domains that are significantly impaired in individuals with developmental coordination disorder.

Most notable among the DSM-5 categories is "other specified neurodevelopmental disorder," which can be specified as "associated with PAE." The section requires explanation of how the identified disorder does not meet the criteria for other neurodevelopmental disorders. The ICD-9-CM code 315.8 recognizes PAE as contributing to developmental disabilities and provides the clinician with the option to invoke DSM-5 in diagnosing outcomes of PAE. By extension, the category "unspecified neurodevelopmental disorder" also serves in equivocal cases to allow for diagnosing outcomes of PAE and allows the clinician to skip over the essential criteria listing the deficits for diagnosis. For instance, it can be applied in a case in which PAE is confirmed and social and occupational dysfunction are identified but specific neurocognitive deficits are not available as standard measurements or are obscured by other pressing mental disorders. Mentioning this diagnosis allows for follow-up as the outcomes of interventions for other coexisting disorders such as anxiety (e.g., panic disorder, generalized anxiety disorder) are evaluated.

Clinically, psychiatrists and mental health professionals accrue significant advantages if they are aware of the disorders within the DSM-5 neurodevelopmental disorders section. Most of the disorders are interrelated in etiology and manifestation. To align with the essential neurocognitive features that support the current DSM-5 criteria, clinicians should identify both the clinical and associated features of the criteria. In clinical situations in which this is unclear or in which subthreshold features are identified, clinicians have the option to request a more comprehensive assessment. This additional step provides information that further categorizes the specific mental disorders or expands the list of differential diagnoses. These steps improve clinical acumen similar to recognizing pervasive developmental disorders associated with mental disorders. Additional social and neuropsychological information may clarify the diagnosis and help to rule out other causes of mental disorders. Studies looking at comorbidity identified high rates of multiple psychiatric comorbid conditions with autism spectrum disorder (Lundström et al. 2015).

Criteria for Further Study: ND-PAE

Although ND-PAE as a diagnosis requires further study, awareness of the criteria is likely to benefit patients and support psychiatrists' skills and practice in caring for individuals affected by the consequences of PAE. The criteria were intended to encompass the behavioral, developmental, and mental health symptoms associated with PAE, and they are appropriate for individuals with or without physical findings (Kable et al. 2016). Although the ND-PAE criteria differ in not necessitating impairment in facial characteristics, weight, height, and head circumference, neurocognitive deficits are pivotal. Referred to as superdomains, self-regulation and neurocognitive and adaptive dysfunction require clinical and standard measurements. Increasingly, the clinical use of the criteria is supported by research showing that these measures identified acceptable numbers of individuals on the FASD spectrum (Sanders et al. 2017).

In a retrospective study, 82 patients previously diagnosed with FASD according to the Canadian diagnostic guidelines were rated according to the new DSM-5 criteria for ND-PAE. Interrater reliability was high, and the ND-PAE criteria (of DSM) overlapped with FASD criteria (of the Canadian diagnostic guidelines) (Sanders et al. 2017). ND-PAE criteria were not as sensitive in subcategorizing patients with FAS and pFAS diagnoses. The methods of the two systems of diagnosis were compared in the study. DSM supports the perspective of clinical judgment, which can introduce some variance when compared with the stricter application of standard deviation of a score on the neurodevelopmental data (for FASD according to Canadian guidelines). Sanders et al. (2017) pointed out that adopting a different threshold for the deviation from the mean and DSM's insistence on an extra domain deficit were the main determinants affecting how the systems compared on sensitivity and specificity. In a different study with 3- to 10-year-old children diagnosed with FAS, a review of the criteria for ND-PAE showed a high rate of endorsed ND-PAE symptoms. Apart from the adaptive criteria being too restrictive, the authors provided evidence for the internal validity of the ND-PAE criteria (Kable and Coles 2018).

When the specific constructs of ARND and ND-PAE were examined among 86 patients diagnosed with ARND (the most prevalent category of FASD diagnosis), Johnson et al. (2018) identified a high sensitivity and specificity between the two sets of criteria. The ND-PAE criteria accurately classified 89.5% of those diagnosed with ARND, suggesting confluence of the diagnostic systems. These results suggest that the high rates of mental health clinicians misdiagnosing patients with outcomes of PAE could be reduced if the clinicians used the criteria to identify those with ND-PAE. ND-PAE seems to offer the optimal option for readily and accurately making the diagnosis. Considering that many people with FASD (mostly undiagnosed) are under the care of psychiatrists and other mental health professionals, ND-PAE is a welcome addition for effective identification. Therefore, future data from mental health settings could be used to support integrating the ND-PAE criteria into the main portion of DSM in the next edition.

Etiological Role of PAE

The weight given to PAE in mental health and neurodevelopmental outcomes remains controversial and is likely to remain so until its exact etiological factors and pathophysiological pathways are fully understood. This understanding may take the form of algorithmic classification and epigenetic formulations. Some have argued that the role of alcohol as an etiological factor was overemphasized and premature for the available level of evidence (McLennan and Braunberger 2017). In the 50 years of alcohol teratogenesis research, the various terms used to describe the outcomes of PAE have contributed to the uncertain role occupied by PAE in mental disorder outcomes. Terms were suggested to explain the subthreshold conditions found in patients who did not fully express the deficits found in those with prototypical FAS. For instance, ARND replaced the ambiguous term "possible FAE" to describe the offspring of mothers who drank significant amounts of alcohol in pregnancy (Stratton et al. 1996). ARND was itself defined as a "complex pattern of behavioral or cognitive impairment…in combination with a history of significant prenatal alcohol exposure" (Stratton et al. 1996, p. 52). It was subsequently subsumed with other diagnostic terms (FAS, ARBD, and pFAS) under the umbrella rubric FASD, which in turn was defined as "the range of effects that occur in an individual whose mother drank alcohol during pregnancy. These effects may include physical, mental, behavioral, and/or learning disabilities with possible lifelong implications" (Bertrand et al. 2004, p. 4).

Whether PAE represents etiological, descriptive, or epidemiological roles in classification is still being researched. This is not unique to PAE and its mental disorder outcomes but is also recognized in other complex disorders. A complex profile is a feature shared specifically in neurodisability due to PAE and generally in other neurodevelopmental disorders. Other shared features include genetic susceptibility, exposure to other substances prenatally, early childhood adversity, residential instability, and chaotic parenting styles. Additionally, delayed recognition and misdiagnosis occur but may be more common in PAE and its outcomes. In mental disorders, disease classification relating to PAE will evolve further.

Embracing Comorbidity

It is natural to want to keep things simple, but the multifaceted aspects of PAE and its related mental disorders hinder this goal. Overlapping clinical features can make diagnosis challenging, and consequent missed diagnoses have been blamed for negative outcomes in patients at the interface of PAE and mental disorders. Because the mental disorders already have recognized treatment modalities and guidelines, patients with mental disorders in the context of PAE could benefit from similar recognized treatments, albeit with some exceptions. Such targeted interventions could also improve patients' functionality, especially when compared with that of patients whose unrecognized conditions receive no treatment. The relationships identified at the interface of mental disorders and the diagnostic outcomes of PAE serve as the pathophysiological underpinnings needed to understand the causes of symptoms and manifestations of dysfunction. Identifying and understanding the biopsychosocial underpinnings of the dysfunction are necessary for prevention, recognition, and intervention. Regarding identification, patients with multiple mental disorders may have specific risk factors that respond to approaches directed at prevention. For instance, the role of trauma and adverse childhood experiences in those with PAE allowed strategies for prevention and specific interventions (Badry and Felske 2013).

Diagnosis Specification

As a result of multiple factors contributing to the etiology of ND-PAE/ FASD and the biopsychosocial complications of PAE in presentation, diagnostic variability continues to be a challenge in the mental health field. Efforts are under way to amalgamate various diagnostic schemes with the goal of developing basic, universally accepted criteria for diagnosis. Because individuals with disabilities resulting from ND-PAE/FASD manifest common signs and symptoms of medical and mental disorders, there is a need to recognize those generally shared symptoms and the signs unique to ND-PAE/FASD. In the meantime, defining phenotypes based on psychological profiles is gaining acceptance for clarifying diagnosis (Taylor and Enns 2018). More symptom-defined clusters may yet assume importance as diagnostic identifiers, and new ways of conceptualizing and delivering treatment may result (Mela et al. 2019). The evolving role of the ND-PAE/FASD diagnosis could be shaped by the experiences of practitioners who use similar protocols in the field of developmental disability. This is relevant given the uniqueness of dual diagnosis in the consequences of PAE and related mental disorders.

It is important that clinicians recognize that lumping or splitting, especially in complex disorders like ND-PAE/FASD, has significant limitations. Some clinicians have attempted to identify common presentations among patients with the overarching diagnosis and then streamline interventions for them, for instance, targeting specific strategies for managing executive function deficits (Coles et al. 2018; Green et al. 2009). These practices have therapeutic value for individuals with such deficits. Given the variability of presentation, however, this approach cannot replace the need for comprehensive diagnostic rigor focused on identifying relevant strengths and weaknesses. This is foundational in informing therapeutic approaches generally. Teams working with individuals who present with mental disorders should adopt a comprehensive stepped approach to recognition and diagnostic specification. Such an approach allows for the gathering of all relevant information relating to the common pathways of mental disorders and ND-PAE/FASD. Contributing factors predisposing to the joint disorders can then be identified easily. Factors such as common genetic loading with a family history of addiction, consequences of trauma, childhood adversity, and psychosocial disadvantage will rise to the top of the list. Other features such as delay in diagnosis and the resulting sequelae may separate ND-PAE/FASD or point to its presence in particular patients.

To complete the diagnostic circle, the clinician identifies the steps associated with reclassifying individuals who have already been diagnosed on the spectrum. There are clusters of symptoms recognized in a group that make them unique. Such symptom profiles, although not used for diagnostic separation per se, serve to guide the understanding of characteristics linked to specific outcomes and interventions. Some patterns include affect regulation problems or impairment in attention. Others may relate specifically to the overarching executive dysfunction (Green et al. 2009). Mental disorder diagnoses accommodate these features easily. A common diagnostic strategy employs algorithmic steps of including or excluding criteria to support one diagnosis or another. When combined with hierarchical thinking, this approach may work well in representing patients with both ND-PAE/FASD and mental disorders.

Clinical Vignette

A 28-year-old woman is referred to a specialist FASD clinic. The process began when her mother, her main support person, read an article about FASD and the commonality of mental disorders. The patient's mother discloses a relatively high quantity of alcohol use during her pregnancy with the patient. The patient is already connected with a mental health clinic and is currently monitored by the outpatient psychiatrists. She manifests inappropriate affect, blunted affect, and negative symptoms and displays bizarre beliefs about radiation coming through her apartment. Consequently, she has changed residences three times in 1 year. Her functioning has deteriorated; she is experiencing weight loss, a reversed sleep pattern, and agitation, and she is exercising poor judgment. She engages in exploitative relationships against her mother's advice. She was fired from her job as a cashier when she made too many mistakes at work.

Red Flags: What Else Could It Be?

The mother's information is significant given the existence of guilt, self-blame, and fear of stigma. The patient's symptoms include poor judgment, being unaware of or not caring about the inherent risk in certain relationships, and a potential math or executive function deficiency, all of which are functionally disruptive and limit her employment prospects. Thought disorder and affect disturbance point to the cognitive and psychotic components of schizophrenia, which is the likely diagnosis. Her impairment in communication, executive function, and academic performance had been unrecognized until her mother's revelation of PAE. Response to antipsychotic medications may be limited, depending on which medication is prescribed. In the existing literature, olanzapine has been shown to produce the better cognitive outcome (Frankel et al. 2006). Some data support the use of aripiprazole and clozapine in patients with the specific consequences of PAE (Hosenbocus and Chahal 2012).

Modifications: What Difference Does Knowledge of PAE Make?

Management of a patient's deterioration requires understanding the contribution of PAE to the clinical picture. If available, a full neuropsychological assessment seeking the level of neurocognitive impairment is indicated. Clinical screenings such as a similarities test, proverb interpretations test, and the Luria hand–motor movement test, along with a Mini-Mental State Examination, provide basic neurocognitive findings. In the absence of a psychologist, occupational therapists can evaluate executive function. Financial competence assessment is also helpful in completely understanding the level of the functional impairment already noted. Once the basic components of the impairment are identified, the patient should be involved in devising a treatment plan.

An FASD-informed treatment method employs modified communication approaches. Focusing on the patient's strengths and providing positive comments and encouragement are a few of the additional strategies not included in the patient's previous treatment. The attitude of the clinician— the patient *won't* perform—will now be changed, based on the identified deficits, to reflect her inability—the patient *can't* perform. A mentor should be identified whose knowledge of the patient's neurocognitive deficits permits a modified approach of teaching skills, checking comprehension, and breaking down plans into manageable steps. The patient's noncompliance will now be viewed as a deficit that requires a supportive and interdependent approach rather than an approach promoting independence, as encouraged in psychiatric rehabilitation practices. Failures in performance should offer opportunities to learn alternate ways of teaching, such as presenting graphical or drawn images. Mentoring and a structure that helps minimize exploitation of the patient, now seen as being unable rather than unwilling to protect herself, is warranted. This vulnerability is a hallmark of her executive function deficits, suggestibility, and risk unawareness. Conversations with the patient's mother that address guilt and shame could increase the patient's self-awareness and self-monitoring. Beneficial results can come from these conversations if they facilitate a more positive relationship and reduce the burden of care and the mother's stress levels. If financial assistance is needed to replace lost wages, clinical measurements revealing adaptive and, likely, intellectual deficits can assist in obtaining disability benefits.

Unifying Diagnostic Classifications

Different diagnostic systems and the heterogeneous nature of the consequences of PAE, coupled with the differing and atheoretical diagnostic approaches to mental disorders, make unification of diagnostic classification very challenging. Achieving the goal of conceptualizing unambiguous, user-friendly, and practical systems of diagnostic classification will require significant effort, but with a patient-centered focus, the process will be highly welcomed, especially in mental health systems. The preferred option may be a single differentiating biochemical test. The existing biomarkers (meconium testing, maternal biochemical status, genetic testing, psychological profiles, and facial dysmorphology) are limited to the specific aspect of the disorder they identify. One advantage in diagnosis is that there is general agreement on the common features that contribute to the identification of individuals with ND-PAE/FASD. To include mental disorders is to consider the points of agreement in the criteria (e.g., evidence of threshold PAE, presence of abnormal growth retardation, neurodevelopmental deficits, and characteristic facial features associated with alcohol exposure). The neurodevelopmental deficits, which are the essential component of the disability, cut across the mental disorder and PAE fields.

Conclusion

Because of their variety and range, many features associated with the consequences of PAE fostered differing systems of classification, which have also been modified over time. A single unified, universally accepted, patient-centered, and clinically useful classification system is desirable and currently being pursued. Strictly sticking to the atheoretical approach to mental disorder classifications will not solve the problems challenging psychiatric nosology of PAE. In our current state of relative ignorance about the mind/brain, we are far from being able to define plausible, stable mechanisms that produce most psychiatric disorders. The intersection of the mechanisms and deficits at the interface of PAE that allow classification in simple forms have advantages for the future. Research should focus on bringing together in a stepwise manner the medical, psychological, and cognitive components of PAE into the classification system.

CLINICAL PRACTICAL APPLICATIONS

- Clinicians should be sensitive and avoid using outdated labels such as *mental retardation*, which can negatively affect the patient.

- The classification systems used for ND-PAE/FASD are many, but they have essentially similar core features.

- DSM-5 also recognizes the role of PAE in developmental coordination disorder, and ADHD.

- In the diagnostic process, both medical and mental (psychological and cognitive) classifications should be considered for individuals with PAE because they inform treatment interventions.

- A suspected diagnosis based on deficits should be used as the roadmap to obtain relevant clinical measures needed to support desired outcomes.

References

American Psychiatric Association: Diagnostic and Statistical Manual: Mental Disorders. Washington, DC, American Psychiatric Association, 1952

American Psychiatric Association: Diagnostic and Statistical Manual of Mental Disorders, 2nd Edition. Washington, DC, American Psychiatric Association, 1968

American Psychiatric Association: Diagnostic and Statistical Manual of Mental Disorders, 3rd Edition. Washington, DC, American Psychiatric Association, 1980

American Psychiatric Association: Diagnostic and Statistical Manual of Mental Disorders, 3rd Edition Revised. Washington, DC, American Psychiatric Association, 1987

American Psychiatric Association: Diagnostic and Statistical Manual of Mental Disorders, 4th Edition. Washington, DC, American Psychiatric Association, 1994

American Psychiatric Association: Diagnostic and Statistical Manual of Mental Disorders, 4th Edition, Text Revision. Washington, DC, American Psychiatric Association, 2000

American Psychiatric Association: Diagnostic and Statistical Manual of Mental Disorders, 5th Edition. Arlington, VA, American Psychiatric Association, 2013

Astley SJ: Diagnostic Guide for Fetal Alcohol Spectrum Disorders: The 4-Digit Diagnostic Code, 3rd Edition. Seattle, WA, University of Washington Publication Services, 2004. Available at: http://depts.washington.edu/fasdpn/pdfs/guide04.pdf. Accessed October 2, 2020.

Astley SJ, Clarren SK: Diagnosing the full spectrum of fetal alcohol-exposed individuals: introducing the 4-digit diagnostic code. Alcohol Alcohol 35(4):400–410, 2000

Badry D, Felske AW: An examination of three key factors: alcohol, trauma and child welfare: fetal alcohol spectrum disorder and the Northwest Territories of Canada: brightening our home fires. First Peoples Child Fam Rev 8(1), 2013

Bertrand J, Floyd RL, Weber MK, et al: Fetal Alcohol Syndrome: Guidelines for Referral and Diagnosis. Atlanta, GA, Centers for Disease Control and Prevention, National Center on Birth Defects and Developmental Disabilities, 2004

Bower C, Elliott EJ, Zimmet M, et al: Australian guide to the diagnosis of foetal alcohol spectrum disorder: a summary. J Paediatr Child Health 53(10):1021–1023, 2017

Chasnoff IJ, Wells AM, King L: Misdiagnosis and missed diagnoses in foster and adopted children with prenatal alcohol exposure. Pediatrics 135(2):264–270, 2015

Chudley AE, Conry J, Cook JL, et al: Fetal alcohol spectrum disorder: Canadian guidelines for diagnosis. CMAJ 172 (5 suppl):S1–S21, 2005

Clarren SK, Astley SJ: The development of the Fetal Alcohol Syndrome Diagnostic and Prevention Network in Washington State, in The Challenge of Fetal Alcohol Syndrome: Overcoming Secondary Disabilities. Edited by Streissguth A, Kanter J. Seattle, WA, University of Washington Press, 1997, pp 40–51

Clarren SK, Smith DW: The fetal alcohol syndrome. N Engl J Med 11:1063–1067, 1978

Coles CD, Kable JA, Taddeo E, Strickland D: GoFAR: improving attention, behavior and adaptive functioning in children with fetal alcohol spectrum disorders: brief report. Dev Neurorehabil 21(5):345–349, 2018

Cook JL, Green CR, Lilley CM, et al: Fetal alcohol spectrum disorder: a guideline for diagnosis across the lifespan. CMAJ 188(3):191–197, 2016

Frankel F, Paley B, Marquardt R, O'Connor M: Stimulants, neuroleptics, and children's friendship training for children with fetal alcohol spectrum disorders. J Child Adolesc Psychopharmacol 16(6):777–789, 2006

Green CR, Mihic AM, Nikkel SM, et al: Executive function deficits in children with fetal alcohol spectrum disorders (FASD) measured using the Cambridge Neuropsychological Tests Automated Battery (CANTAB). J Child Psychol Psychiatry 50(6):688–697, 2009

Hosenbocus S, Chahal R: A review of executive function deficits and pharmacological management in children and adolescents. J Can Acad Child Adolesc Psychiatry 21(3):223–229, 2012

Hoyme HE, May PA, Kalberg WO, et al: A practical clinical approach to diagnosis of fetal alcohol spectrum disorders: clarification of the 1996 Institute of Medicine criteria. Pediatrics 115(1):39–47, 2005

Hoyme HE, Kalberg WO, Elliott AJ, et al: Updated clinical guidelines for diagnosing fetal alcohol spectrum disorders. Pediatrics 138(2):e20154256, 2016

Johnson S, Moyer CL, Klug MG, Burd L: Comparison of alcohol–related neurodevelopmental disorders and neurodevelopmental disorders associated with prenatal alcohol exposure diagnostic criteria. J Dev Behav Pediatr 39(2):163–167, 2018

Jones KL, Smith DW: Recognition of the fetal alcohol syndrome in early infancy. Lancet 302(7836):999–1001, 1973

Jones KL, Smith DW, Ulleland CN, Streissguth AP: Pattern of malformation in offspring of chronic alcoholic mothers. Lancet 1(7815):1267–1271, 1973

Kable JA, Coles CD: Evidence supporting the internal validity of the proposed ND-PAE disorder. Child Psychiatry Hum Dev 49(2):163–175, 2018

Kable JA, O'Connor MJ, Olson HC, et al: Neurobehavioral disorder associated with prenatal alcohol exposure (ND-PAE): proposed DSM-5 diagnosis. Child Psychiatry Hum Dev 47(2):335–34, 2016

Kendler KS: Explanatory models for psychiatric illness. Am J Psychiatry 165(6):695–702, 2008

Landgraf MN, Nothacker M, Heinen F: Diagnosis of fetal alcohol syndrome (FAS): German guideline version 2013. Eur J Paediatr Neurol 17(5):437–446, 2013

Lundström S, Reichenberg A, Melke J, et al: Autism spectrum disorders and coexisting disorders in a nationwide Swedish twin study. J Child Psychol Psychiatry 56(6):702–710, 2015

Mattson SN, Foroud T, Sowell ER, et al: Collaborative Initiative on Fetal Alcohol Spectrum Disorders: methodology of clinical projects. Alcohol 44(7-8):635–641, 2010

May PA, Gossage JP, Smith M, et al: Population differences in dysmorphic features among children with fetal alcohol spectrum disorders. J Dev Behav Pediatr 31(4):304–316, 2010

McLennan JD, Braunberger P: A critique of the new Canadian fetal alcohol spectrum disorder guideline. J Can Acad Child Adolesc Psychiatry 26(3):179–183, 2017

Mela M: Accommodating the fetal alcohol spectrum disorders in the Diagnostic and Statistical Manual of Mental Disorders (DSM V). J FAS Int 4:1–10, 2006

Mela M, Coons-Harding KD, Anderson T: Recent advances in fetal alcohol spectrum disorder for mental health professionals. Curr Opin Psychiatry 43(4):328–335, 2019

O'Connor MJ: Mental health outcomes associated with prenatal alcohol exposure: genetic and environmental factors. Curr Dev Disord Rep 1:181–188, 2014

Sanders JL, Breen RE, Netelenbos N: Comparing diagnostic classification of neurobehavioral disorder associated with prenatal alcohol exposure with the Canadian fetal alcohol spectrum disorder guidelines: a cohort study. CMAJ Open 5(1):E178–E183, 2017

Stratton K, Howe C, Battaglia F (eds): Fetal Alcohol Syndrome: Diagnosis, Epidemiology, Prevention, and Treatment. Washington, DC, National Academies Press, 1996

Taylor NM, Enns LN: Factors predictive of a fetal alcohol spectrum disorder diagnosis: parent and teacher ratings. Child Neuropsychol 25(4)507–527, 2018

Tough SC, Clarke M, Clarren S: Preventing fetal alcohol spectrum disorders: preconception counseling and diagnosis help. Can Fam Physician 51:1199–1201, 2005

Watkins RE, Elliott EJ, Wilkins A, et al: Recommendations from a consensus development workshop on the diagnosis of fetal alcohol spectrum disorders in Australia. BMC Pediatr 13:156, 2013

Wise J: Guidance on fetal alcohol syndrome aims to improve diagnosis and treatment in Scotland. BMJ 364:1396, 2019

PART V

Treatment

CHAPTER 13

Pharmacological Intervention

WHAT TO KNOW

The dearth of pharmacological studies addressing ND-PAE/FASD affects the level of guidance provided for prescribing psychotropic medications.

Stimulants are the most prescribed and studied psychotropic medications in ND-PAE/FASD, followed by antipsychotics, antidepressants, mood stabilizers, and α-adrenergic agonists.

There is emerging evidence that aggressiveness in ND-PAE/FASD responds to risperidone.

The neurocognitive deficits associated with PAE can be grouped into four clusters (hyperarousal, hyperactivity, affect dysregulation, and cognitive inflexibility), which can be a substrate for psychotropic medications.

Repetitive transcranial magnetic stimulation with its generative potential for white matter is heralded as a possible intervention for ND-PAE/FASD.

The complex and comorbid conditions inherent in persons with ND-PAE/FASD require a high level of expertise and skill of mental health clinicians. Over the five decades that the disorder has been recognized, more efforts have been directed at characterizing its manifestation and long-term prognosis. In the 1990s, research on the concepts and efficacy of intervention started with biopsychosocial interventions. A pair of randomized trials of stimulants involving those diagnosed with FASD initiated the human pharmacological studies (Oesterheld et al. 1998; Snyder et al. 1997). Before then, study of the metabolic effects of alcohol on pregnant mothers and offspring in animal models to whom psychotropic medications had been administered dominated the extant science. Alcohol was then noted to reduce the excretion of psychotropic medications (chlorpromazine), and decreased blood alcohol clearance rates occurred when benzodiazepines and phenothiazines were also administered (Patten et al. 2014). Alcohol inhibits hepatic alcohol dehydrogenase. The effects of several classes of medications on patients diagnosed with ND-PAE/FASD have now been studied in mostly retrospective case series (Peadon et al. 2009). The level of evidence for biological and psychopharmacological intervention is insufficient to propose specific guidelines (Mela et al. 2018). However, wide individual variations in neurocognitive deficits imply that the current level of evidence allows for individual approaches in selecting effective medications. Until the level of evidence changes, medication use for patients with ND-PAE/FASD should be guided by existing principles for the use of psychotropic medications in individuals with other developmental disorders (Ji and Findling 2016).

Using pharmaceutical agents to treat individuals with ND-PAE/FASD depends on the orientation of the health care clinic, knowledge of the prescriber, and goals and purposes of the treatment. Diagnosis-based, rather than impairment-based, systems of care limit the prescription of agents to mainly those with a formal diagnosis. Generally, this indicates a higher threshold of difficulty because insistence on fulfilling the diagnostic criteria informs that type of treatment. Family physicians or general practitioners, psychiatrists, social workers, psychologists, and pharmacists have varying prescribing privileges. The knowledge base of these mental health professionals ranges from basic to advanced to proficient levels of expertise and experience with psychopharmacological agents. Given that prescriptions specific for PAE outcomes are off-label, special and enhanced expertise about the neurology and pathogenesis of ND-PAE/FASD are a requisite for patient care. In this chapter, I review the existing research studies on all psychotropic medications prescribed to patients with ND-PAE/FASD and their responses and the adverse consequences. Given the dearth of research in the field, a model combining a decision tree and prescription principles and practice, as used in other neurodevelopmental disorders, is proposed. The ultimate goal is to exhaust available social, behavioral, and environmental interventions before prescribing specific medications.

Many of the symptoms manifested in individuals with ND-PAE/FASD, either alone or comorbid with other mental disorders, are amenable to psychotropic medications. Patients present with anxiety, mood, and behavioral symptoms. Although it may be logical, psychotropic medications should be used cautiously for the plethora of psychological and mental disorder symptoms, with a view toward using current evidence specific to the population, focusing on the most debilitating symptoms, and ensuring close monitoring and adjustments in a patient-centered manner. Ultimately, the goals of treatment are to enhance function and, as much as possible, well-being. When the risks and benefits of medications are weighed, the emphasis and dependence on medication will vary depending on which consideration (risk or benefit) takes precedence. The relationship between the prescriber and the patient is pertinent to and serves to enhance compliance, safety, and functional outcomes.

Pretreatment Factors of Note

In this chapter, I focus on what to do, especially pharmacologically, when a person has been diagnosed with the consequences of PAE. However, it is clinically astute for mental health professionals to be sensitive to behaviors that may implicate the neurocognitive deficits of ND-PAE/FASD, especially when the subject has not yet been diagnosed or is in the clinical process of obtaining a diagnosis. Mostly, the patient is attending clinical settings where the professional is focused on other mental health problems (depression, anxiety, atypical dysfunction, and the concern of others about the patient), not necessarily the consequences of PAE. Suspicions of the effects of neurocognitive deficits are increased when patients' behaviors appear inconsistent with the primary reason they were referred to the mental health system (Substance Abuse and Mental Health Services Administration 2014). Such is the case when patients present with unusual complications of treatment, when they manifest behavior consistent with their expressed desire for treatment and behavior that interferes with the same treatment. Deficits from PAE cause patients to show apparent and irrational noncompliance, including nonattendance at care settings (Grant et al. 2013). These should inform the need to explore the reasons of the behaviors in the context of neurocognitive deficits. For instance, poor planning ability related to executive dysfunction should be suspected if a patient repeatedly fails to attend or is late to appointments. Impulsivity may be suspected when patients abruptly discontinue medication as a protest for an unrelated matter. Patients with high verbal expression and poor comprehension abilities may fail to execute instructions communicated to them, and patients may be construed as noncompliant if they do not follow through with instructions. Instructions are usually given in multiple, and these may be thought understood because the recipient acceded; however, the patient may be experiencing slow information processing with or without memory difficulties. Common indicators, such as recalcitrant behavior, impulsive actions, and evidence of poor judgment, should prompt a closer review of the origin of the initial referral symptoms or unexplained behaviors. Assessment of the deficits may provide sufficient basis and guidance for clinicians to modify current strategies, especially by eschewing ineffective and traditional strategies.

Screening for the consequences of PAE could help select individuals for treatment, and there are recommended tools for identifying indicators of neurocognitive deficits arising from PAE. Current evidence does not support a single or uniform tool for use in all settings; most of the existing tools apply only to the specific context in which they were developed and are not universally predictive. Screening tools for children, indigenous populations, and probationers, for example, are used with the populations for whom they were developed (Goh et al. 2008). Until more accurate tools are identified, signs of neurocognitive deficits can be observed and are noted when exercising a high clinical acumen. To improve the recognition of ND-PAE/FASD, certain historical and familial indicators are helpful in guiding the decision to pursue a full interdisciplinary assessment. The astute clinician should, in any event, seek out information indicating a maternal history of alcohol use disorder; a personal history of poor attachment, which may be the result of neglect during childhood or residential instability associated with involvement with the child welfare system; and the need for academic support through special education classes. The cumulative features should inform the conduct and completion of a standardized assessment, which remains the most reliable and valid means available to identify and intervene in these complex situations. The outcome will depend on whether the assessment is conducted by clinicians adhering to nosology of mental disorders or ND-PAE/FASD.

Goals of Treatment and Therapeutic Working Alliance

Treatment to achieve patient-centered goals should be the ultimate purpose for assessment. This can be threatened when impulsive, irrational, and simplistic consequences of neurocognitive deficits of PAE interfere with the goals and processes of intervention. Treatment-interfering behaviors, as they are known, include actions and behaviors that pose a risk of harm to self or others. As products of neurocognitive disability, individual or collective interfering symptoms must be interrupted as a matter of first principle.

Well-informed treatment should also address potentially destabilizing factors, such as homelessness and adverse social determinants of health (unemployment, lack of financial support, failed accommodation of the deficits, ongoing victimization), and factors that threaten the safety of the therapeutic relationship. Clinicians should follow principles that establish safety and guarantee collaborative therapeutic interactions.

Pharmacological treatment is one of many strategies to support people with PAE who are manifesting mental disorder consequences. Stabilizing many factors is not only complementary to pharmacotherapy, it is foundational to its success. For instance, ongoing substance use by a patient prescribed medications (e.g., stimulants) impedes treatment because it also contributes to perpetuating the same neurocognitive and psychological deficits identified for correction. Use of illicit substances is associated with chaotic living, which contributes to noncompliance and resistance. Directing efforts toward managing substance use is pivotal for any expected benefit from psychotropic medications. Efforts should involve engaging caregivers to play supportive roles in the various aspects of psychosocial care. Such care participation from significant others should be invited early in the treatment process. Management should include efforts to protect patients and prevent persistent abuse; adverse childhood experiences and abuse were found to occur four times more often in people with PAE than in those in the general population (Price et al. 2017; Totten 2010). Focusing on reducing the impact of past trauma also mediates the beneficial effects of medications. This exploration of abuse serves as a process by which patients feel trusted, safe, accepted, and open to experience in therapeutic relationships. This in turn creates an atmosphere conducive to introducing medication treatment.

Every treatment relationship is challenged by the extent of the boundaries expected. First, the clinician should recognize the learning style of the patient with ND-PAE/FASD, which will facilitate maintaining appropriate boundaries within which the therapeutic working alliance will thrive. The clinician should regularly explain and review the boundaries of the therapeutic relationship and the patient's relationships with others. Next, specific boundary training should be included in therapy sessions because one of the negative outcomes a patient may experience is exploitation. If such exploitation involves giving his or her medications to others, the patient is deprived of the medication's benefits. This can occur because of the patient's susceptibility to suggestions from other, more cognitively abled persons. Patients should be guided to identify characteristics and responses of associates that point to insincere friendship and ulterior motives. Strategies that help patients to withdraw safely and access help from the clinical team members should be taught. The clinician should focus on reducing impulsive reactions that stem from impaired judgment and provide exercises to strengthen good decision making. Because cognitive deficits diminish insight, repeated roleplays should be used to act out desired responses, such as how to respond to invitations to indulge in alcohol and illicit substance use or to requests for the patient's medications (Grant et al. 2013). Visual presentation of information also accommodates deficits associated with poor verbal learning skills and should be employed regularly. Individual patients who have memory deficits are better off with techniques incorporating written material, cues to recall, and use of technology to aid recall. In a typical case management context directed at supporting patients, comprehensive efforts should provide mentors, access to programs providing financial support, and guardianship or a financial administrator for the assessed patient.

When these interpersonal and environmental factors are adequately addressed, the chances of success with psychotropic medications are improved. The patient and supportive caregivers are well informed, and the various complicating features are stabilized. Thus, the foundation for psychotropic medication use is made viable.

Practical Pharmacological Treatment of ND-PAE/FASD

Clinical Vignette

A 40-year-old man recently discovered that he was adopted at birth. He expresses feeling abandoned, and his grief leads to a suicidal attempt. He previously received diagnoses of schizoaffective disorder, bipolar disorder, borderline personality disorder, panic disorder, and dependent personality traits. He is under the care of his family doctor and an addiction therapist (he was using alcohol to cope with distress and was drunk when he tried to drive his car into an oncoming truck in his suicide attempt). When he survived, he was so disappointed that he began swallowing his medications until the police arrived to rescue him. When placed in self-help groups for rehabilitation and addiction treatment, he reports that he does not want to go. He was diagnosed with static encephalopathy (a term indicating a history of PAE but with a milder form of clinical manifestations) 20 years earlier. At that time, he was described as impulsive and aggressive and showing poor awareness of boundaries.

When he brings in the medications he used in his overdose attempt, they include sodium valproate (1,500 mg), aripiprazole (15 mg), clonazepam (3 mg), prazosin (4 mg), and mirtazapine (30 mg). He reports he was recently taking methylphenidate (30 mg), but the doctor discontinued it because he was misusing (crushing and snorting it) and diverting (selling to others in exchange for favors). The interactions of these medications were reviewed. The rationale for the use of each medication should be anchored on specific symptom clusters.

Hyperarousal explains a group of symptoms characterized by excessive and increased physiological and psychological arousal as a protective response to feeling unsafe. Prazosin could have been prescribed for that, given its usefulness for PTSD and nightmares resulting from past trauma. *Hyperactivity*, a common manifestation of ADHD, is an unusual and abnormal state of increased activity and stimulation, such that the affected person is easily excitable and impulsive. Methylphenidate could have been prescribed for this cluster of symptoms. Misuse and diversion among alcohol- and drug-dependent patients is not uncommon, but discontinuing methylphenidate without a system of support around the patient can contribute to impulsive behaviors, including self-harm and suicide attempts.

Other medications are prescribed based on manifested symptoms. Rational pharmacology warrants that neural correlates inform choice of medications (Table 13–1). *Affect dysregulation* encompasses the inability of affected person to modulate and moderate their affective experiences and responses to acceptable emotional levels to be adaptive and goal directed. Clonazepam may have been prescribed for anxiety and panic. The mood stabilizer sodium valproate is indicated for affect dysregulation. Another important cluster to consider may be inferred by the use of aripiprazole. *Cognitive inflexibility* is the cluster of symptoms that describes a person's inability to modify tasks and behaviors in response to the changing environment; the strategies the person employs are maladaptive and difficult to modulate without changing the rigidity of certain concepts that person holds. The PAE-informed approach adopts a parsimonious explanation for the psychological deficits; medications that have been proven effective with similar conditions are recommended.

The use of medications to treat FASD and its consequences has been traced and shown to evolve over time; focus was initially on ADHD-type symptoms, then on symptomatic relief, and currently on ligand-specific clusters (Mela et al. 2019). The rationale for using psychopharmacological agents can be guided by the expected response of specific brain regions to neurotransmitters (Tyrer and Bateman 2004). The proper practice of off-label prescription implies that doses, monitoring, and changes adhere to the official standard guidelines for each medication. However, standard doses produce side effects in patients with neurodevelopmental disorders. Monitoring these patient closely should enhance clinicians' abilities to detect side effects. The patient may complain about unusual symptoms. When the clinicians attend carefully to spoken and unspoken concerns, the correct problems are isolated. Those problems can then be linked to the consequences of PAE. Pharmacists with knowledge of PAE support patients better. Following up on lost medication, using various ways to communicate with patients, confirming patients understand instructions, and contacting patients

TABLE 13–1. Proposed clusters and pathogenesis of ND-PAE related to psychotropic medication use

DOMAINS/ CLUSTERS	CLINICAL FEATURES	BIOLOGICAL PATHOGENESIS	RECOMMENDED LIGANDS
Autonomic hyperarousal	Irritability Hypervigilance Insomnia Anxiety and tension Anger Agitation Aggression Reduced pain threshold	Noradrenergic activation of the autonomic nervous system Hypothalamic-pituitary-adrenal axis abnormality	First-line: α-adrenergic agonist Second-line: SSRIs
Neurocognitive: hyperactivity	Restless movement Impulsiveness Inattention Executive dysfunction	Dopaminergic and noradrenergic abnormality	First-line: Amphetamine-based stimulant Second-line: Other stimulant and nonstimulant with noradrenergic and dopaminergic effect
Cognitive inflexibility	Low frustration tolerance Poor social skills Poor reasoning Poor reality testing Poor abstraction Poor perspective taking	Abnormalities in prefrontal cortex, basal ganglia, and anterior cingulate gyrus Sensitized mesolimbic dopamine system	First-line: Atypical neuroleptic Second-line: Other atypical neuroleptic
Mood dysregulation and anxiety and depression	Mood swings Excitability Anxiety Depression	Serotonergic deficits Gap junction abnormalities	First-line: Mood stabilizers Second-line: SSRIs
Others	Specific and nonspecific Combination of above features	Multiple explanations	First-line: Adjunct, choline supplementation, minocycline

Note.   SSRIs=selective serotonin reuptake inhibitors.

via electronic devices provide the requisite supports. The frequency of visits should be individually fixed and guided by factors such as having a mentor, supportive caregivers, level of cognitive impairment, level of risk behaviors, and treatment-interfering or life-threatening behavior. Although community care is preferable to institutional care, there are times when protection from self or others and risk to others may necessitate admission to the hospital. In such a context, anxiety becomes an important indicator of distress leading to disturbed behavior because the majority of patients do not like to be confined.

Overall, the best effective care will result if clinicians on a multidisciplinary team share need-to-know information freely and apply principles that view disability as an opportunity to learn and correct functioning. Some patients are resistant due to cognitive inflexibility and will not consider medications even if previous treatment yielded positive results. Occasionally, testimonies of successful nonmedication treatment by others increase the patient's resolve to not consider or comply with psychotropic medications. If the risk outweighs the benefit of doing nothing, a patient may require involuntary treatment with medications. Preferably, this is the last option available to the clinician, and, ideally, the impasse occurred at the beginning of relationship building with the patient. Local mental health laws should guide the approach that is least onerous and restrictive. Attempting various approaches to garner cooperation may even involve doing nothing and having the patient hear from others that they are better when taking, as opposed to not taking, the medication. Videos of others in a similar situation and visual representation of people who made improvements in their health may appeal to the resistant patient's desire to change and to accept treatment.

Service Delivery Relevant to Treatment of ND-PAE/FASD

Mental health teams and addiction treatment teams have evolved and are now interdisciplinary in nature and function. Such teams provide a possible framework to innovate in comprehensive assessment of the consequences of PAE. Psychologists, social workers, and psychiatrists, as well as other mental health practitioners on a team, are assets beneficial to the comprehensive process of FASD diagnosis through a mental health lens (Coles et al. 2016). Adopting the approach of delivering services to individuals with ND-PAE/FASD through the existing mental health system is bound to increase the diagnostic capacity and to scale up specialized skills to benefit the team and the patient. Not all jurisdictions have as many professionals as team members. The alternative to trained PAE specialists in the mental health system is to source competent teams specializing in the comprehensive assessment of PAE. There are specialized clinics in tertiary, rural, and community settings that fit this model (see Chapter 20, "Clinical Relevance of Fetal Alcohol Spectrum Disorder in the Mental Health System"). Referral to experts is similar to requesting a second opinion when a more comprehensive assessment is needed to confirm the suspicion of the cognitive deficits, which can occur when consulting with an individual with autism or Down syndrome presenting in the regular mental health system. Another similar referral is called for when individuals with schizophrenia need assessment and rehabilitation as a result of cognitive deficits. An appropriate and well-rounded assessment should identify both strengths and weaknesses that are pivotal to ensuring targeted intervention. This fosters a strength-based approach in intervention. These specialized diagnostic teams are increasing (Cook et al. 2016) and are combining data and joining efforts to make reasonable evidence-based advances in the field.

Other Indications for Pharmacotherapy

In recognition of fetal toxicity and the deficits associated with the nutritional problems of PAE, biological prevention and intervention studies were initiated. Antioxidants, essential amino acids, and vitamins were proposed as replacements for the missing products from oxidative stress that were linked to deficits. In preclinical studies, choline was associated with amelioration of deficits, including epigenetic/molecular changes and gross motor, memory, and executive function deficits (Akison et al. 2018). Human studies employed, for example, a double-blind control trial of choline supplementation in pregnant mothers with heavy alcohol consumption. Improved adherence to the essential nutrient choline, irrespective of maternal education, intellectual function, depression, nutritional status, or alcohol use, was significant in confirming acceptability of this "promising" treatment (Jacobson et al. 2018). More research found additional beneficial results from clinical studies of choline administered postnatally to include improvement in processing speed and executive function (Wozniak et al. 2015). Improved nutrition remains a protective factor, and because nutrient deficiency in PAE can be corrected, this line of research has the potential to help especially in the preschool age range (Georgieff et al. 2018).

Sleep problems in various forms have been associated with PAE. Reticular activating system dysfunction, arousal deficits, and sensory processing problems especially have contributed to severe problems (Hanlon-Dearman et al. 2018). Side effects of medications, poor adherence to routine, and adverse consequences of trauma also contribute to sleep problems. Psychotropic medications are advised as a last resort (Ipsiroglu et al. 2015). Effective behavioral and psychosocial interventions actively search to uncover the multiple unrecognized causes of sleep problems. Only by understanding the multifactorial mechanisms can the biological treatment make sense. In a recent review, Hanlon-Dearman et al. (2018) identified specific PAE-induced neurotoxic effects on sleep architecture, circadian physiology, and respiratory control. There is, then, a cascade of social, functional, and interpersonal consequences that jointly perpetuate the sleep problems. It is therefore crucial that the factors beyond the particular individual (e.g., poor sleeping environment, cold, noise) be corrected first before introducing medications as a last resort. Using medications will depend first on what the likely cause of the sleep problem is. There is also an age-dependent variation in the approach. A central sleep-deficient system, peripheral sensory processing, and structural obstructive causes may be different for different age groups. Altered arousal responses, for instance, were reported during sleep in alcohol-exposed infants, and older subjects showed sleep fragmentation associated with neuromuscular abnormalities affecting airway muscles (Troese et al. 2008; Wills et al. 2006).

The teratogenic damage to the suprachiasmatic nucleus was identified in preclinical research; it is critical to the circadian rhythm and contributes to reducing the sleep-wake neurotransmitter GABA (Hanlon-Dearman et al. 2018). Thus, enhancing the function of GABA is a rational approach to treating sleep disorders associated with PAE. GABA neurotransmitter dysfunction is the basis for some of the apoptotic changes observed in PAE-induced hyperarousal. Psychological approaches for reducing hyperarousal, including a regular sleep pattern, mindfulness, creative catharsis, vigorous exercise, and eye movement desensitization, are available for use with those with ND-PAE/FASD. At the same time, hyperarousal was reduced by α-adrenergic agonists in a few studies (Ozsarfati and Koren 2015). Guanfacine and clonidine were reported to facilitate dopamine and norepinephrine neurotransmission, which produced sleep-inducing benefits by reducing hyperarousal (Calles 2008). Melatonin has also been favorably recommended in addition to basic sleep hygiene (Hanlon-Dearman et al. 2018). In older individuals, zopiclone, mirtazapine, trazodone, and tryptophan are likely to be effective and may also produce fewer side effects.

Review of Psychotropic Drug Use

Findings from two systematic reviews (Mela et al. 2018; Peadon et al. 2009), about a decade apart, confirmed the slow progress made in researching and reporting the effect of psychotropic drug use in individuals with the neurocognitive deficits of ND-PAE/FASD. To date, available evidence of two crossover randomized trials and mostly retrospective case series is insufficient to guide treatment. The patient populations of the studies included were small (total 329), and so it was impossible to conduct a statistically useful power calculation. Too wide a range of medications was used in the studies, which precluded drawing any inference concerning specific benefits of the medications. Little progress has been made in funding clinical trials since the last controlled study over two decades ago.

In the available research, stimulants were the most prescribed and studied of all psychotropic medications in subjects with ND-PAE/FASD. Given the demonstrated damage of PAE on catecholamine and other neurotransmitter (i.e., dopaminergic, noradrenergic, serotonergic, cholinergic, glutamatergic, and histaminergic) systems, using psychotropic medications will likely continue to attract attention and, hopefully, research. Foundational to this is an effort to identify and understand the pathophysiology of PAE in order to effectively target interventions. Stimulant use, especially amphetamine salt–based use, was premised on the finding that D_1 receptors of the mesocortical pathway were dysfunctional in individuals with PAE (Cheng et al. 2018; O'Malley and Nanson 2002). Table 13–1 shows the sites where pathogenesis relates with the recommended medication on the basis of the receptor affinity for the drugs on combined deficits. Some approaches recognize executive dysfunction as the target for treatment (Hosenbocus and Chahal 2012).

The role of antipsychotics in treating patients with ND-PAE/FASD really began as a counterintuitive research finding when positive outcomes in social skills were found in those treated with risperidone and olanzapine (Frankel et al. 2006). The outcome was better for the patients taking antipsychotics alone than for those taking stimulants alone or both stimulants and antipsychotics. Consequently, the addition of risperidone in a case series of patients taking several medications produced clinical improvement in behavioral symptoms (Ozsarfati and Koren 2015). In other childhood developmental disorders, such as conduct disorder, ADHD, and autism spectrum disorder, combining an antipsychotic with stimulants (Knecht et al. 2015) produced additive benefits and modulated behavioral problems in several studies. Effective responses were obtained with olanzapine and risperidone in those with the consequences of PAE in improving social skills functioning, reducing short-term aggressiveness, and treating features of conduct disorder, which are the specific challenges that also interfere with other treatments. Most of the studies reported were carried out in young people (Knecht et al. 2015; Ozsarfati and Koren 2015). It is not clear how adults will respond, given the increasing functional deficit with age and additional comorbid difficulties. A case series of two patients showed significant changes in psychotic symptoms among patients with ND-PAE/FASD who were treated with clozapine. Monitoring is crucial and must be done proactively. The quality of psychotic symptoms can be distressing, and with their poor coping resources, patients may be more sensitive to feeling overwhelmed in managing symptoms to improve function.

Antidepressants studied in a few patients effectively produced positive responses by reducing depressed mood. For instance, in a retrospective trial of 11 patients treated with sertraline, 82% of patients showed "marked improvement" (Coe et al. 2001; Mela et al. 2018, 2019). Mood stabilizers (carbamazepine, valproate sodium, and oxcarbazepine) were reported as useful in patients with mood dysregulation and for some with seizure disorders.

Researchers have suggested that, with adequate funding, the norepinephrine reuptake inhibitors atomoxetine and reboxetine should be evaluated, given their receptor-reactivity profile. Findings from these studies will expand the knowledge of these medications' mechanisms of action and enhance the incorporation of psychotropic medications into ND-PAE/FASD treatment.

Dosing of Psychotropic Medications in ND-PAE/FASD

In determining the exact dosage needed to treat a patient with ND-PAE/FASD, prescribers should consult the prescribing guidelines for their jurisdiction. The compendium for pharmaceutical specialties provides a range of dosages for the different medications but no dosing indication approved by licensing agents. Worldwide, these agencies, such as the U.S. Food and Drug Administration, approve and monitor the efficacy and safety of medications. Prescribers should, therefore, be acquainted with the validated and approved dosages of each of the psychotropic medications according to their jurisdiction's national or local formulary. The British National Formulary and the U.S. Pharmacopeia National Formulary are examples of such resources. For those with a history of medication sensitivity or those naïve to psychotropic medications, a safer lower-dosage (one-half or one-third of the recommended dosage) approach should be considered and offered. For instance, in the use of sertraline for an adult patient with major depression in the context of PAE, a dosage of 25–50 mg should be initiated and titrated up.

Once prescribed, the focus of care then shifts to regular assessment of the drug's effects—benefits and adverse events—from several sources, including close family members. If the patient is determined to be intolerant, the medication can be discontinued or the dosage decreased to manage the adverse reactions from the offending medications. Depending on the available support, a patient may receive an increased dosage once tolerance to the side effects is achieved and some benefit is registered with the medication. As suggested for developmental disorders, the approach of *target dosing*, in which a particular dosage of medication guides prescription, is inappropriate for those with ND-PAE/FASD. Instead, the clinician from initiation stage onward should regularly and frequently appraise the risk-benefit ratio of the medication. This will determine whether it is adjusted, continued at the same dosage, or discontinued for a different medication (Ji and Findling 2016). This is an example of when the importance of involving the pharmacist becomes crucial.

Future Use of Psychotropic Drugs

Medications with mind-altering effects are indicated for the comorbid mental conditions or other symptom clusters common in ND-PAE/FASD. Stimulants and other psychotropic medications have yielded a level of evidence sufficient to recommend the development of a decision tree. Instead of the algorithm being definitive for practice, the level of evidence supports use of the algorithm for gathering data on efficacy. For treatments to be effective, they should have specific molecular or neurobiological targets. This will, it is hoped, develop with better characterization of the comorbid conditions. Such profiles should be shaped by epigenetic findings that uncover therapeutic targets. The future choice of psychotropic medications for use in those with ND-PAE/FASD will depend on the type and nature of outcomes algorithms yield in those treated in a semisystematic fashion.

Although not specifically pharmacological approaches, neurofeedback, repetitive transcranial magnetic stimulation, and deep cranial stimulation used to achieve neuromodulation are being heralded as potential treatments for ND-PAE/FASD. Initially used to treat cortical excitability in seizure patients with FASD, repetitive transcranial magnetic stimulation can potentially increase nerve conductivity. A few protocols for studying its efficacy in the treatment of children with FASD have been proposed, and results are awaited.

Conclusion

The use of medications—intentionally, or perhaps, inadvertently—for those with ND-PAE/FASD has been around since the disorder was initially characterized. The principle of using ligands that are sensitive to neurotransmitter changes, based on the current level of PAE damage to neurotransmission, aligns with the like pathogenesis of other mental disorders for which similar reasoning occurs. At the current time, rational pharmacology focused on clusters of commonly inherited symptoms allows the addition of psychotropic medications and other nonpsychotropic medications for patients who preferably have received adequate psychosocial interventions. There is a definite need to use a decision tree approach in which a risk-benefit appraisal for prescribing, starting at a low dosage, is preferred over target dosing. Research is needed to identify better alignment of indicators and specific molecules for managing mental and dysfunctional presentations. As a last resort, medications complement existing strategies of building relationships, establishing realistic expectations, and responding to individual strengths to enhance function.

CLINICAL PRACTICAL APPLICATIONS

- Instead of achieving a required target dose, the risk-benefit ratio of the medication should guide dose adjustment in patients with ND-PAE/FASD (starting low and going slow).
- Clinicians should observe indications of impulsivity, risk taking, and executive dysfunction, which will affect prescribing practices.
- To support therapeutic collaboration during prescribing, interfering and destabilizing factors such as self-harm, substance use, and homelessness assume a clinical focus and significance.
- The pharmacist, by supporting efforts to enhance compliance, communication, and safe use of medications, becomes a vital member of the multidisciplinary team.
- Video testimonies of successful use of psychotropic medications can serve to enhance compliance in patients whose cognitive inflexibility affects their attitude toward medication use.
- Using a decision tree, taking into account the ligands responsive to psychotropic medications, should be considered for a staggered introduction of psychotropic medications.

References

Akison LK, Kuo J, Reid N, et al: Effect of choline supplementation on neurological, cognitive, and behavioral outcomes in offspring arising from alcohol exposure during development: a quantitative systematic review of clinical and preclinical studies. Alcohol Clin Exp Res 42(9):1591–1611, 2018

Calles JL, Jr: Use of psychotropic medications in children with developmental disabilities. Pediatr Clin North Am 55(5):1227–1240, 2008

Cheng Y, Wang X, Wei X, et al: Prenatal exposure to alcohol induces functional and structural plasticity in dopamine D1 receptor-expressing neurons of the dorsomedial striatum. Alcohol Clin Exp Res 42(8):1493–1502, 2018

Coe J, Sidders J, Riley K, et al: A survey of medication responses in children and adolescents with fetal alcohol syndrome. Mental Health Aspects of Developmental Disabilities 4(4):148–155, 2001

Coles CD, Gailey AR, Mulle JG, et al: A comparison among 5 methods for the clinical diagnosis of fetal alcohol spectrum disorders. Alcohol Clin Exp Res 40(5):1000–1009, 2016

Cook JL, Green CR, Lilley CM, et al: Fetal alcohol spectrum disorder: a guideline for diagnosis across the lifespan. CMAJ 188(3):191–197, 2016

Frankel F, Paley B, Marquardt R, O'Connor M: Stimulants, neuroleptics, and children's friendship training for children with fetal alcohol spectrum disorders. J Child Adolesc Psychopharmacol 16(6):777–789, 2006

Georgieff MK, Tran PV, Carlson ES: Atypical fetal development: fetal alcohol syndrome, nutritional deprivation, teratogens, and risk for neurodevelopmental disorders and psychopathology. Dev Psychopathol 30(3):1063–1086, 2018

Goh YI, Chudley AE, Clarren SK, et al: Development of Canadian screening tools for fetal alcohol spectrum disorder. Can J Clin Pharmacol 15(2):e344–e366, 2008

Grant TM, Brown NN, Graham JC, et al: Screening in treatment programs for fetal alcohol spectrum disorders that could affect therapeutic progress. Int J Alcohol Drug Res 2(3):37–49, 2013

Hanlon-Dearman A, Chen ML, Olson HC: Understanding and managing sleep disruption in children with fetal alcohol spectrum disorder. Biochem Cell Biol 96(2):267–274, 2018

Hosenbocus S, Chahal R: A review of executive function deficits and pharmacological management in children and adolescents. J Can Acad Child Adolesc Psychiatry 21(3):223–229, 2012

Ipsiroglu O, Berger M, Lin T, et al: Pathways to overmedication and polypharmacy: case examples from adolescents with fetal alcohol spectrum disorders, in The Science and Ethics of Antipsychotic Use in Children. Edited by Di Pietro N, Illes J. London, Elsevier, 2015, pp 125–148

Jacobson SW, Carter RC, Molteno CD, et al: Feasibility and acceptability of maternal choline supplementation in heavy drinking pregnant women: a randomized, double-blind, placebo-controlled clinical trial. Alcohol Clin Exp Res 42(7):1315–1326, 2018

Ji NY, Findling RL: Pharmacotherapy for mental health problems in people with intellectual disability. Curr Opin Psychiatry 29(2):103–125, 2016

Knecht C, de Alvaro R, Martinez-Raga J, Balanza-Martinez V: Attention-deficit hyperactivity disorder (ADHD), substance use disorders, and criminality: a difficult problem with complex solutions. Int J Adolesc Med Health 27(2):163–175, 2015

Mela M, Okpalauwaekwe U, Anderson T, et al: The utility of psychotropic drugs on patients with fetal alcohol spectrum disorder (FASD): a systematic review. Psychiatry and Clinical Psychopharmacology 28(4):436–445, 2018

Mela M, Coons-Harding KD, Anderson T: Recent advances in fetal alcohol spectrum disorder for mental health professionals. Curr Opin Psychiatry 32(4):328–335, 2019

Oesterheld JR, Kofoed L, Tervo R, et al: Effectiveness of methylphenidate in native American children with fetal alcohol syndrome and attention deficit/hyperactivity disorder: a controlled pilot study. J Child Adolesc Psychopharmacol 8:39–48, 1998

O'Malley KD, Nanson J: Clinical implications of a link between fetal alcohol spectrum disorder and attention deficit hyperactivity disorder. Can J Psychiatry 47(4):349–354, 2002

Ozsarfati J, Koren G: Medications used in the treatment of disruptive behavior in children with FASD: a guide. J Popul Ther Clin Pharmacol 22(1):e59–e67, 2015

Patten AR, Fontaine CJ, Christie BR: A comparison of the different animal models of fetal alcohol spectrum disorders and their use in studying complex behaviors. Front Pediatr 2:93, 2014

Peadon E, Rhys-Jones B, Bower C, Elliott EJ: Systematic review of interventions for children with fetal alcohol spectrum disorders. BMC Pediatr 9:35, 2009

Price A, Cook PA, Norgate S, Mukherjee R: Prenatal alcohol exposure and traumatic childhood experiences: a systematic review. Neurosci Biobehav Rev 80:89–98, 2017

Snyder J, Nanson J, Snyder R, et al: A study of stimulant medication in children with FAS, in The Challenge of Fetal Alcohol Syndrome: Overcoming Secondary Disabilities. Seattle, WA, University of Washington Press, 1997, pp 64–77

Substance Abuse and Mental Health Services Administration: Addressing Fetal Alcohol Spectrum Disorders (FASD) (Treatment Improvement Protocol [TIP] Series 58, HHS Publ No SMA 13-4803). Rockville, MD, Substance Abuse and Mental Health Services Administration, 2014.

Totten M: Investigating the linkages between FASD, gangs, sexual exploitation and woman abuse in the Canadian Aboriginal population: a preliminary study. First Peoples Child Family Rev 5(2):9–22, 2010

Troesc M, Fukumizu M, Sallinen BJ, et al: Sleep fragmentation and evidence for sleep debt in alcohol-exposed infants. Early Hum Dev 84(9):577–585, 2008

Tryer P, Bateman A: Drug treatment of personality disorder. Advances in Psychiatric Treatment 10:389–398, 2004

Wills LM, Swift JO, Moller KT: Craniofacial syndrome and sleep disorders, in Sleep: A Comprehensive Handbook. Edited by Lee-Chiong TL. Hoboken, NJ, Wiley, 2006, pp 551–560

Wozniak JR, Fuglestad AJ, Eckerle JK, et al: Choline supplementation in children with fetal alcohol spectrum disorders: a randomized, double-blind, placebo-controlled trial. Am J Clin Nutr 102(5):1113–1125, 2015

CHAPTER 14

Psychological Treatment

WHAT TO KNOW

The variables associated with successful interventions are resilience, hope, and a willingness to change.

Psychological interventions, including trauma-informed care, counseling, individual therapy, and comprehensive support and supervision, are individualized and patient centered and involve multiple systems of care.

Generic or specialized centers for assessment and treatment of ND-PAE/FASD, begun mostly out of necessity, innovate to achieve the goal of addressing outcomes.

Psychological interventions adopt the principles of correcting deficits by initiating techniques that address affect regulation, executive dysfunction, and impulsivity in addition to providing practical support for the patient and caregivers.

Technology and computer-based interventions may transform the interventional approach for correcting diverse cognitive deficits.

For many individuals with deficits associated with PAE, outcomes are unfavorable. Not only have their deficits gone unrecognized by mental health clinicians with whom they have interacted, they have been subjected to unproven psychological interventions. The mental health system provides, especially in the case of adults, unmodified treatments that have been adopted from other disorders or treatment for comorbid conditions. Because of the previous lack of diagnostic classification to specify the consequences of PAE, associated symptoms are attributed to diagnosable mental disorders, which are assumed to be primary. Informed clinicians who employ psychological interventions recognize the long-term consequences of PAE and, because they are aware of the neurocognitive deficits, aim to remedy those or modify their approaches to accommodate those deficits. The ultimate goal is to improve function and rehabilitate patients diagnosed with the consequences of PAE. By providing appropriate care, the PAE-informed mental health professional becomes a potent catalyst for achieving this goal.

In this chapter, I adopt principles necessary for incorporating existing and emerging innovative treatments that benefit patients. The discussion stresses the relevance of preventing harm to the patient caused by a lack of awareness of deficits and nonmodification of techniques. Individual patient-centered approaches that apply general, yet particularly relevant, interventions are gaining ground in the field. One section in this chapter describes treatments developed for and especially applicable to children and adolescents with ND-PAE/FASD. Technology is having an impact on new treatments, and so research findings are presented on existing computer gaming and video treatments.

Principles of Psychological Interventions

The neurocognitive deficits of PAE and psychosocial factors in the individual inform the development of effective treatments. For psychological interventions to be effective, patients should be competent in the language of instruction, capable of information recall, and proficient in implementing learned information and strategies. With sufficient capacity, the affected person is then able to implement the concepts of therapy and generalize them to other relevant settings. These psychological interventions are much needed for patients and families, but their process, content, acquisition, and success are limited by deficits in cognitive functions (Pei et al. 2016). For that reason, a number of principles guide interventions, and clinicians are better placed to assist patients if they adhere to those.

Recognition of the existence of neurocognitive deficits in settings outside the field of developmental disorder requires a heightened level of suspicion to identify signals that point to PAE. On the basis of these signals, clinicians should request a complete assessment of the extent of cognitive deficits and strengths in the individual. With or without such a wealth of information, which usually supports the treatment plan, the patient's abilities are best aligned with realistic and modified expectations. Approaches to learning, whether academic or skill-based, are best provided as simplified and within a strength-based structure, which includes support and supervision. The method of supervision, usually termed mentoring, facilitates self-direction and enhances the safety of the individual and those in the circle of influence. Research has uncovered the positive role of the informed mentor and therapist, which is realized when the individual's willingness to change is recognized, hope is instilled, and resilience is reinforced (Pei et al. 2016). Although not exactly researched in PAE, *scaffolding*, in which the support person is with the patient during a task, offering assistance as needed, and gradually withdraws only as the patient progressively shows independence, is indicated for this strength-based approach.

Although these principles are general and applied to most interactions of mental health professionals with different age groups of patients, a few factors are identified as pertinent to special populations. Some of these factors are derived from findings of surveys involving mothers raising children, adult women with substance use disorders (Rutman 2016), and offenders in the community (Pei et al. 2016; Tait et al. 2017). For instance, by recognizing the high level of trauma in substance-using and cognitively impaired women, patient-centered accommodations based on principles of safety and relationship were recommended as foundational to successful intervention. Modifications are based on the disability identified. Nonjudgmental communication and stigma-reducing first-person language are a few of the recognized approaches (Rutman 2013). Individualized and flexible approaches are needed, especially in programs where group therapy is the mainstay of treatment. During individual skills training sessions, therapists should follow up to check for real understanding of the concepts presented in the group setting. Overall, these principles combine research findings and expertise in the field to propose interventions relevant to the goals collaboratively set by the clinician and patient to achieve maximum functioning in various settings. This assessment of learning pervades all aspects of communication with the patient.

Considerations for Service Delivery

With more than 90% of individuals with FASD reported to have a concurrent mental disorder, approaches involving mental health interventions are inevitable. However, the application of these traditional interventions, unmodified, is frequently unsuccessful or even harmful (Anderson et al. 2020; Tait et al. 2017). The observed negative outcomes of criminal involvement, suicide, and a shortened life expectancy have been documented and stem from gaps in care. The appropriate care needed by patients should be consistent with the identified deficits and be responsive to the vulnerability of those at the interface of ND-PAE/FASD and mental disorder.

Delivering representative and optimal care to individuals affected by the adverse consequences of PAE requires a systematic approach. Highly specialized service models with experts in comprehensive assessments and intervention for individuals with PAE are few. To respond at a supportive level for the large number of affected patients, the mental health system should innovate to provide services tailored to PAE treatment; these could be an add-on highly specialized service or one complementary to the general mental health system. Patients formally diagnosed with ND-PAE/FASD traverse general health services and general mental health and addiction services. They are expected to be overrepresented in child, adolescent, and forensic mental health services. A lifespan approach also means that clinical offerings must address variations in age, gender, and culture and supply specific psychological interventions directed at different groups of patients.

Interventions are determined by the mode and severity of the clinical features, deficits, and adverse consequences. Interventions also depend on the ancillary care needs and the location of patients, whether they are in an ambulatory, residential, or institutional setting. In severe life-threatening cases, institution-based patient care in general, specialty (child and adolescent, liaison, and forensic), or rehabilitation facilities is needed. The acute services in a hospital, for instance, deliver care with the objective of the patient moving from the most intense service, transitioning through intermediary steps, and settling in a rehabilitation service preferably in the community. Transitions across developmental ages and from institution-based care are recognized pressure points that the system needs to respond to in order to support the patients' trajectories (Brown et al. 2012).

The recommended services for patients with ND-PAE/FASD incorporate existing evidence and common expert practice. Combining the two approaches offers the best patient benefit. To intervene psychologically and select and support the most appropriate care, clinicians need knowledge of the patient's circumstances. Practice-based approaches with emerging evidence include trauma-informed care, counseling, individual therapy, and comprehensive support and supervision. These essential components of intervention also have a preventive role when together they reduce negative outcomes (Rutman 2016). Furthermore, interventions that embrace harm reduction principles or actively enhance improvement in symptoms and function are psychologically aligned with the recognized deficits of PAE. To offer specific psychotherapy and counseling, therapists rely on the patient's extent of verbal expression and communication when choosing a therapy model. Thus, special attention should be paid to ensure adequate exchange of information and understanding. Group therapy is rarely the most desirable option given the complexity and variation of abilities.

Models of Assessment and Intervention Clinics

ND-PAE/FASD is multifaceted; thus, treatment should be patient centered and individualized and involve multiprofessional and multisystem pathways. Uniquely to individuals with neurocognitive manifestations, the identification, assessment, and diagnosis occur in a variety of settings by multiple professionals at different levels of expertise. Identification and assessment form the essential diagnostic process, which also assumes a significant therapeutic role. This role begins with a fuller understanding of the person when deficits are adequately evaluated. The development of a few clinics provides a framework for others to consider in their jurisdictions about how best to introduce psychological intervention. The secret for any successful delivery of services includes collaboration between relevant stakeholders and data-driven intervention with evaluation and funding support.

A pilot project was initiated following the experience of a clinical team with diagnosing and supporting a few individual patients. This developed from the strong and fruitful collaboration between the interested health professionals and members of an FASD advocacy group in the community, which led to a grant application. A 3-year grant supported the development of services to assess and diagnose more adult patients. Through evaluation of the project, some challenges with the process were recognized. How to identify the right professionals with the right expertise to diagnose adults and what to do considering the developmental disability of diagnosed individuals when it comes to treatment were among the challenges. Insufficient training on aspects of developmental disorder, especially from PAE, was noted as an impediment to the applied intervention (Olson et al. 2009). To intervene, diagnosis was needed, but this turned out to be more complicated than diagnosing and intervening with children. Adults were identified by a mosaic of social issues. There were increased reports of traumatic head injury, alcohol and drug use, and justice-related and mental health problems. Teams desiring to initiate an intervention service should carefully consider the challenges frequently encountered. These should be guideposts for navigating obstacles to care and supportive clinical pathways (Anderson et al. 2020).

Understanding the disability and reframing the patient's behavior and treatment informed by this understanding are essential to supporting psychological approaches. Adult brain-based behavior without that understanding can be misconstrued as resistance, denial, noncompliance, and acting out or as features associated with personality disorders. In a helpful replacement interpretation, statements were suggested in place of common misconceptions of brain-based deficits. In place of viewing the patient as lazy, not trying, and not caring, clinicians may choose to adopt the view that a patient affected by negative outcomes of PAE was indeed trying hard and was tired of failing but unable to show the requisite feelings. This might involve an assumption that the patient's *won't* is better viewed as a *can't*. A clinician in a countertransference state of assuming "the patient is trying to irritate" might alter his or her view and see the patient as having difficulties remembering (Grant et al. 2013; Rutman 2016).

When interventions are modified to suit patients' specific situations, they find it easier to accept and use the strategies. Treatment progress is achieved by adopting a positive reinforcement perspective. Attendance may be enhanced if incentives fit with the patients' desires and interests. Patients require a structured routine that fits their schedule. When schedule disruptions are reduced, anticipated, and better predicted, the irritating misbehaviors associated with such changes are minimized. Patients are supported and learn to negotiate and cope better with change. Clinicians should recognize that memory problems, poor organization, and poor planning, combined with time pressure, contribute to patients' obvious dysfunction. Any psychological intervention should recognize that PAE causes slow information processing. To overcome that, the clinician should learn a helpful strategy to apply in any interaction: When a patient is given information and is expected to respond or make a decision, the informed clinician intentionally guides the patient to take time to contemplate and analyze the information. This will prevent making a hasty decision when the information has not even been comprehended. The resulting benefits are reduced anger, improved patience, and adequate use of time, which are helpful and assist the patient in replicating and generalizing learned skills and strategies. This strategy arises from the clinician's knowledge of brain-based deficits (Rutman 2016).

Repetition of skill-based learning and pictorial representations are great accommodations for the person with PAE. Reality-based or personal examples rather than abstract concepts also facilitate knowledge acquisition and practice. Instead of being asked to add numbers, the patient can be asked to calculate the sum of real-life examples, such as monetary items. The patient can choose items from an advertising flyer, for example, and calculate their total cost rather than laboring over addition worksheets.

Court diversion in youth and adults and interventions in children's mental health and education engagement follow the establishment of diagnostic services. The evaluation component allows research findings to inform service development. Given that resources remain scarce, grant funding and using a pilot model are currently the most successful approaches for most services. In one study, a group of legal practitioners and community advocates collaborated to initiate an intervention for those with ND-PAE/FASD in the court system. Both youth in another province and children in a university teaching hospital received care based on models developed on the tenets of community mobilization, collaboration, and alternative arrangements that are less dependent on government funding (Coles et al. 2018; Flannigan et al. 2018; Longstaffe et al. 2018).

Existing Types of Services for ND-PAE/FASD

The FAS Diagnostic and Prevention Network began in 1993 as a single clinic in Seattle, Washington, sponsored by the Centers for Disease Control and Prevention to manage patients with PAE. Following the clinical description of FAS, a multidisciplinary team comprising pediatricians, social workers, and psychologists began the task of providing a range of services. Clinics have expanded across the state; they involve the screening, diagnosing, surveilling, intervening, preventing, and training aspects of the consequences of PAE. Through a network of clinics supported by legislation and funding, this specialized project diagnosed by far the largest number of patients with FASD (3,000). The diagnostic process is standardized using the four-digit code (Astley and Clarren 2000). Evaluation of the project came in the form of research studies, cost analysis, and, recently, genetic studies (Hemingway et al. 2018). Other services have arisen from funded research projects. The Collaborative Initiative on Fetal Alcohol Spectrum Disorders provides high-quality research findings from a service delivery model. The model of clinical research allows hypothesis generation and examines the effectiveness of interventions (Mattson et al. 2010).

Services for Children and Adolescents

Most FASD diagnostic clinics focus on children and adolescents. The level of specialization varies by jurisdiction and expertise. Diagnosis of and intervention with neonates and preschool-age children form part of a mandate from the Centers for Disease Control and Prevention at the Emory Neurodevelopment and Exposure Clinic in Atlanta, Georgia. This clinic treats children as young as those in the neonatal period. Services evolved initially from a primarily PAE-related diagnostic clinic (Fetal Alcohol and Drug Exposure Clinic); currently, children from birth through 21 years are served. The services are directed to patients with a history of prenatal exposure to alcohol, drugs, and other substances. Operated by members of a multidisciplinary team, genetic, neurodevelopmental, and psychological testing, as well as intervention and research, are core activities of this academic center.

In another child diagnostic center, a list of recommendations for those diagnosed with FASD was compared with a list for those not diagnosed. The older the child, the more likely mental health interventions were to be recommended. The research was also helpful because it identified education, anticipatory guidance, family support, and safety as the core recommendations given to those diagnosed (Pei et al. 2017). Individual patients are best served in clinical models where meaningful recommendations accompany the multidisciplinary efforts and form the basis for psychological interventions, such as provision of mental health, addiction, and counseling services. Social interventions addressing concerns such as housing, mentoring, employment, and financial support are also contained in the practical recommendations.

FASD Diagnostic Center

Most children diagnosed with FASD receive assessment, diagnosis, and some support services in specialized diagnostic centers. Some are located as stand-alone clinics, whereas others are part of existing child and adolescent services. Tool kits have been developed to facilitate recognition and management of ND-PAE/FASD. Adult diagnosis is relatively new, becoming established almost a decade after child diagnostic clinics were established. Some clinics have evolved and are responsible for all ages of individuals throughout the lifespan. Other clinics start as child-only diagnostic clinics, but out of necessity, they branch out into adult diagnosis. The number of clinics specialized in diagnosing adults is increasing, and unique findings related to adults are being discovered. The range of interventions varies by jurisdiction and expertise. In a rural setting, diagnosis, special intervention, quality assurance, and support services have expanded over the two decades (McFarlane 2011). As mentioned, unique research findings among adults with mental health symptoms in a clinic were reported (Pei et al. 2017). These results inform the kinds of interventions available to patients. An example of specialized intervention may be legal in nature, such as a group of experts undertaking a special assessment of individuals on death row. Although assessment focused, the recommendations of these FASD experts have been influential in revoking some death sentences of inmates with FASD (Brown et al. 2018).

In 2017, an FASD-specific diagnostic service for adults was established. The LVR clinic, established at the Department of Psychiatry and Psychotherapy, is part of the hospital of the University of Duisburg-Essen in Essen, Germany. Results from the clinic have provided a unique perspective, including the use of psychiatric instruments of assessment. The impact on policy can be appreciated because these findings, if replicated, can be compared with other clinics in other regions and could help determine assessment standards. Economic costs are important, because a sustainable service means patients have access to intervention strategies. It is conceivable that many clinics may be initiated if the process, economic, and intervention outcomes serve as the impetus for other jurisdictions to emulate the steps required to actualize clinic development and advance interventions. There is some evidence that by having many such centers collecting the same clinical information, large databases of information on ND-PAE/FASD assessment and intervention will shape research and practice. In turn, the search for diagnostic standardization is more likely and so is standardized intervention. Equally important, standard treatment protocols can be developed and evaluated. These are essential for outcome-based treatment improvement.

Clinical Vignette

A female student at a local university is referred to a clinic because she is failing her first-year courses. Her psychological assessment shows a deficit in executive function, which translates into significant difficulties with finishing tasks. Her language, memory, and attention domains are equally impaired, and along with a confirmed history of PAE, she is diagnosed with ND-PAE/FASD. She is behind in her work, and despite threats to withdraw from courses, she demonstrates no changes. In therapy, she insists that she will not take any medications. As a teenager she was treated involuntarily with haloperidol injection because she was in an agitated state and uncontrollable, and she developed significant painful dystonia and severe akathisia as a result.

The patient's current treatment includes sleep hygiene to support learning and concentration in the classroom. To improve her functioning, it is essential that she receive accommodations in school. The case manager calls the university's office for student accommodation for advice on how to support the patient. The essential component of the treatment strategy is the process of analyzing a number of steps. Figure 14–1 shows the progression of thinking and actions that can directly support the patient. Stage I calls for a high index of suspicion. In Stage II, the case manager should ensure that all strategies to obtain a comprehensive assessment lead to actions known to help patients, such as realistic expectations (Stage III) and support and supervision (Stage IV).

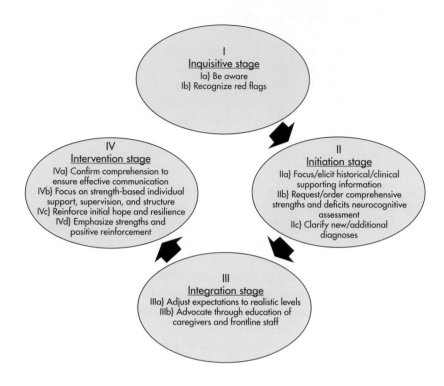

FIGURE 14–1. Essence of treatment modification.

Psychological Interventions and Strategies

Individual strategies to enhance positive outcomes are the mainstay of intervention in PAE and its mental disorder consequences. Attending to the social environment and supporting individual functioning and capacity are part of the requisite biopsychosocial treatment. In planning treatment, the goal, outcome, and prognosis are linked to understanding the extent of the disorder. This is achieved with adequate and comprehensive assessment. The outcome of the assessment is a list of recommendations proposed to address the identified deficits. These recommendations also identify targets for intervention that in turn should be efficacious and cost-effective. Diagnosis as intervention is a well-known concept that implies that the diagnostic process unveils important treatment targets and hidden deficits. Ideally, these deficits, although current, should previously have been identified and corrected. Intervention for cancer serves as one comparative example to understand the strategies for intervention. Cancer treatments incorporate the essential deficits of the disease state, e.g., type of cancer, stage and spread of the disease, target of treatment, and known response; these essentials inform treatment. Similarly, knowing the types of neurocognitive deficits, current comorbid conditions, and targets for intervention in FASD, revealed via the diagnostic process, are essential for effective interventions.

For the intervention to be most effective, goals are set. This involves minimizing the discrepancy between the patient's ability and the therapist's expectations. Proper diagnosis provides the correct level of realistic and modified expectations. The deficits identified through the diagnosis are the guidepost to apply strength-based interventions. If strength-based interventions are uniformly taught and applied, therapists will develop effective means of helping patients. Beyond symptoms, wider psychosocial correlates are targeted for intervention. From a psychological perspective, treatment targets are wider, involving factors that range from solutions to decrease criminal involvement to solutions for improving positive outcomes. Varied outcomes were reported in a number of research studies. For instance, in a socialization research paradigm, improved self-esteem was demonstrated among indigenous youth following a theater arts program. Increased school participation, enhanced reading ability, curtailed addictions, targeted mental health interventions, and instilled hope and resilience fostered by spiritual and cultural endowment have also been reported (Keightley et al. 2018; Pei et al. 2016) as aligning with psychological interventions.

Communication Specific to Psychological Intervention

The backbone of the therapeutic alliance—through which interventions are formulated and delivered—is communication. The recognized communication deficits of individuals with PAE arise from a combination of the various effects and weights of receptive language, expressive language, inattention, and memory problems. Varied manifestations occur, but most times, the picture of ND-PAE/FASD is complex (Proven et al. 2014). Recognizing these communication problems, information must be presented as simple, concrete, and easy to follow. Impaired individuals need skills to help manage the quantity of sentences at rates that can be better understood. Without such skills, benefits are lost even at counseling sessions because the patient is unable to assimilate the information presented verbally. Well-developed interventions focus on improving memory so patients are not left trying to fill their memory gaps with fabrications. By understanding the neurocognitive diversity of patients, therapists intervene with strategies intended to allow the individual patient sufficient time for decision making and to reduce distractions in the patient's surroundings. Such approaches represent a valid modification to correct identified deficits in the speed of information processing and in intellectual prowess. They promote assimilation of information in counseling or psychotherapy. Real understanding in the context of communication cannot be premised on the mistaken assumption that an impaired person, who says the information was understood, actually did understand. Low self-esteem and not wanting to look stupid are explanations of why miscommunication is frequent (Grant et al. 2013). To support the patient and guarantee understanding, a gentle and tactical evaluation of communication is required. Without embarrassing the impaired individual, the therapist can request that the individual explain in his or her own words what he or she understood from what was spoken. Patients who can adequately explain what was said from their own perspective demonstrate better and enhanced comprehension.

Communication is a two-way process. Supporting comprehension minimizes misunderstanding. As a result, instructions, information, and suggestions in therapy are applied and so better optimized. Other benefits for the patient, and the intervention method, are supporting the cognitive exercises of shifting, balancing, and comparing information. Only with the proper handling of information, including analysis, will patients be better able to make informed decisions and self-regulate behavior. These prosocial qualities depend on supported communication skills (Brown et al. 2012).

Informal Methods of Communication

Informal methods are available such that the learning environment cues particular responses. Therapy can take place while walking with patients or completing a task, such as gardening. This removes the perception of a classroom and makes it less likely that patients will be bothered by being thought of as stupid, thus perpetuating a self-fulfilling prophecy. As the saying goes, some patients, like some youth, believe it is better to be "bad" than "stupid." The advantage of the nonstructured environment for learning is that it serves other nonformal intervention purposes also. Patients use natural surroundings like gardens for grounding in affect regulation relating to trauma intervention. They often communicate more freely without the exigencies of classroom rules.

Family Intervention Programs

The family intervention approach began with the evaluation of the role of the family in the outcomes of children diagnosed with ND-PAE/FASD. Aspects of the caregiving environment and family function were extracted and integrated to develop the framework necessary to enhance elements of care for the child and the caregivers. Early in the establishment of the family intervention approach, it was recognized that the adoption of a lifelong perspective in support of developmental and family management was relevant for future positive impact.

The coaching program is an example of an intervention for caregivers and families. The essential components involve mentoring, teaching about FASD, and educating families about accessible resources. In evaluating the effectiveness of this program, researchers identified some psychological benefits. Participants experienced reduced caregiver stress, achieved goals, and were more satisfied. These benefits also had positive ripple effects on the diagnosed children.

Traditional family intervention approaches found to be effective in mental health practice can be modified and adopted for patients with PAE and its effects. In addition to education, family training and specific stress-reducing approaches will benefit children and adults. *Expressed emotion*, defined by its characteristic attitudes of excessive criticism, hostility, and emotional overinvolvement of the patient's family and caregivers, is best viewed as a toxic factor in the patient's care. Interventions that ameliorate expressed emotion have the potential to enhance more positive outcomes. It follows that patients with ND-PAE/FASD and their families and caregivers need this psychological intervention. Research is still needed to more reliably evaluate this strategy.

Multicomponent interventions, comprising in-house parental behavioral training with sessions targeting behavior problems of the child, have been systematically studied. Positive outcomes in the child specifically related to emotion regulation, self-esteem, and anxiety and improvement of parenting efficacy were found.

Enhancing Protective Factors

Psychologically addressing the influences likely to produce negative outcomes can be viewed as a form of intervention. Approaches for reducing harm include management of parental substance use and the levels of violence in the household. In essence, focusing on the negative effect of poor social determinants of health is a necessary treatment approach. Childrearing practices should be acknowledged and matched with the needs of the child. Early diagnosis and the creation of a nurturing, stable, stimulating, and structured childrearing environment are factors that enhance positive outcomes. Adequate nutrition and an enriched environment for the child with ND-PAE/FASD have been associated with improved results and fall within the recommended types of psychological interventions.

Preventive Psychological Treatment

The role of psychological interventions in reducing harm to the fetus cannot be overemphasized. Genetic, familial, cultural, and relational factors contribute to women drinking alcohol during pregnancy (Coons 2013). Mothers who drink during pregnancy have been shown to have more adverse life experiences predisposing them to major mental disorders. A majority were found to have been victims of sexual abuse and to have high rates of mental disorders (Astley et al. 2000). Active case finding and planned interventions have potential positive preventive benefits. Astley et al. (2000) stated the following: "A FAS diagnostic and prevention clinic can be used to identify women at high risk for producing children damaged by prenatal alcohol exposure. Primary prevention programs targeted to this population could lead to measurable reductions in the incidence of FAS" (p. 509). Prevention of perinatal depression has received attention in this regard. After reviewing the risks and benefits of psychological service–based and pharmacological interventions, referral to and provision of counseling in the form of cognitive-behavioral therapy and interpersonal therapy were judged beneficial to women with current or at high risk of developing perinatal depressive conditions (U.S. Preventive Services Task Force 2019).

Recommendations of counseling interventions for perinatal depression can be applied to women with a high risk of perinatal alcohol consumption. No current accurate screening tools exist to identify such women, but evidence shows that the risk of developing perinatal depression, which occurs in one out of seven women, is associated with long- and short-term negative consequences and bears resemblance to the risk factors for women drinking during pregnancy. The risk factors associated with perinatal depression reported by the U.S. Preventive Services Task Force (2019) are

> personal or family history of depression, history of physical or sexual abuse, having an unplanned or unwanted pregnancy, current stressful life events, pregestational or gestational diabetes, and complications during pregnancy (e.g., preterm delivery or pregnancy loss). In addition, social factors such as low socioeconomic status, lack of social or financial support, and adolescent parenthood have also been shown to increase the risk of developing perinatal depression." The U.S. Preventive Services Task Force 2019 found limited or mixed evidence that other studied interventions such as physical activity, education, pharmacotherapy, dietary supplements, and health system interventions were effective in preventing perinatal depression. (p. 582)

Essentially, intervening at the maternal prepregnancy and pregnancy stages makes a lot of psychological sense for the development of a prospective offspring. Efforts to identify at-risk women and to intervene may not exactly be a treatment for the consequences of PAE, but much depends on these approaches to protect fetuses and prevent negative outcomes. In a study of a group of high-risk women, in which women with the consequences of PAE were overrepresented, this approach was clinically useful (Astley et al. 2000; Velasquez et al. 2013).

Psychological Modification

Functional improvement in ND-PAE/FASD depends on interventions that target specific deficits or apply traditional interventions in modified and cognitively flexible approaches. Potential successful outcomes are limited if all neurocognitive deficits are not elicited through comprehensive assessment. Positive outcomes are better aligned with interventions that adopt a lifespan perspective, from childhood to the elderly phase of life.

Specific Treatment for Neurocognitive Deficits

Among the many brain domain deficits, a few are amenable to direct intervention related to PAE damage. Self-regulation, executive function, and impulse control are a few treatment targets for which interventions have been developed. Although piloted and studied in populations initially diagnosed with ND-PAE/FASD, it is safe to propose that, given the trajectory of those with consequences of PAE in developing mental disorder, there is a positive mental health role for these interventions.

Alert is a program that teaches the affected patient self-regulation skills. Patients are taught to categorize arousal at three levels (high gear, low gear, and just right), based on the vestibular and somatosensory systems that control self-regulation. They use five modalities (looking, touching, moving, listening, and putting something in the mouth) to shift and control their level of arousal. Neurobehavioral outcomes that were improved by the program in controlled studies included organization, metacognition, naming, and affect recognition (Wells et al. 2012). Targeted emotional problem-solving skills are among the best results of Alert. A posttreatment MRI study (Soh et al. 2015) also found increases in brain grey matter after 12 weeks of Alert treatment. Larger studies (Kapasi et al. 2020; Layer and Benson 2020) have been conducted in schools and child clinics, with improvement shown in neurocognitive deficits. The effectiveness of the Alert treatment for FASD was further supported when a randomized control trial compared treated 8- to 12-year-olds with a wait-list control group (Nash et al. 2018). Alert improved functional integrity in the neural circuitry for behavioral regulation in children with FASD. Using functional MRI, the treatment group showed posttreatment changes in the prefrontal, temporal, and cingulate regions (Nash et al. 2018). Studies like these need additional replication to illuminate the direction of interventions with high neurocognitive domain specificity.

MILE, or Math Interactive Learning Experience, recognizes the math deficits in the academic achievement problems associated with ND-PAE/FASD and is a manualized program for young children, their parents, and teachers. Comparison with control subjects (e.g., for 6 weeks of individual graphomotor [handwriting] skills) showed significant benefits for MILE (Coles et al. 2009). This was replicated in 4- to 10-year-olds in a different context, and significantly greater changes in math achievement again were recorded compared with the contrast group (Kully-Martens et al. 2018).

A treatment target in a complex multifaceted disorder such as ND-PAE/FASD requires a combined metacognitive strategy addressing several cognitive domains. The manualized intervention GoFAR (focus and plan, act, and reflect) was developed for that purpose. GoFAR targets the domains of problem solving, behavior control, attention, and adaptive function. This approach meets the integrative framework recommendation for comorbid disorders in ND-PAE/FASD. Because mental health clinicians are able to administer the program, it is accessible for their comorbid patients. These domains are directly related to PAE. So far, the results from a number of studies have shown benefits in improved daily skills and behavior. Evidence now includes randomized controlled studies. Researchers found improved metacognition in attention, adaptive, and behavior domains among GoFAR subjects who also showed improved effortful control of behavior (Coles et al. 2015, 2018; Kable et al. 2016; Nash et al. 2015, 2018; Soh et al. 2015). GoFAR has repeatedly shown advantages in participant self-regulation (Coles et al. 2018).

The Parent-Child Assistance Program (PCAP) is a mentoring/case management and professional training program. It is conceptualized as an adjunctive intervention in other social and health care sectors, but this program is directly applicable and essential in ND-PAE/FASD treatment. In PCAP, the at-risk mother is matched with an experienced staff member for a protracted period (2–3 years). Positive outcomes have been reported in both child and mother (POOLE). PCAP also helped prevent mothers from having additional offspring with ND-PAE/FASD. Mental health professionals regularly encounter disenfranchised and vulnerable pregnant alcohol- and substance-using mothers in their practice. This presents an opportunity to promote appropriate intervention for those high-risk, difficult-to-engage mothers. PCAP is highly effective (Denys et al. 2011).

Supportive and Daily Skills Training

When the goal is to help delay the speed of responding without thinking, instruction through pictorial representation and roleplay should be considered to guide psychological interventions. Patients able to understand are taken through various scenarios and questioned about how they would react. The counseling sessions encourage patients to apply the colors of the traffic light as reminders for controlling impulsive acts. "Driving" through life, the patient is shown how a decision is made as the "car of issues" approaches a light. The first act is to stop (as with a red light) all activities occasioned by issues pushing for a decision. Instructions are given to inhibit responses during this stage. The yellow light is imagined as a contemplative phase in which the patient considers various possible actions he or she may take. This stage should prompt the generation of many options for dealing with the problem at hand. Usually, over the waiting period of seconds or minutes, the patient is instructed to generate options in preparation for acting on one of them. The patient is encouraged after some time has elapsed to decide on the most reasonable option just as the imagined traffic light turns to green. The idea is that action is permitted only after thoughtful consideration rather than on impulse.

These decision scenarios are presented during the session, and the three-component traffic light model is rehearsed. A past impulsive act with negative outcome is reconstructed and discussed. As an example, a probation officer denies a patient's request to stay out past curfew to visit her boyfriend, who is leaving the city for a 6-month mission trip. Because her boyfriend's departure is set for the next day, she wants to spend time past curfew with him. In the past, an immediate disagreement with the parole officer would lead to assuming the risk of going without permission, staying out past the curfew, and damning the consequences. During the counseling session, cognizant of her PAE-related neurocognitive deficits, the parole officer's denial is equated with a stress that calls for a decision. The patient is then encouraged to imagine the red light that comes on. This signals stop; all responses cease for a while. The next stage to consider is the yellow light zone in which the patient is encouraged to generate possible ways for dealing with the impasse with the parole officer. With the guidance of the clinician, the patient can consider a range of actions: asking if the boyfriend can come to see her instead; asking to speak to the officer's supervisor; viewing 6 months as easily passable and staying put; or electing to go, bearing the consequences of violating a condition of probation and challenging the decision of the authorities. Finally, the patient imagines the green light as she chooses what action to take, based on a well-thought-out decision exempt from impulsivity.

During that roleplay of scenarios and examples of challenges, the patient's emotions are closely observed and identified by the clinician. Another critical intervention is to teach the patient how to identify specific emotions. This is relevant, given the poor emotional control described in those with PAE. By understanding the specific emotions experienced, the patient learns how to exert control by distraction, catharsis, and acceptance. The ability to control emotions is greatly needed for such confrontational interactions; otherwise, any irrational response has multiple layers of consequences, ones that the patient's cognitive deficits prevent him or her from understanding or accepting. Helping the patient identify the emotions being experienced reduces confusion over emotion types. Identifying the correct affect (e.g., anxiety, sadness, anger, irritation) will facilitate the patient's adoption of interventions for emotional control. Visual images displaying different emotions have been used to train cognitively impaired individuals about the classification and meaning of specific emotional experiences and how to respond to them.

Patients struggling with task initiation and planning also receive instructions and roleplay, based on a list of identified personal strengths and weaknesses. In planning to successfully complete a task, a list of the steps in the process should be generated by the clinician and patient. They should be broken up into manageable steps to engender confidence in initiating and completing those steps. Obstacles to getting started and persevering should be listed and strategies to overcome them stated. Patients should be given guidance on deciding when to initiate the chosen action in order to overcome procrastination and poor task completion. Self-evaluation minimizes frustration because patients are guided to align expectations with their actual abilities. Praise and encouragement are essential elements that support successful initiation and planning strategies. Acknowledging something constructive and incorporating humor during sessions are necessary to maintain positive responses and behavior modification.

Another manifestation of neurocognitive deficit is inflexibility, which leads to an inability to learn from mistakes, deal with uncertainty, and problem solve. Individuals with PAE may misunderstand a joke, leading them to misinterpret the other's intent and exhibit a response that is out of sync. Patients demonstrate inflexibility when they repeatedly arrive late to appointments; when, in spite of advice, they keep company with the same negative crowd that contributed to difficulties; or when they become aggressive when made to switch from one situation to another. This is often dubbed "having a hard time with change." The opportunity to learn from new and different activities, which are associated with negative emotions, especially irritation and anger, is lost. In roleplays, patients can be encouraged to complete tasks that have no actual right or wrong perspective. By flipping coins and guessing in unpredictable games, the patient learns how chance can allow new and unexpected events in the array of solutions.

When a cognitively impaired patient has to change case workers or stop seeing a familiar mental health therapist, the patient can become emotionally disturbed. This again is linked to the pervasive tendency to be inflexible. The patient and therapist should collaboratively generate a list of reasons that explain why the familiar therapist must be changed. Reasons for staff change or absence may include transferring due to illness in the family, returning to school to upgrade knowledge, being at risk from a gang, moving to start a family, and needing rest for self-care. Usually, such a list will not immediately alleviate the distress; however, reemphasized over time, the patient may gradually become reconciled and, eventually, with control of emotion and support accept these reasons. In practice, one might identify an activity in which the patient desires sameness, for example, going for lunch at the same restaurant. Clinician and patient should generate a list of risks and benefits of going to the same place, presenting the worst case scenario compared with the best possible outcome and other potential outcomes within that range. Visualizing the extremes facilitates flexibility by creating an interval prospectively open to a range of possibilities. A similar model is to suggest that the risks are too great and encourage the patient to consider how to manage them. Even though these in-session tasks may be easily completed, they do not become part of a repertoire until they are carried out in real-life practice.

Other skills that should be taught are problem solving and social skills. Problem-solving strategies using events from daily life are helpful. Patients should imagine a friend who is having a particular challenge and, playing the role of confidant, should generate solutions to serve as advice to this friend. Practically, they should be taught to identify the specific problem and then generate and write or draw out a list of possible solutions. For each solution, patients should be asked to consider the advantages and disadvantages. Finally, they should be encouraged to select the most favorable option, identify any possible obstacles, and consider what to do about those obstacles if they arise in the future. If the first option hypothetically fails, they should consider what the next best plan should be. Patients are known to benefit from improved social skills. These essential behavior patterns enable individuals to maintain appropriate boundaries during interactions with others. Patients learn to make appropriate comments and avoid compromising actions because of poor awareness of an action's cause and effect (Frankel et al. 2006; O'Connor et al. 2006).

Computer Games for Neurocognitive Deficits

With advances in technology, several computer games are now available for patients with ND-PAE/FASD. These games can be played individually or used in roleplay sessions during therapy. The goal is to mitigate the effects of CNS dysfunction associated with ND-PAE/FASD. Generally, computer games allow repeated attempts to achieve success, motivate efforts to improve, and contain built-in reinforcement systems via commendation. Additionally, they are an attractive forum for most patients. By eliminating negative comments even in failure, patients' self-esteem is preserved and task completion is more likely. Most of the tests have levels of difficulty adjusted to performance, stimulating internal self-evaluation as a means to improve performance. Using these games opens the possibility of translating success from one context to another, perhaps generalizing improvement in PAE-related symptoms to other mental disorder symptoms.

In patients with ADHD, for instance, task prioritization and time management were improved by using mobile personalized and interactive games (Avila-Pesantez et al. 2018). Improvement in symptoms of inattention in response to playing a number of video games was also noted (Kerns et al. 2010; Strahler Rivero et al. 2015). Using a three-dimensional model with built-in feedback and a video game modified from a NASA-developed pilot instruction program, patients with ADHD have achieved varying levels of success (Pei and Kerns 2012; Zuberer et al. 2015). There is no reason these strategies cannot be applied to patients diagnosed with consequences of PAE and mental disorder. The targeted symptom and potential neurocognitive basis for the change should guide the selection and development of effective platforms. Inhibition, cognitive control, attention, executive functions, and memory constitute correlates with specific gaming indications applicable for patients with PAE. It has been proposed that children with less comorbidity and better cognitive ability have a better chance of success; however, even adult brains are subject to neuroplasticity, and given the benefits of cognitive remediation, functional improvement is still possible.

Computer-based interventions can guide a patient by objectively displaying choices—choices that can improve safety, activities of daily living, and relationships. Self-guided, free of blame and grade, such games provide a means of supporting individual effort and motivation. The use of technology such as texting and social media is popular as a way of communicating with those more likely to forget if nontechnological approaches were used. A caseworker can text to check with a patient about how compliant he or she has been; this form of "gentle stalking" can be successful. Clinicians can text reminders for medical or supervision appointments and medication compliance or help the patient to utilize the calendar reminder options on most mobile devices.

Conclusion

Having an intervention goal is a better way to evaluate improvement in care and assess how efforts directed at producing positive outcomes are measured. Goals should consider whether interventional efforts contribute to the acceptance, care, and rehabilitation of patients and the management of the consequences of PAE. Psychological treatment is individualized and flexible, fueled by a strong and dynamic relationship between patient and therapist. So much depends on this relationship because psychological interventions affect all facets of care. Innovative technology and specific targeted treatments are worthy of consideration.

Social interventions, such as mentoring and providing appropriate support, structure, and supervision, can be combined with medications specific to ND-PAE/FASD. Medications do not contradict but can complement psychological interventions. Emerging evidence of the positive effect of current psychological interventions for children and parents or caregivers of children with FASD is promising. Evidence is still emerging for adults and special groups (Pei et al. 2016). These evidence-based interventions dispel the notion that there is no treatment for FASD. Interventions for children with added benefits for parents, sleep strategies specific for individuals with ND-PAE/FASD, and programs to improve math, cognition, reading, affect regulation, safety, and executive function are areas in which good results have been noted (Kully-Martens et al. 2018; Petrenko et al. 2017). Some of the research has been replicated and is informing current clinical practice.

CLINICAL PRACTICAL APPLICATIONS

- Psychological interventions should strive to reduce stigma, be non-judgmental, be supportive, and use supervisory mentoring for patients with ND-PAE/FASD.

- Where individual therapy is unavailable, therapists should use group sessions as a last resort for patients with ND-PAE/FASD and follow up to ensure true understanding of the material presented in the group.

- Clinicians in forensic, child, and adolescent services should expect a high rate of PAE-induced neurocognitive deficits and use modified approaches to fit the identified deficits.

- Goal setting is a uniquely pivotal step in treatment because it incorporates realistic and modified expectations at the outset.

- Clinicians should ask patients to relay information imparted to them in their own words to confirm comprehension as a means of facilitating effective communication.

- Praise, encouragement, and humor are essential counseling skills in caring for the patient and reducing caregiver stress.

References

Anderson T, Mela M, Rotter T, Poole N: A Qualitative investigation into barriers and enablers for the development of a clinical pathway for individuals living with FASD and mental disorder/addictions. Canadian Journal of Community Mental Health 38(3):43–60, 2020

Astley SJ, Clarren SK: Diagnosing the full spectrum of fetal alcohol-exposed individuals: introducing the 4-digit diagnostic code. Alcohol Alcohol 35(4):400–410, 2000

Astley SJ, Bailey D, Talbot C, Clarren SK: Fetal alcohol syndrome (FAS) primary prevention through FAS diagnosis: II: a comprehensive profile of 80 birth mothers of children with FAS. Alcohol Alcohol 35(5):509–519 2000

Avila-Pesantez D, Rivera LA, Vaca-Cardenas L, et al: Towards the improvement of ADHD children through augmented reality serious games: preliminary results, 2018 IEEE Global Engineering Education Conference (EDUCON), Tenerife, 2018, pp 843–848

Brown J, Haun J, Zapf PA, Aiken T: FASD and competency to stand trial (CST): an exploratory review, in Ethical and Legal Perspectives in Fetal Alcohol Spectrum Disorders (FASD). Edited by Jonsson E, Clarren S, Binnie I. Cham, Switzerland, Springer, 2018, pp 201–227

Brown NN, Connor PD, Adler RS: Conduct-disordered adolescents with fetal alcohol spectrum disorder: intervention in secure treatment settings. Crim Just Behav 39(6):770–793, 2012

Coles CD, Kable JA, Taddeo E: Math performance and behavior problems in children affected by prenatal alcohol exposure: intervention and follow-up. J Dev Behav Pediatr 30(1):7–15, 2009

Coles CD, Kable JA, Taddeo E, Strickland DC: A metacognitive strategy for reducing disruptive behavior in children with fetal alcohol spectrum disorders: Go-FAR pilot. Alcohol Clin Exp Res 39(11):2224–2233, 2015

Coles CD, Kable JA, Taddeo E, Strickland D: GoFAR: improving attention, behavior and adaptive functioning in children with fetal alcohol spectrum disorders: brief report. Dev Neurorehabil 21(5):345–349, 2018

Coons KD: Determinants of drinking during pregnancy and lifespan outcomes for individuals with fetal alcohol spectrum disorder. J Dev Disabil 19(3):15–29, 2013

Denys K, Rasmussen C, Henneveld D: The effectiveness of a community-based intervention for parents with FASD. Community Ment Health J 47(2):209–219, 2011

Flannigan K, Pei J, Rasmussen C, et al: A unique response to offenders with fetal alcohol spectrum disorder: perceptions of the Alexis FASD Justice Program. Canadian Journal of Criminology and Criminal Justice 60(1):1–33, 2018

Frankel F, Paley B, Marquardt R, O'Connor M: Stimulants, neuroleptics, and children's friendship training for children with fetal alcohol spectrum disorders. J Child Adolesc Psychopharmacol 16(6):777–789, 2006

Grant TM, Brown NN, Graham CJ, et al: Screening in treatment programs for fetal alcohol spectrum disorders that could affect therapeutic progress. Int J Alcohol Drug Res 2(3):37–49, 2013. Available at: http://www.ijadr.org/index.php/ijadr/article/view/116. Accessed October 1, 2019.

Hemingway SJA, Bledsoe JM, Davies JK, et al: Twin study confirms virtually identical prenatal alcohol exposures can lead to markedly different fetal alcohol spectrum disorder outcomes-fetal genetics influences fetal vulnerability. Adv Pediatr Res 5:23, 2018

Kable JA, Taddeo E, Strickland D, Coles CD: Improving FASD children's self-regulation: piloting phase 1 of the GoFAR intervention. Child Fam Behav Ther 38(2):124–141, 2016

Kapasi A, Pei J, Kryska K, et al: Exploring self-regulation strategy use in adolescents with FASD. Journal of Occupational Therapy, Schools, & Early Intervention, September 23, 2020

Keightley M, Agnihotri S, Subramaniapillai S, et al: Investigating a theatre-based intervention for indigenous youth with fetal alcohol spectrum disorder: exploration d'une intervention basée sur le théâtre auprès de jeunes autochtones atteints du syndrome d'alcoolisme foetal. Can J Occup Ther 85(2):128–136, 2018

Kerns KA, Macsween J, Vander Wekken S, Gruppuso V: Investigating the efficacy of an attention training programme in children with foetal alcohol spectrum disorder. Dev Neurorehabil 13(6):413–422, 2010

Kully-Martens K, Pei J, Kable J, et al: Mathematics intervention for children with fetal alcohol spectrum disorder: a replication and extension of the math interactive learning experience (MILE) program. Res Dev Disabil 78:55–65, 2018

Layer L, Benson J: Children With fetal alcohol spectrum disorder (FASD): outcomes from the application of an adapted alert program. Am J Occup Ther 74(4 suppl 1):7411515359, 2020

Longstaffe S, Chudley AE, Harvie MK, et al: The Manitoba Youth Justice Program: empowering and supporting youth with FASD in conflict with the law. Biochem Cell Biol 96(2):260–266, 2018

Mattson SN, Foroud T, Sowell ER, et al: Collaborative initiative on fetal alcohol spectrum disorders: methodology of clinical projects. Alcohol 44(7-8):635–641, 2010

McFarlane A: Fetal alcohol spectrum disorder in adults: diagnosis and assessment by a multidisciplinary team in a rural area. Can J Rural Med 16(1):25–30, 2011

Nash K, Stevens S, Greenbaum R, et al: Improving executive functioning in children with fetal alcohol spectrum disorders. Child Neuropsychol 21(2):191–209, 2015

Nash K, Stevens S, Clairman H, Rovet J: Preliminary findings that a targeted intervention leads to altered brain function in children with fetal alcohol spectrum disorder. Brain Sci 8(1):E7, 2018

O'Connor MJ, Frankel F, Paley B, et al: A controlled social skills training for children with fetal alcohol spectrum disorders. J Consult Clin Psychol 74(4):639, 2006

Olson HC, Oti R, Gelo J, Beck S: "Family matters:" fetal alcohol spectrum disorders and the family. Dev Disabil Res Rev 15(3):235–249, 2009

Pei J, Kerns K: Using games to improve functioning in children with fetal alcohol spectrum disorders. Games Health J 1(4):308–311, 2012

Pei J, Leung WSW, Jampolsky F, Alsbury B: Experiences in the Canadian criminal justice system for individuals with fetal alcohol spectrum disorder: double jeopardy? Can J Criminol Crim Just 58(1):56–86, 2016

Pei J, Tremblay M, McNeil A, et al: Neuropsychological aspects of prevention and intervention for FASD in Canada. J Pediatr Neuropsychol 3:25–37, 2017

Petrenko CLM, Pandolfino ME, Robinson LK: Findings from the families on track intervention pilot trial for children with fetal alcohol spectrum disorders and their families. Alcohol Clin Exp Res 41(7):1340–1351, 2017

Poole N, Schmidt RA, Green C, Hemsing N: Prevention of fetal alcohol spectrum disorder: current Canadian efforts and analysis of gaps. Subst Abuse 10(suppl 1):1–11, 2016

Proven S, Ens C, Beaudin PG: The language profile of school-aged children with fetal alcohol spectrum disorder (FASD). Canadian Journal of Speech-Language Pathology & Audiology, 37(4)268–279, 2014

Rutman D: Voices of women living with FASD: perspectives on promising approaches in substance use treatment, programs and care. First Peoples Child Fam Rev 8(1):107–121, 2013

Rutman D: Becoming FASD informed: strengthening practice and programs working with women with FASD. Subst Abuse 10(suppl 1):13–20, 2016

Soh DW, Skocic J, Nash K, et al: Self-regulation therapy increases frontal gray matter in children with fetal alcohol spectrum disorder: evaluation by voxel-based morphometry. Front Hum Neurosci 9:108, 2015

Strahler Rivero T, Herrera Nunez LM, Uehara Pires E, Amodeo Bueno OF: ADHD rehabilitation through video gaming: a systematic review using PRISMA guidelines of the current findings and the associated risk of bias. Front Psychiatry 6:151, 2015

Tait CL, Mela M, Boothman G, Stoops MA: The lived experience of paroled offenders with fetal alcohol spectrum disorder and comorbid psychiatric disorder. Transcult Psychiatry 54(1):107–124, 2017

U.S. Preventive Services Task Force: Interventions to prevent perinatal depression: US Preventive Services Task Force Recommendation Statement. JAMA 321(6):580–587, 2019

Velasquez MM, von Sternberg K, Parrish DE: CHOICES: an integrated behavioral intervention to prevent alcohol-exposed pregnancies among high-risk women in community settings. Soc Work Public Health 28(3–4):224–233, 2013

Wells AM, Chasnoff IJ, Schmidt CA, et al: Neurocognitive habilitation therapy for children with fetal alcohol spectrum disorders: an adaptation of the Alert Program. Am J Occup Ther 66(1):24–34, 2012

Zuberer A, Brandeis D, Drechsler R: Are treatment effects of neurofeedback training in children with ADHD related to the successful regulation of brain activity? A review on the learning of regulation of brain activity and a contribution to the discussion on specificity. Front Hum Neurosci 9:135, 2015

CHAPTER 15

Critical Success Factors

WHAT TO KNOW

Successful clinics are composed of clinicians with a selected and well-coordinated set of skills who adopt a panoramic and lifelong perspective for patients with ND-PAE/FASD.

Successful prevention programs should involve a wide scope of healthy behavior rather than a circumscribed target of PAE and should be transferable across cultures.

Understanding an individual, especially the manifestation of deficits, involves knowledge of the physiological and psychological developmental trajectory.

The accepted standard of care includes a focus on quality of life based on patient- and family-centered goals.

Trauma is a unifying concept in mental disorder and PAE; addressing trauma is pivotal in any intervention.

The common language guide (Looking After Each Other Project 2017) recognizes the various terminologies of PAE and attempts to usher in a dignified and consistent approach to sharing information among participants and sectors that engage those with ND-PAE/FASD.

Recognizing and understanding deficits associated with PAE are pivotal aspects of success in each patient.

WHAT TO KNOW

Patients' willingness to change, resilience, and hope are critical success factors.

In this chapter, I examine factors and strategies that have positively contributed to the development of the interface between PAE, its outcomes, and mental disorder. Mental health professionals work in multiple settings, but no matter where they practice, their goals in supporting patients usually align with the outcomes patients themselves desire. To be effective, mental health professionals should support strategies and programs that enhance quality of life, ensure interdependence, and are socially responsible and inclusive. The sections in this chapter discuss the intersecting factors of success on which it is crucial for clinicians to base their intentions and services.

Examples of Success Factors in Clinics

The clinical pathway that enables success in patients starts from the point of referral and initial engagement with services of care. The patient who navigates the services and system for diagnosis and intervention meets professionals already prepared with a set of skills. The multidisciplinary clinic is the most densely packed system of care. Its successes have been based not on location but on clinicians collaborating with the patient's referral goals. McFarlane and Rajani (2007) provided an analysis of the critical factors and challenges to the success of FASD diagnostic clinics in rural areas specifically and all diagnostic clinics generally. Critical factors include team selection and coordination as well as the development and management of the team. A commitment to client/family–focused services and the establishment of cultural connections within the community are also identified as important features of a diagnostic clinic model. Mental health professionals seeking to replicate critical successes should select team members with the appropriate skills for interdisciplinary collaboration.

Strategies for Reducing Stigma

Knowledge is power. Experience is more powerful. Training and education of providers and working together to achieve a reduction in the negative attitudes toward alcohol use during pregnancy and its effect as manifested in offspring require concerted efforts. Sources of stigma may be different for medical professionals than for the general public. Efforts have been successful in identifying specific candidates who are most vulnerable to stereotyping, prejudice, and discrimination among those with ND-PAE/FASD (Corrigan et al. 2019). Identifying these vulnerable individuals is helpful in determining successful antistigma interventions. Such interventions should focus on contact-based rather than education-based strategies (Corrigan et al. 2017). When patients interact directly with people whose fears have been heightened because of myths they have heard about PAE, the experience offers a better potential for a change of attitude than hearing or learning about the person affected by PAE from others. Many successful stories of people living with the consequences of PAE surprise listeners and dispel stereotypes. Events in which a team composed of the person with lived experience, a caregiver, a front-line provider, and a clinician or researcher engage with various audiences, practically and in person, should be promoted.

Engaging in Prevention and Education

Public and group education aimed at reducing stigma has produced minimal societal results in specifically reducing alcohol use during pregnancy. There are a few exceptions. Where there are documented benefits, the health message was broad enough to target women of childbearing age (Hankin 2002). Critical success was identified when preconception counseling was targeted and messages were combined with other health-specific strategies (Tough et al. 2005). Counseling a woman about the healthy aspects of sobriety— long life, a healthy liver and heart—represents a more attractive message than one restricted to drinking during pregnancy. The CHOICES program—which addresses high-risk women by offering them contraception to avoid becoming pregnant while still drinking—was evaluated, and several successful strategies were identified (Johnson et al. 2015). In addition, brief, short-term interventions with female students and those who are at high risk of having a PAE-affected child continue to be relevant, critical, and successful methods for clinicians to adopt. Public messaging has received relatively little traction in addressing stigma related to the byproducts of PAE or the apathy of professionals who specifically ascribe mental disorders to those with PAE to include them in the mental health system. Recently, the ability of CHOICES to reduce alcohol-exposed pregnancies in indigenous women was discovered (Symons et al. 2018). This followed cultural and linguistic alterations to accommodate the population (Hanson et al. 2017). This hugely successful program therefore is showing wide acceptability and is ready for knowledge generalization across cultures (Niccols et al. 2010).

A successful targeted education is proposed based on its impact in other fields. Having the right and authority of lived experience to speak to colleagues will fall on those who have developed an interest in the interface. Those educators, researchers, and clinicians have an exquisite sense of awareness of what transpires in the mental health field and the field of PAE. They provide insights capable of impacting service development as well as changing practice among their colleagues. This type of peer-directed information sharing should occur in national organization workshops and conferences. These occasions situate appropriately the information, questions, and evaluations of the material presented. Only through such avenues can adequate engagement of professionals be successfully harnessed for the benefit of the patient. The interrelatedness of the fields of PAE and mental disorders supports the success of individuals by inviting professionals and specifically mental health professionals to assume responsibility of care by contributing their skills, which are so well aligned with comorbid work. This is advocacy, a role ascribed to all clinicians and invaluable in engaging both one's colleagues and decision makers.

Importance of Diagnosis in Improving Outcomes

Because the diagnostic process is elaborate and resource dependent, evaluating its utility and determining its success-enhancing qualities are important. Generally speaking, the critical success factors of diagnosis are related to the cost-benefit ratio. As with most things, the disadvantages have to be weighed against the advantages. Clinicians have reported that they do not probe for a history of PAE because it has stigmatizing connotations, adds nothing to the intervention, and is an expensive venture. Some patients do not recover from the daunting effect of knowing harm came to them because of their mother's "choice." Failing several times in life and finally recognizing yet another major failure during the extended diagnostic psychological testing have been reported as stress inducing. Patient responses have been severe, including diminished self-esteem and suicidal behavior. Blame and guilt are well described and serve to discourage others from going through the diagnostic process.

Notwithstanding the disadvantages noted, the advantages of diagnosis portend positive consequences because diagnosis is the entry point for accessing services and qualified experts responsible for those services. Diagnosis provides an explanation and potential preparedness for difficulties not yet encountered. It is the "advance notice" that may play an essential role in acquiring much-needed help and support from health care, school, and social services. If interventions are scarce, treatment of FASD can benefit from strategies used in similar conditions such as autism, ADHD, and other intellectual disabilities. Early diagnostic identification leads to and facilitates effective intervention. Interventions can be focused and directed to specific deficits and domains, for example, social skills training, rehearsal training for memory deficits, and strategies for correcting deficits in communication, math, and affect regulation. Interventions can also be general, supporting healthy life decisions for the person with ND-PAE/FASD.

Over time, mental diagnoses have become more fashionable and desirable. Public campaigns and antistigma programs in which celebrities identify with highly stigmatized disorders continue to effectively influence the general acceptance of disorders. For instance, the progress and success made in the acknowledgment of HIV/AIDS, major depressive disorder, and traumatic encephalopathy are connected to antistigma programs. Acknowledgment of ADHD, for example, was accepted as positive in enhancing effective treatment and future goals (Statens Beredning för Medicinsk Utvärdering 2013). Viewing diagnosis as a positive thing is supported by many social forces, and increasing visibility and acceptance in society are critical success factors. In international conferences, people diagnosed with FASD proudly attend and present to the audience on their personal experiences. The culture of relating to lived experiences in clinical and research endeavors is a reality of modern society. The improvements patients derive from interventions are only possible because diagnosis identifies strengths, triggers services, and explains behavior and its causes. In addition, early diagnosis was shown to be a protective factor for the adverse effects of PAE in the long run (Streissguth et al. 1996).

Importance of Psychology and Physiology of Brain Development

Although puberty and adolescence overlap in timing, they are not synonymous. To relate to the adolescent, the clinician needs to view the gradual transitions from childhood to adulthood through soft events (e.g., development of self-esteem, puberty-related changes). Awareness that peer-directed socialization, novelty seeking, and risk-taking behaviors characterize this developmental phase helps promote success in care. Some patients with ND-PAE/FASD can only be understood when their behaviors are translated into the appropriate age category. An adult who responds in the care setting with noncompliance and repeated early dropouts from programs may be displaying arrested development from an earlier age. This may be understood if the person experienced multiple caregivers because of short-lived residential placements. That is why knowing the basis for a behavior in light of the developmental trajectory and level of physiological maturity is essential for successful treatment.

Mental health professionals chart these phases and help parents and family accept and support the adolescent's ontogenetic shifts. They may also explain adult behaviors that have adolescent precursors. Because prominent neural interconnectivity, especially in the prefrontal cortex, correlates with certain neurobehavioral features in adolescence, this knowledge and its application in clinical care become more critical. Appropriate and time-specific neuronal pruning and plasticity are foundational to this knowledge. Neurodevelopmental delays central in FASD depend on the role of PAE in effecting the maturing of neural interconnectivity. Higher IQ protects cognitive development. Individuals with FASD are characterized by slower maturation. The consequence of this is that abstract reasoning develops and appears late in development. Adolescents with FASD are doubly disadvantaged; they manage stress poorly and experience a delay in their decision-making ability. It is therefore not surprising to experience a later-in-life manifestation of decisional deficit because of a vulnerability to the stresses and strains of everyday living, which leads to risk taking.

To contribute to positive outcomes, it is essential for the clinician and for those who support the person affected by PAE to understand these crucial physiological and psychodevelopmental trajectories.

Role of Culture in ND-PAE/FASD

Meaning-making through interpretive understanding of the interaction of PAE and mental disorder extends beyond demographic variables of the patients. Clinicians adopt an understanding framework for the patients they care for but always in political, ethnic, cultural, and socioreligious contexts. Values and beliefs about inheritance, choice, clinical expression, and therapeutic efficacy mean that PAE and mental disorder come together at a "melting point" of interpretations. The patient situated within this multi-pronged framework most often is influenced by caregivers' and clinicians' knowledge and experience. The accuracy of that experience is implied but not necessarily proven. In the future, successful treatment will rely on relaying the cumulative knowledge about PAE and mental disorder while reducing myth and misinterpretation. The beneficent acts of doctors and health care workers should, as a matter of social continuity, intersect with the patients' clinical expectations. The politics of alcohol and PAE can affect the understanding of its relationship with mental disorder. Deconstruction of myths and being mindful of racial and cultural politics, especially from an historical perspective, help to avoid blame and reinforce resilience in interventions. Imbalance in the role of gender and cultural empowerment may be mistaken, and the result could pose a risk of assigning ND-PAE/FASD to the sector of society apportioned the weight of the inequality. In reality, modifying professional bias and social inequalities can transform existing negative outcomes and bring about an improved quality of life.

Reflecting on and critically reviewing the slow progress of accepting the ND-PAE/FASD diagnosis especially within the mental health fields are essential for successfully providing services to those who have lived with misdiagnoses. Stigma reduction through open conversation about PAE is a positive step toward increased access to maternal histories. When the obstacles of obtaining the history of PAE are overcome, success in diagnosis and treatment will be guaranteed. The important contextual factors that emerge in clinical presentations should be identified. Clinicians can then recognize and validate patients' different sources of support, levels of understanding of problems, and the previous interventional steps taken. Only then, can the mental health specialist reinforce individual-centered outcomes and goals. Holistic health for people with ND-PAE/FASD demands such innovative approaches to improve health outcomes.

Removing Barriers to Health

The compartmentalization of mental and behavioral health from physical health is now a recognized barrier to optimum health. Other obstacles high on the list of policy-related barriers to care include limited insurance coverage, treatment dependent on diagnosis, lack of access, and fragmentation of care. Considering the need to streamline services and make them user-friendly, an integrated service with a navigator or mentor for the person with ND-PAE/FASD offers the best option for facilitating services. Of course, such health care assistants should be well informed about the link between neurocognitive deficits and the required interventions for managing them. If the treatment of people experiencing the disadvantages associated with PAE is to be successful, the system should ensure quality care through the use of these navigation advocates or mentors.

Trauma-Informed Care

Health care systems that recognize the relevant contributions of the various factors affecting health are inherently successful. In ND-PAE/FASD, this should take the form of strategies to influence recognition, policy change, and clinical interventions regarding trauma. There have been advances in the prevention of mental disorder; controlling adverse childhood events has the potential to eliminate a sizable portion of the direct and indirect causes, and this benefit extends to ND-PAE/FASD. Given the weight of evidence for a relationship between adverse childhood experiences and all forms of mental disorder, prevention should be a logical and sound approach to addressing global mental health (Mersky et al. 2013). Table 15–1 shows the essential components for comprehensive care.

TABLE 15–1. Essential care principles (4 Rs)

Recognition of neurocognitive deficits

Relationship building and sustenance (therapeutic working alliance)

Realistic and modified expectations

Realization of trauma

Preventing childhood trauma involves treating toxic stress. In turn, and critical to success, trauma intervention will greatly improve the health of future generations. Successful initiatives seek to enlighten the public about the lifelong impact of trauma caused by abuse, neglect, and maltreatment. Correcting household dysfunction during childhood should be supported by deliberate, diligently evaluated policies. Data on adverse childhood experiences should be collected, and the information derived from such data should be shared in the appropriate quarters to influence policy. Some effective campaigns used a multifaceted approach to demonstrate the importance of caring and building trusting relationships within the family in decreasing the impact of childhood trauma (Substance Abuse and Mental Health Services Administration 2014). Similar approaches are necessary if pivotal goals in prevention and intervention are to be reached.

Role of Common Language

Qualitative research shows that misdiagnosing the effects of PAE contributes to negative consequences (Anderson et al. 2020). Many inappropriate terms and mislabels are applied to those with ND-PAE/FASD by mental health professionals who are oblivious to the neurocognitive deficits. Patients who forget their appointments are viewed as acting deliberately and are either threatened with exclusion or actually excluded from services. Without awareness of PAE-induced inflexibility, impulsive and aggressive acts can be construed as antisocial in nature. Patients who cannot keep their stories straight, even if this is a result of impaired comprehension arising from slow information processing, are labeled as dishonest or manipulative. Patients are said to have brain damage, meaning they need an "extra" or "new" brain. These are some of the difficulties that highlight how using the wrong language contributes to misrepresentation of individuals with ND-PAE/FASD. These inconsistent and sometimes diametrically opposed representations demand a fundamental awareness of PAE deficits and adoption of a unified terminology and nonstigmatizing language.

Related to unifying ideas, strategy and policy changes came about when the use of a common language was proposed for addressing those with ND-PAE/FASD. The person-first language guide (Looking After Each Other Project 2017) stemmed from the principle of patient dignity: individuals are said to be affected—not afflicted—with a neurodevelopmental disability. These token initiatives are not insignificant for policy change and societal influence on the strength-based approach that is necessary for future success in the field. Communities who speak the same language are more connected, and ensuring common ground in communication across sectors (parents, teachers, educators, clinicians, and individuals with lived experiences) portrays solidarity for the principles outlined to regulate activities in health care. Overall, such positive messaging contributes to the recognition of the resilience of individuals, which is a component for moving the field in a positive direction. It serves to minimize how language perpetuated discrimination and stereotyping.

Red Flags: What Else Could It Be?

The interval between and timeliness of recognizing warning signs and responding with a comprehensive assessment holds critical success factors. Research findings should guide clinicians to attend to aspects of the patient interview relevant to identifying PAE and its consequences. A family history of maternal chronic liver disease, poor life choices, residential or outpatient addiction therapy, alcohol-related incarceration, and alcohol-related cause of death are suggestive of PAE. Although more difficult to assert, history of sexual abuse, domestic violence, and self-harm or suicide attempt in the patient's mother are also indicative. Other relevant findings are records of poor academic achievement. Learning difficulties that cause the patient to require special education are usually related to PAE. Learning difficulties are closely linked with high rates of behavioral problems. These, in turn, affect school performance and may be the indirect reason to require special education or may contribute to dropping out of school.

The many principles for optimum care are based on work with individuals who are easily misunderstood. In the mental health system, clinicians need to have a broad conception of how neurocognitive deficits manifest in the clinical environment. It is that recognition that is the foundation of a strong working

TABLE 15–2. Strategies for effective one-on-one interactions

Maintain an attitude of respect and kindness.

Speak directly in the first person.

Use visual forms: diagrams, lists, demonstrations, visual analogue scale.

Use roleplay and reverse roleplay.

Ask nonleading questions.

Play to the patient's strengths.

Use repeat strategy for long-term memory enhancement.

Combine "restriction with permission."

Prepare and plan ahead for changes.

Write instructions in the patient's words.

Recognize that mistakes are learning points.

Choose a stress-free room or location.

alliance with the patient with neurocognitive deficits, who is likely to be misinterpreted. As a result, the clinician is best placed to adopt realistic and modified expectations of the patient (see Table 15–1). Table 15–2 lists ideas for vital strategies to help with communication during counseling, assessment, and supportive therapies. These strategies and directly addressing trauma experience are necessary critical success factors in clinical encounters.

Role of Team Consultation

Behavioral disturbance with high risk of harm preoccupies caregivers and demands the expertise of mental health professionals. Ill-equipped clinicians who adopt traditional approaches and assume that patients are choosing bad behaviors respond negatively. These modalities add nothing useful to the intervention, suggest negative reinforcement for those behaviors, and insist on cognitive-behavioral modification. These approaches then frustrate the patients, caregivers, and clinicians. They yield poor results and harm the misunderstood patient. The first step in adopting the appropriate intervention is to recognize the behavioral problems associated with neurocognitive impairments. These red flags can point to the level of assessment needed to determine the severity of the deficits. The information linking neurocognitive deficits with the behavioral problems is relevant for the empathic understanding of the person. This information also informs the use of strategies with the best chance of success and functional improvement.

A universal principle to adopt when caring for a behaviorally disturbed person is that relationship building is crucial. The clinician–patient relationship is the foundation of a long-term process to understand the patient's strengths, appreciate the contribution of past experiences to the current manifestation, and instill hope to facilitate the required change. Through the relationship, strong bonds are formed, and tasks are initiated and maintained at a level of persistence that enables the accomplishment of collaboratively set goals. These are the essential components of a good therapeutic working alliance. Such a relationship facilitates the patient's access to the clinician's expertise. Clinicians are more effective if they collaborate with patients and adopt an attitude of readiness to learn from them, as well as guiding the intervention. Embracing measured and realistic expectations of the patient, which entails matching the behavior with the neurocognitive deficits, delivers the first benefit to both patient and clinician. It is not about lowering the level of patient competence or expectations of what the patient can do; it is about supporting success by playing to the patient's strengths. This approach requires that the expectation will not deplete the patient's neurocognitive resources for displaying acceptable behavior. Highly successful teams also address the consequences of trauma in the patient.

The value of team consultation and having an informed diagnosis is demonstrated in the following vignette.

Clinical Vignette

A 15-year-old school dropout expresses distress by repeatedly self-harming (wrist slashing using either a razor blade or a pin). She also abuses alcohol and solvents. She was diagnosed with ND-PAE/FASD at the age of 13 after she left school and ran away from home (at the time, she lived with her mother and stepfather). Over the past year, she has visited the child and adolescent psychiatry emergency room more than 100 times. Her mental disorders include reactive attachment disorder, oppositional defiant disorder, unspecified feeding or eating disorder, conduct disorder, borderline personality disorder, panic disorder, polysubstance use disorder, and ADHD. The most life-threatening behaviors (self-harm and alcohol and solvent use) were creating challenges for the team managing her care. She displays significant noncompliance and therapy interference by losing her medication and repeatedly going to a pharmacy to buy or steal mouthwash. She frequently goes to the emergency room, intoxicated from drinking mouthwash, and asks to be admitted to the adolescent psychiatric ward. Opinions about how best to manage her care are diverse. The family insists she should be in an extended-stay facility for psychiatrically disturbed adolescents. The psychologist drafts and recommends a behavioral modification program with a cognitive-behavior therapy component. The plan contains significant consequences for recurrent behavior problems. The social worker recommends referral to an eating disorder center capable of managing the wrist-cutting behavior, and the psychiatrist elects to consult with a specialist with an interest in PAE.

The current therapy approach seems ineffective, and the team's frustration level is significant. The team is split, and tensions are running high. The specialist sees the team dysfunction and fast-tracks a consultation with a PAE expert. The specialist's first recommendation is respite care for the primary team. A secondary team (the specialist along with experts with a PAE-based approach) reviews the previous neuropsychological reports completed 2 years earlier after the diagnosis of ND-PAE/FASD. Their recommendations incorporate those previous findings and the current clinical manifestation of challenging behaviors. This is based on the understanding that "diagnosis may result in more realistic expectations for the future and the adoption of compensatory strategies" (Grant et al. 2013).

The patient clearly has not grieved the loss of function in the 2 years since she learned about the ND-PAE/FASD diagnosis and the impact of PAE on her life. She is angry with her mother for separating from her father and for admitting to drinking alcohol during pregnancy, which she was told caused her poor performance in school. She is isolated at school and loses confidence when she is the target of bullying by other students. She wants to be popular, but her struggles with her school subjects and poor social skills preclude that. These factors gave rise to self-defeating, risk-unaware, and life-endangering behaviors. She cannot be trusted with the medications (methylphenidate, risperidone, citalopram, and zopiclone) that she overdosed on.

The recommended management starts with the assignment of a mentor with expertise in ND-PAE/FASD. At the outset, relationship building centers on meeting where the patient likes to go, which is the city central bus stop. The staff finds a self-expressive nonacademic arts program for youth and enrolls the patient. She calls off many meetings a few minutes before the mentor is due to arrive. Some meetings that she cancels seem to actually be due to poor recall and disorganization; however, other cancellations appear deliberate. The mentor is relentless about calling her, accepting the "apologies" offered, and rescheduling new appointments. With the mentor relationship tested and found to be stable over a 6-month period, the patient begins to reach out to the team using text messages and Snapchat. A strategy to avert solvent use flows from the understanding that whenever she is distressed because someone puts her down, the first source of relief that she turns to is the pharmacy. Initially, she tried to obtain the prescribed medication that relieves distress. However, she was told by the pharmacist that she did not have a prescription and could not receive medication without a doctor's review. She became upset, saw a bottle of mouthwash, snatched it, and drank it. She was conditioned to go to the same pharmacy, sometimes disguised, in order to obtain the mouthwash.

The mentor initiates a plan that teaches the patient how to rate her level of distress (with 10 being the worst level of distress on a visual analog scale). When her distress reaches 3, she is guided to consider texting the mentor as her first response. She loses many objects, but she seems to hold on to her phone very well. The mentor also enlists a colleague as a secondary contact person. The patient occasionally "fires" the mentor, and the secondary person becomes the "favorite" person for a while. The mentor also teaches her to count to 10 whenever she feels like going to the pharmacy. By stopping to count, the patient learns to delay her actions, which prompts texting to the mentor. This concept is termed *restriction with permission* (see Table 15–2); it is a replacement process. The patient who is told not to do something should be told to do something else in place of what would have been done.

Although information is communicated in a way that the patient shows she understands, she is asked to relay her true understanding of the plan in her own words. The initial execution of the plan is unsuccessful for the first 3 weeks, and several episodes of intoxication occur. The patient is able to describe in a learned problem-solving approach why she is not texting. Collaboratively, the mentor and patient agree on specifically timed goals, and the patient begins to reach out by text whenever she has a problem. The rates of emergency room visits are reduced, and compliance with medication is made possible through an innovative approach. The patient loves a TV program about cats, and the program also links to various pictures of cats on the internet. She sets a notification alert on her phone that sounds like cats mewing to signal when she is expected to take her medications.

Various outcomes for this patient were improved, and the team saw the value of the principles (e.g., relationship building, realistic expectations, and modified approaches) used by the specialists. The different approaches were generalized and transferred so that transition of care back to the primary team after the patient stabilized was successful. The mentor was the only constant figure because of jurisdictional issues. Future efforts should address transition to adulthood, reestablishment of the right educational environment, and method of tutelage. Ongoing support to combat the patient's addiction was based on managing distress and thus eliminating the need for solvents and alcohol. Sensitivity to the possibility of trauma (bullying and abuse) is worthy of special consideration. The essential components for success are now under the purview of the primary treatment team: support, supervision, mentoring, and structure, along with the adoption of easy-to-follow communication strategies.

The mentor occupies an invaluable and central role, functioning to connect the patient with essential services, which the patient may be unable to access without hand-holding by an experienced person. Navigating the health care system is complicated enough for neurotypical people; the cognitive deficits of patients with PAE make this even more difficult. Their inability to navigate such a complex system can be misunderstood as lack of interest or recalcitrance. A mentor serves multiple purposes, including being a conduit to services and professionals. A mentor also promulgates the essentials of the best practice guide on FASD to those interacting with the patient in the health and social sectors (Pei et al. 2018; Figure 15–1).

Research and Evaluation

Without an evolving, innovative, and change-amenable discipline, any progress is likely to be temporary or permanently stymied. Efforts to put devel-

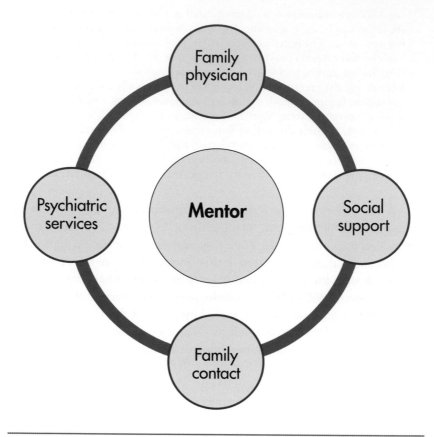

FIGURE 15–1. Critical central role of the mentor in relation to health professionals and patient support.

opments and advancements in ND-PAE/FASD through a research and evaluation process should be unrelenting. The speed of technological advancement demands no less. The evaluation process should include the cost-benefit analysis of services, investments, and research in the field. Economic studies reviewing social returns on investment are indispensable for advancing the field.

Funding research that recognizes the immediate knowledge translation reasoning (applicably practical and implementable) should be patient centered and patient oriented and should engage the family. This type of research stands the chance of precipitating change along life transitions. It is the vital link for changing outcomes in successful ways. Already some benefits are accruing to individuals as common principles for success have been proposed in the field.

Conclusion

To be effective in achieving results in the management of patients with ND-PAE/FASD, clinicians should emphasize understanding and supporting the patient. Understanding ranges from the reason why brain development was arrested to the manifestations of patient behavior vis-á-vis the current diagnosis. If frustration or failure characterized previous involvement with services, vulnerable patients need a different approach, one that recognizes the effect of trauma on the person and relies on an informed mentor and therapists who modify their expectations of the patient to realistic levels. Research and critical review are essential for progress to occur in the field.

CLINICAL PRACTICAL APPLICATIONS

- Stigma about ND-PAE/FASD among mental health professionals is strong, but interacting with affected persons provides an opportunity for a change of attitude and allows more informed synergistic alliances.

- Mental health professionals should employ advocacy roles to influence clinical, management, and policy outcomes related to ND-PAE/FASD.

- Ensuring the standard of care means that efforts are directed at obtaining a diagnosis that identifies strength and deficits and without which ineffective intervention and negative outcomes are likely.

- By minimizing stigma in clinical practice, clinicians likely obtain more accurate clinical information and thus empower disenfranchised patients with ND-PAE/FASD.

- Silos of care (medical, mental, and social) should be abolished in favor of integration of services guided by well-informed mentors.

- Successful care begins with recognizing deficits and building relationships with patients.

- Responding to trauma and adopting realistic expectations sustain treatment successes.

References

Anderson T, Mela M, Rotter T, Poole N: A Qualitative investigation into barriers and enablers for the development of a clinical pathway for individuals living with FASD and mental disorder/addictions. Canadian Journal of Community Mental Health 38(3):43–60, 2020

Corrigan PW, Lara, JL, Shah BB, et al: The public stigma of birth mothers of children with fetal alcohol spectrum disorders. Alcohol Clin Exp Res 41(6):1166–1173, 2017

Corrigan PW, Shah BB, Lara JL, et al: Stakeholder perspectives on the stigma of fetal alcohol spectrum disorder. Addict Res Theory 27(2):170–177, 2019

Grant TM, Brown NN, Dubovsky D, et al: The impact of prenatal alcohol exposure on addiction treatment. J Addict Med 7(2):87–95, 2013

Hankin JR: Fetal alcohol syndrome prevention research. Alcohol Res Health 26(1):58–65, 2002

Hanson JD, Nelson ME, Jensen JL, et al: Impact of the CHOICES intervention in preventing alcohol-exposed pregnancies in American Indian women. Alcohol Clin Exp Res 41(4):828–835, 2017

Johnson SK, Velasquez MM, von Sternberg K: CHOICES: an empirically supported intervention for preventing alcohol-exposed pregnancy in community settings. Res Soc Work Pract 25(4):488–492, 2015

Looking After Each Other Project: Language Guide: Promoting Dignity for Those Impacted by FASD. Manitoba, Canada Northwest FASD Partnership, 2017. Available at: https://www.fasdcoalition.ca/wp-content/uploads/2016/10/LAEO-Language-Guide.pdf. Accessed October 5, 2020.

McFarlane A, Rajani H: Rural FASD diagnostic services model: Lakeland Centre for fetal alcohol spectrum disorder. Can J Clin Pharmacol 14(3):e301–e306, 2007

Mersky JP, Topitzes J, Reynolds AJ: Impacts of adverse childhood experiences on health, mental health, and substance use in early adulthood: a cohort study of an urban, minority sample in the U.S. Child Abuse Negl 37(11):917–925, 2013

Niccols A, Dell CA, Clarke S: Treatment issues for Aboriginal mothers with substance use problems and their children. Int J Ment Health Addict 8(2):320–335, 2010

Pei J, Tremblay M, Poth C, et al: Best Practices for Serving Individuals With Complex Needs: Guide and Evaluation Toolkit. Alberta, Canada, PolicyWise for Children & Families, in collaboration with the University of Alberta, 2018. Available at: https://canfasd.ca/wp-content/uploads/2018/09/Best-Practices_June12018.pdf. Accessed October 3, 2020.

Statens Beredning för Medicinsk Utvärdering: ADHD—Diagnostik och behandling, vårdens organisation och patientens delaktighet. En systematisk litteraturöversikt (SBU Rep No 217). Stockholm, Statens Beredning för Medicinsk Utvärdering (SBU), 2013

Streissguth AP, Barr HM, Kogan J, Bookstein FL: Understanding the Occurrence of Secondary Disabilities in Clients With Fetal Alcohol Syndrome (FAS) and Fetal Alcohol Effects (FAE): Final Report to the Centers for Disease Control and Prevention (CDC) (Tech Rep No 96-06). Seattle, University of Washington, 1996

Symons M, Pedruzzi RA, Bruce K, Milne E: A systematic review of prevention interventions to reduce prenatal alcohol exposure and fetal alcohol spectrum disorder in indigenous communities. BMC Public Health 18(1):1227, 2018

Substance Abuse and Mental Health Services Administration: Understanding the impact of trauma, in Trauma-Informed Care in Behavioral Health Services (Center for Substance Abuse Treatment, Treatment Improvement Protocol [TIP] Series 57, HHS Publ No SMA 13-4801). Rockville, MD, Substance Abuse and Mental Health Services Administration, 2014

Tough SC, Clarke M, Clarren S: Preventing fetal alcohol spectrum disorders: preconception counseling and diagnosis help. Can Fam Physician 51:1199–1201, 2005

PART VI

Special Populations

CHAPTER 16

Special Issues in Children and Adolescents (the Young)

WHAT TO KNOW

Policy should be enacted to ensure substitute caregivers (foster and adoptive parents) are trained on the implications of and interventions with children and adolescents with ND-PAE/FASD.

Comprehensive diagnostic assessment in and of itself, by identifying both strengths and deficits, constitutes a protective factor against lifelong negative outcomes of PAE.

Neurobiological understanding of the manifestations of PAE offers a parsimonious diagnostic formulation when multiple diagnoses are possible.

Executive function deficits are at the core of the major PAE manifestations and related mental disorders.

Children and adolescents make up a special population of those diagnosed with ND-PAE/FASD. Early delays in milestone development, school adjustment issues, and early development of negative outcomes from the effects of PAE create challenges in caring for these patients. In this chapter, I lay out the special issues and disorders that complicate the development of a young person with ND-PAE/FASD. Sleep problems, instability, and adverse childhood effects are a few of these. Critical to development is the role of education, including special education, in ameliorating the deficits of PAE, and strategies to improve learning are outlined. I stress the importance of having the family represented and engaged in the care plan because the family unit, which sometimes is a modified, nonbiological one, is crucial for stability and development. I also describe the advancement made so far in developing various treatments (individual, family-based, technological, and psychological) for this special population, with the possibility of generalizing some of them to other populations of individuals with PAE.

Clinical Vignette

A 15-year-old is suspended from school for disruptive and aggressive behavior and persistently failing to complete homework assignments with no good reason. This occurs despite several warnings from his teacher. He demonstrates conduct disorder symptoms (e.g., rule breaking, lying, stealing), low mood, and irritability. He began smoking marijuana about 4 weeks prior to the consultation, stating that it helps with sleep. He is accused of breaking and entering a pharmacy that sells medical marijuana but has not been charged.

Past history shows two previous contacts with professionals at 3 and at 8 years old. At 3 years old, he was described as a "difficult sleeper," insisting on placing his head and chin on a cold wet blanket, which he took to bed. This was the only thing that got him to sleep. At that time, his parents were separated. The custody arrangement meant he moved repeatedly between his mother's and father's residences. Both parents had different routines. He was at the time described as more anxious after he witnessed several physical assaults his mother endured. Instead of going to bed, he would stay awake and wait with the babysitter until his mother returned from work at 10 P.M. As a result of all these changes, his routine was unpredictable. His mother, usually tired, occasionally would allow him to watch TV until very late. At times, she caved in regarding his insistent requests to sleep in bed with her, instead of in his bed in his own room. This happened especially when he could not get to sleep, staying up late into the night. At times during the night, he was said to get up, scream fearfully and loudly, and then appear lifeless. His father did not report similar problems. His parents were not able to look after him for the next 5 years because of their ongoing alcohol use. He had various living arrangements and was placed in two different foster homes. The first arrangement broke down after 3 months because the foster parent used excessive physical punishment.

At 8 years old, he was again living with his mother in a social services housing project. His sleep problems continued, and he would watch TV late into the night. He was noisy at night, playing loud music and occasionally banging excitedly on the wall. This disturbed and infuriated the neighbors, and so his mother sought help to avoid being evicted. He was described as hyperactive, involved in bullying behavior with other boys in school, and unable to sit still in class; his grades continued to fall. His doctor at the time tried prescribing methylphenidate (Ritalin), which he partially complied with. The medication was said to worsen his symptoms of hyperactivity, irritability, and disturbed sleep.

Red Flags: What Else Could It Be?

The past history of encounters with health services is vital in understanding this patient. The current clinical presentation is likely to lead to a diagnosis of major depressive disorder, PTSD, and conduct disorder (Table 16–1). He has a short history of cannabis use but not sufficient to meet criteria for a disorder. The early account of disturbed sleep leading to prolonged nocturnal problems could be thought of as related to a mood problem, a reaction to parental discord, witnessing violence, and residential instability, which he faced at the time. Behavioral problems may be viewed as insomnia related or misclassified as the precursor of conduct disorder. Later on, disturbed sleep can contribute to daytime behavior problems in school. Clinical features, such as parental backgrounds and the patient's challenging behaviors, should attract the clinician's attention and lead to identifying more red flags (Table 16–1). Another perspective involves viewing this presentation via the lens of neurodevelopmental disability, with peak problems occurring at the time of the two points of contact with mental health services. If that perspective is considered, the two points of clinical contact best fit a stress-diathesis model (Hellemans et al. 2010). In such a case, neurodisability is a foundational vulnerability that, when impacted by stress, creates the manifested symptoms. Knowledge of neurocognitive deficits helps explain some indicators such as pervasive sleep problems, misunderstanding of agitated behavior by past clinicians, parental reinforcement of difficult behaviors, and parental absence. Exacerbated by residential instability, a neurocognitive deficiency can suggest the consequences of PAE and serve as distant red flags. Failing grades should prompt functional assessment of cognition to identify the effect of neurocognitive dysfunction. The potential contribution of poor sleep to developmental issues should become clearer when an adequate review of the patient's sleep pattern is undertaken. Such a review would identify the link between disruptive behavioral problems and poor quality of sleep.

Although not always a direct factor, a history of parental alcohol use, as reported in the vignette, especially at levels described as causing dysfunction, suggests a strong possibility of prenatal dysfunction including PAE (Singal et al. 2017). Other prenatal risk factors reported in the literature are malnutrition, stress, and smoking. Instability of residence from an early age can arise when foster parents of an apprehended child do not understand the origin of neurocognitive behavioral deficit. More commonly, behav-

TABLE 16–1. Clinical information indicating PAE in children

Alcohol use in both parents

Parental dysfunction associated with alcohol use

Early exposure (experienced or witnessed) to traumatic events

Significant and early onset of sleep disturbance

Mood instability indicative of affect dysregulation

Misperception of cold and heat, indicative of sensory processing problems

Easily diagnosable with a mental disorder(s) (conduct, night terrors)

Unsuccessful foster care placement and residential instability

Behaviors suggestive of conduct disorder

ioral problems are accentuated when parents apply, albeit mistakenly, child-rearing practices commonly used in neurotypical children. Expecting to get a predictable response, parents get exasperated trying to manage or discipline a child or adolescent with the neurocognitive deficits of PAE. Smoking cannabis as a sleep aid appeals to youth even in the absence of scientific evidence. Unfortunately, the risk of demyelination in young people is real. Most research on the age of onset of alcohol and substance use among those with PAE reports an early onset age, usually 12 years of age (Lange et al. 2013, 2017). Early use of cannabis increases the risk of a number of disorders. Thus, even a short history of use, as reported for the youth in the vignette, warrants a full review. By evaluating the nature, extent, severity, and response to the trauma the patient experienced or witnessed, a potential diagnosis of PTSD could be considered and clinically supported. It is noteworthy that the rates of adverse childhood experiences in those with PAE are estimated to be four times the rate in the general population (Frankenberger et al. 2015; McQuire et al. 2020). Patients presenting with substance use and behavioral problems are also likely to have a list of strengths discoverable during an assessment. Should these red flags be the reason for diagnosing ND-PAE/FASD in the youth, care should be taken to use strategies that cater to the identified deficits. What is important is that mental health clinicians attend to these atypical manifestations with a perspective that considers PAE when red flags are present.

Modification of Care: What Difference Does ND-PAE/FASD Make?

Given the possible number of diagnoses in the patient, ND-PAE/FASD offers a parsimonious explanation of the manifesting disruptive behavior

(Glass and Mattson 2017). Sleep problems related to PAE involve prenatal damage to sleep centers and behavior problems accentuated by childhood adversity. Assessment that confirms the diagnosis should apply modified approaches for treatment. Subtle yet effective steps contribute to the appropriate clinical modifications to support patients (Table 16–2). Strategies should accommodate the patient's impaired processing speed, deficit in communication, affect regulation, hyperactivity, and sleep problems (Bertrand and Interventions for Children with Fetal Alcohol Spectrum Disorders Research Consortium 2009). Allowing a pressure-free interval after a question gives the adolescent an opportunity to respond according to his experience and ability—not playing to the audience and repeating what he thinks they want to hear from him. Improving communication in this way can reduce irritability and impulsive responses from the patient and support empathy for caregivers and teachers. Sleep interventions recognize that the expectations for recovery and efforts to succeed are shared by the support team and not solely placed on the patient alone. This requires a strong and positive supportive relationship with the patient.

TABLE 16–2. Knowledge-based modifications for different approaches to ND-PAE/FASD

Adaptive communication style

Responsive sleep solutions

Appropriate level of empathy

Measured expectations of the youth

Attention to youth use of illicit drugs

Alternative wellness-focused strategies

Rational pharmacotherapy

Multiprofessional collaboration

A modification of expectations is necessary to facilitate understanding and collaboration. By reducing the pressure on the patient, the increased risk of stress-induced substance use for coping will be curtailed. In addition, this modified approach contributes to managing sleep and behavioral problems. The treatment team and patient should develop a program that includes good sleep hygiene, a bedtime routine, and pre-sleep rituals. Anxiety management, choice of an α-agonist (e.g., clonidine, guanfacine), psychoeducation, and collaboration with caregiver are unique approaches to be applied to cognitively impaired individuals. Specific to ND-PAE/FASD, occupational therapy assessments for sensory processing difficulties and establishing a functional analysis of behavior are essential steps in modification and management. The value of recognizing the PAE red flags is that application of ineffective standard strategies used with neurotypical individuals can be prevented (see Table 16–2).

Melatonin has been suggested as effective both in correcting sleep inversion and improving sleep induction. Dosing should start low and be increased slowly, while comparing benefits and risks (Ipsiroglu et al. 2015). Symptomatic treatment of hyperactivity and impulsivity may not be necessary with improvements obtained using melatonin. Alternatively, pharmacological agents can help reduce depressive symptoms, including insomnia. Cannabis use should be discouraged through psychoeducation, counseling, and parental supervision, and with sleep improvement, the patient may be encouraged to quit using, especially when use has been short-term.

The results of comprehensive assessment offer the significant advantage of knowing the extent of deficits, as well as the patient's strengths. These are the building blocks for corrective approaches to behavior problems, developing individual education plans, and monitoring progress. The description of the neurocognitive profile is really the asset for improving functional abilities and promoting a more stable development (Hagan et al. 2016). Mental health professionals dealing with a similar patient may come from different specialties (forensic, adolescent, or substance use). The essential components for understanding—full assessment, targeted communication, and interagency collaboration—should be applied by all team members and viewed with an awareness of the uniqueness of the neurodisability of individuals with PAE.

If a specific criminal matter arises, for example, the argument can be made that impulsivity, as part of the neurocognitive deficit, contributed to criminal justice involvement, and this should mitigate culpability. Options available to the legal team depend on the community resources and services available. Court diversion programs and referral to and involvement with intensive community supervision and mentoring support are relevant for good outcomes. Successful mentoring is more likely if undertaken by an organization with staff who has established skills in managing those with similar deficits, using protocols that employ the patient's strengths. The assessment result can function as a protective factor, influencing the life trajectory of the youth with ND-PAE/FASD to minimize long-term negative outcomes in adulthood, including outcomes of other diagnosable mental disorders. Treatment modification informed by the recognition of indicators of PAE completes the circle of appropriate care, harm prevention, and functional improvement from a lifelong perspective. Mental health professionals, caregivers, and patients seek such outcomes. Without detection of red flags, these positive outcomes are unlikely.

Executive Function Differences in ADHD and ND-PAE/FASD

Among children with the consequences of PAE, ADHD is the most frequent comorbid diagnosis (Fryer et al. 2007; Streissguth et al. 2004). The overlap of etiology, clinical manifestation, and treatment of children with FASD and ADHD contributes to, in some cases, diagnostic uncertainty and treatment delay. Alcohol-exposed children with ADHD are suspected of having varying and inadequate responses to stimulants compared with those not so exposed. So identifying patients with ADHD with a history of alcohol exposure has clinical utility, which relates to facilitating early diagnosis, improving treatment, and ameliorating the effects of secondary disabilities (Kingdon et al. 2016). The hallmark deficit in neurodevelopmental disorders with executive dysfunction is shared in ADHD and FASD. Executive dysfunction in both conditions characteristically manifests as hyperactivity, inattention, impulsivity, poor judgment, and failure to consider consequences (Kingdon et al. 2016).

Clinically, the highly comorbid relationship of ND-PAE/FASD and ADHD has benefited from existing research, especially on the most significant deficit. Still, differences reported in the varying executive function skills exist, but, overall, moderate effect sizes in deficits compared with normal children are more standard. A few helpful findings relate to the breakdown of higher-order executive, memory, and attention skills. In individuals with ND-PAE/FASD, the most prominent expression of impairment included behavioral disinhibition and disorganization. Also, compared with typical children, patients with ND-PAE/FASD manifested large effect deficits in planning, fluency, set-shifting, and working memory. The reported deficits in attentional vigilance and inhibition control were only moderately affected (Kingdon et al. 2016).

Helpful to the mental health professional, patients with nondysmorphic FASD who are commonly encountered in the mental health system show overall differences in executive function compared with control subjects. These moderate effects were, however, not different from patients with FASD with dysmorphic features. Additionally, those with dysmorphic FASD differed significantly in the deficits related to planning, fluency, and set-shifting. A meta-analysis examined the executive function differences of those with ADHD and those with the consequences of PAE. Overall, the latter showed more persistent planning, fluency, and set-shifting deficits than patients with ADHD alone. Patients with deficits from PAE were found to be impaired, to be older, to show more dysmorphia, and to have greater IQ differences (Khoury and Milligan 2019; Tsang et al. 2016).

Still, these findings are preliminary and require validation. In the mental health system particularly, screening children not yet diagnosed with ND-PAE/FASD, especially the nondysmorphic type, is necessary because identifying them by other means is unreliable. There are no clinically effective differences to apply. Dysmorphia is not differentiated based on executive function differences, and so it cannot be a reliable screen. Furthermore, it means that obtaining a valid neuropsychological profile should not be compromised as an important component of assessment. More studies are needed to ensure that these neurocognitive features can distinguish between clinical subgroups.

The current level of evidence was best summarized following the meta-analytic finding in which Kingdon et al. (2016) stated:

> Taken together, these data provide evidence that on a group level, FASD does not produce an identical cognitive profile to ADHD. Specifically, FASD is associated with a larger magnitude of executive deficits than ADHD on a group level, and more consistent impairments in planning, set-shifting, fluency, and possibly working memory. Thus, attention and executive function deficits in FASD may represent a different underlying etiological pathway than those observed in ADHD, which may mandate a different approach to treatment. (O'Malley and Nanson 2002, pp. 12–13)

Issues Emanating From School

Pooled estimates of FASD in school children range from 3% to 16% (Lange et al. 2018; May et al. 2018; Popova et al. 2019). In those attending school and in foster care, the rate of PAE is about fourfold higher than the rate in the general population (Fuchs et al. 2010). The school environment can reveal many consequences of PAE. Cognitive and academic dysfunction, psychological disorders, behavioral problems, and difficulties with independent living are commonly found in those affected. These directly impact functioning at school. It is therefore important to engage teachers in identifying those struggling with the PAE-induced difficulties. Teachers are complimentary support team members whose awareness of strategies for instructing students with PAE-induced neurocognitive deficits is essential for school success.

PAE causes deficits in memory, comprehension, and abstract thinking, skills necessary for learning. Children have strengths that can be channeled for learning in their unique ways. Teachers need to know through appropriate functional assessment what those strengths entail. In the case of ND-PAE/FASD, creative approaches are needed to fulfill criteria for and acquire support for special education.

The finding of neurocognitive deficits provides a rationale for advice from treatment team members about the nature of the teaching environment conducive to learning, preferably one free of distracting objects and clutter. Recommendations to teachers should direct them to break down and simplify steps to task completion, using visual rather than verbal presentations and offering generous praise and support for students (Carpenter 2011). Using role-play and storytelling are effective methods for working with learning deficits. Instructions capitalizing on the sensory strength and various sensory pathways assist individuals in learning. Diversity in neurocognitive function calls for individualized learning plans informed by assessments completed by a multidisciplinary team of specialists.

Child and Adolescent Issues in Communication

Functional and social communication, by promoting the exchange of information and connecting with others, is an essential ingredient of well-being and quality of life for children and adolescents. Communication difficulties are common in individuals with ND-PAE/FASD and other neurodevelopmental disorders and can serve as a prompt to request more comprehensive assessments. In specific language impairment and autism spectrum disorder, cognitive variables (i.e., working memory, language, and executive function) correlate with a person's ability to communicate. Specific to ND-PAE/FASD, communication difficulties characterized by deficits in receptive and expressive language increase the risk for learning and behavioral problems. These manifest as communication, emotional, and behavioral disorders, which unfortunately are common in children and youth heavily exposed to alcohol prenatally. ND-PAE/FASD may thus be suspected when parents report the patient is having trouble maintaining conversation, answering questions, and staying on topic in the context of neurobehavioral disorders (Glass and Mattson 2017). Patients with ND-PAE/FASD share deficits in speech discrimination and comprehension with individuals with other specific language impairment. Separating these deficits requires professional support, but parents can be taught how to communicate with their children. Clinicians can also learn from parents what approaches yield the best exchange of information between parents and the affected children. Combining these methods with existing PAE-informed communication styles, clinicians can improve the likelihood of effective treatment and positive relationships and outcomes.

Focus on the Family Unit

Issues special to children are relevant to mental health professionals; challenges and success in the clinical presentation of a particular patient cannot be separated from the familial background. To support the family and child or youth, the mental health professional should adopt a lifetime approach, starting with the first contact between the diagnosed child and the family. Scenarios of adoptive, foster, biological, and other relatives and their needs are depicted in the following vignette, which covers a range of issues: school, friendship, medications, and overall transition to adulthood:

Clinical Vignette

A 32-year-old mother decides to pursue a second adoption, a sibling of her 9-year-old son, who was recently diagnosed by a multidisciplinary team with ND-PAE/FASD. The team has a contract to diagnose and treat six children in a catchment area and has a 2-year waiting list. The child psychiatrist is responsible for both siblings (the child being adopted is 7 years old) and must consider several issues that arise during consultation with this mother and her sons. Both sons are diagnosed with ADHD and reactive attachment disorder. During the clinical assessment, it becomes apparent that the child being adopted has feeding problems and is losing excessive weight. He is described as hyperactive and inattentive in class. The mother notices that something is wrong and is afraid to go through the challenges of obtaining diagnosis and support; she remembers the experience with her older adopted son. It will be at least 2 years before an appointment with the specialist team can occur, and she expresses anxiety over going with the "wrong" diagnosis as happened previously. Her older son struggled to understand her, and he was misunderstood in his various schools.

Her younger son fails to meet normal developmental milestones and behaviors, sleep issues are frequent, and he reports abuse in a previous foster home and is now struggling with nightmares and mood problems. The woman's immediate goals are to learn modified communication approaches to help her sons, to learn to manage the experience of differences between her sons, to deal with emotional conflict and to "keep sane." She also wants to find peer support. She reveals to the child psychiatrist how petrified she was when she noticed signs of abnormalities in her younger son. She considers putting off the adoption, but ultimately, she decides to proceed.

Approach to Complicated Cases

A few strategies are useful in cases such as the one outlined in the vignette. A sympathetic professional helped this mother during the diagnosis of her 9-year-old. Similar empathetic support through such a relationship should be emulated. There are no shortages of issues and concerns. The clinician collaborates with the family to develop goals and apply current evidence on family interventions, school support, and effective individual techniques. In general, additional targeted and appropriate interventions include family therapy, referral to an expert mental health specialist/psychiatrist, substance use support for parents, and support from foster and adoptive families with knowledge of the manifestations and risks associated with prenatal exposure to multiple substances (Leenaars et al. 2012). Other avenues of assistance are direct interventions for postnatal trauma, enhancing the quality of parent–child interaction, strengthening of maternal affection and attachment, advocating for placement stability, teaching modified ways of communicating, and fostering adaptive and safe functioning. The clinician should think about issues in school with teachers and students who interact with the boy. FASD-informed interventions include these (e.g., stability of placement, attachment, positive parent–child interaction), and many more may be accessed if there are special services in the locality (see Chapter 14, "Psychological Treatment"). An online support group may offer additional help. These services make the whole family the focus of intervention, not just the mother or the sons.

Other treatment strategies require attending to the deficits identified. Interventions should target self-regulation and executive function early. Financial support can be accessed, and efforts should be directed at planning future transitions into adolescence and adulthood. Counseling the mother and using the findings of comprehensive assessments to direct appropriate care are critical success factors. The comprehensive components of support to the child-parent unit are listed in Table 16–3.

TABLE 16–3. Components of professional support for dyad of child and parent

Prepare for "bad news" while providing support.

Appreciate the parent's role in the diagnostic process.

Sensitively interpret and process reactions (e.g., emotional, relational).

Reduce negative experience (blame and shame).

Point out resilience and hope.

Explain causation with biopsychosocial paradigm.

Describe path of care and system.

Identify essential peer support.

Offer commitment to work for positive outcome.

Provide opportunities to explain and debrief.

Plan for transitions and treatments.

Challenges of Families and Caregivers

The misdiagnosis and misclassification of patients with PAE and its mental disorder outcomes were associated with lack of knowledge in the field of ND-PAE/FASD (Chasnoff et al. 2015; Cook et al. 2018). The absence of a diagnostic system to identify patients with the disorder also accounted for misclassification. Until the current diagnostic criteria for ND-PAE/FASD were published in 2013 (with the exception of a very short period in the 1980s; see Chapter 1, "History of Fetal Alcohol Spectrum Disorder and Mental Disorders") (American Psychiatric Association 2013), clinicians had no means of focusing on the construct of the mental disorders originating from PAE. Among other diagnoses commonly ascribed to those with PAE in the child and adolescent mental health system are neurodevelopmental, internalizing, and externalizing disorders. These diagnoses were selected because they were the only options available to diagnosticians. Reactive attachment disorder, conduct disorders, oppositional defiant disorder, and PTSD were reported among the most frequently encountered (mis)diagnoses from DSM (Chasnoff et al. 2015; Dubovsky 2009; Weyrauch et al. 2017). Others included neurodevelopmental disorders offered as a multiaxial diagnosis (e.g., intellectual disorder), a coexisting spectrum of disorders (e.g., language and reading disorders), and completely incidental disorders (e.g., Tourette's syndrome, autism spectrum disorder). Other professionals adopted the view that the disorders with which they labeled patients were treatable, whereas FASD was viewed as having no treatment (Anderson et al. 2020; McLennan and Braunberger 2017). Regularly offering these non-PAE diagnoses was the practice of several clinicians in the child and adolescent mental health system. Pediatricians with a special interest in learning disability and FASD and family members criticized this practice, suggesting it was perpetuated because of the ease of prescribing medications, even if the indications for prescribing were misplaced.

One of the implications of this regular and frequent practice of offering multiple diagnoses to patients with PAE and its sequelae of mental disorders is that it violated the parsimonious principles and practice of diagnosis (Glass and Mattson 2017). Offering multiple diagnoses perpetuates a seemingly irrational method of thinking about diagnoses when they coexist in the absence of a recognized diagnostic model or system. For many years, an opportunity was missed. Adopting the role of PAE and its sequelae produces a more cogent and coherent explanation for the diverse presentations. Such explanatory approaches and adopting a lifelong perspective are more helpful in managing patients and supporting families.

The short-term treatment approaches with medications were ineffective in managing all the emerging PAE outcomes (Mela et al. 2018; O'Malley and Rich, 2013). At times, psychosocial supports were terminated after a certain age, usually the age at which adult services assume care. Reduction or termination of support has been linked to poor outcomes, including criminal involvement, for many individuals with unrecognized PAE and mental disorder (Streissguth et al. 2004). With protracted disability and caregiver stress, these families encountered and reported a heavier burden of care. The experiences of parents who were surveyed about their experience of raising children with the neurocognitive consequences of PAE should guide mental health professionals in planning care for patients. Parents reported that they regularly confront professional ignorance and limited knowledge. They have to fight hard to access services, and they still are blamed for causing the disabilities, increasing their feelings of responsibility (Mukherjee et al. 2013; Whitehurst 2012). These parental experiences should inform the necessary changes to optimize care (Mukherjee et al. 2013).

Family-Based Influences on Brain Development Affected by PAE

Although deficits are regularly determined in those with PAE, strengths identified during assessments are the backbone of care planning. Both deficits and strengths are based on neurological correlates, which inform the clinical manifestations of PAE, as well as the effective interventions. Brain development is influenced by the consequences of PAE and related factors such as family adversity, trauma, and early onset of substance use in the adolescent. As such, clinical assessment should focus on eliciting all relevant factors that contribute to brain development. Some factors cause disruption of neural circuits, whereas others support normalization of function (Georgieff et al. 2018). The clinician who adopts a lifelong perspective will identify prenatal, perinatal, and postnatal contributors to brain development. Among these factors, PAE, which functions directly as a neurotoxic factor, should be recognized. PAE also indirectly insinuates distress during pregnancy and is a red flag for many other factors relevant to brain development. For instance, PAE regularly coexists with poverty, poor nutrition, additional polysubstance use, domestic violence, and poor access to care. These all make important contributions to the mechanisms of brain damage specifically and brain development in general. Recognizing the weight of PAE in the development of a particular individual has implications for diagnosis, intervention, and prevention. For instance, the value of diagnosis based on PAE, is the recognition of important protective factors and the rallying of support and intervention for the individual. Diagnostic processes identify the negative trajectory, explain the complexity at the core foundation of multiple etiologies (malnutrition, trauma/adversity, head trauma, effect of solvents and illicit substances on cognition and behavior, and toxic stress), and serve as red flags for an investigation of maternal mental health (Singal et al. 2017).

Parents react differently at the time of diagnosis. Clinicians support families competently when they are sensitive to the wide range of reactions. Directly, clinicians provide the brain-based explanation geared toward the need expressed by the parent(s). Indirectly, the astute and sensitive mental health professional is a safety net, providing helpful information and resources, wise counsel, and advocacy. The clinician owes the parents or caregivers a candid explanation of the nature of the disability. That explanation should be based on current knowledge of causation, expected course, available treatment, and sources of intervention. Knowledge of the complex, yet uncharted, system that the patient will navigate contributes to the self-evaluation and commitment of the caregiver that will be needed for the lifelong journey ahead. Supporting a child or adolescent with PAE is stressful and can lead to burnout, but it can become easier with an understanding of the disorder. The mental health professional's ability to provide informed support flows from his or her willingness to understand the expressed needs of parents and caregivers.

Evidence now exists about how families navigate the diagnosis and management of their children and youth diagnosed with intellectual disability (Watson et al. 2011). Parents who care for children with ND-PAE/FASD rated public and professional support as positively helpful (Coons et al. 2018). Some families of children with ND-PAE/FASD identified their strength in caring as coming from observing their children's achievement and the professional help they received to support their children. These motivators were further analyzed among 84 caregivers using semistructured interviews. Coons and colleagues (2018) used the family adjustment and adaptation response model and identified unique, yet similar, experiences of family challenges, meaning-making, and adaptation strategies among respondents. In further analysis of these responses, the authors identified components of the model of adjustment and adaptation. They reported that parents desired "understanding FASD and advocating on their child's behalf, day-to-day adaptation, transformational outcomes, as well as the importance of informal and formal supports" (p. 157). Thus, the brain-based explanation and the guiding role of the professional cannot be overemphasized.

Counseling Parents About the Effect and Outcomes of PAE

Although information on the mechanisms of developing FASD is still insufficient, parents appreciate details such as timing, quantity of alcohol, protective factors, and genetic composition that contribute to the development of ND-PAE/FASD. Access to such information may be helpful in reducing the detrimental effect of the news of the disability. Parents surveyed described hearing about the consequences of PAE in their children as the "most frightening and confusing pieces of information" (Beckman and Beckman Boyes 1993). Parents may be at a considerable disadvantage when they learn of the ND-PAE/FASD diagnosis because they may have already been on a tortuous path marked by underdiagnosis and misdiagnosis, which is common with FASD (Chasnoff et al. 2015).

In addition to the awareness of their child's impairment and the challenges their child will face, parents who were interviewed identified coexisting issues. They reported encountering a lack of professional knowledge about FASD and a lack of support for families. They described their experience as a journey in which they had to "fight, battle, and struggle." Many respondents pointed out multiple causes of familial anxiety associated with the disparate and inadequate recognition and understanding of FASD and the disjointed nature of the services, if available at all (Whitehurst 2012).

Any intervention with a chance of success in children and adolescents should be based on the idea that the family is a protective unit. It is important to be factual with parents so that guilt and self-blame are reduced and managed appropriately. Parents should be afforded the opportunity to ask questions and learn about the impact of alcohol on their offspring. Explaining the teratogenic effect of alcohol may include describing the mechanism(s) through which alcohol affects normal development of the embryo and precipitates the resulting clinical features. Many people do not know that alcohol, which is consumed socially in many communities, is a teratogen. Unanswered questions remain on the effect and role of the father's use of alcohol in conception and pregnancy.

Parents need to understand the variability in how the disorder manifests and the reasons for the differences. A diagnosis usually conveys to the layperson a shared commonality in the presentation of features. However, the spectrum used to describe FASD has a double-edged effect. It conveys the different ways that the disorder manifests, such as physical versus mental or cognitive features. At the same time, it erroneously suggests that severity is on a scale, without accounting for the baseline deficit that characterizes the disorder. Impairment ranked below the third percentile in three neurocognitive domains is the essential criterion for diagnosing FASD. That level of impairment is significant enough to raise the level of care above many of the recognized mental disorders in which one domain may be so impaired. Organs widely affected by PAE (e.g., brain, liver, gut, skin, ears) should be identified, and the information should be communicated to the parents so they can anticipate and attend to the consequences of impairment.

Parents, biological or substitute, occupy an important role in supporting the young person with ND-PAE/FASD. Parents' advocacy for their children in accessing appropriate care depends on the information they receive about the deficits of their children. As a major and lifelong intervention necessary for those with the diagnosis, counseling and support should take into account the gaps identified, such as lack of information by professionals and lack of FASD targeted services. Table 16–4 lists the effective programs and approaches for family counseling used with children who manifest the consequences of PAE. Alleviating negative feelings and supporting the efforts of the parents along with the important strategies found to be effective in parenting practices should be comprehensively employed.

Effective counseling and family therapy take into account emotions associated with events during the gestation of the affected child. Some mothers do not become aware of their pregnancy until quite late. Other mothers stop drinking once they find out they are pregnant. Pregnancy produces different emotional states and reactions that must be processed in the context of the parent's psychological makeup. Surrogate parents also experience and express a range of emotions, including those related to the late discovery of the circumstances of alcohol use in the lives of their children. Clinicians should be ready to deal with the consequences of misidentification, missed diagnosis, erroneous multiple diagnoses, and misguided treatment. Some parents have only one child with ND-PAE/FASD in a family with other typically developing children. Other parents have multiple children with the same deficits or have even adopted twins with ND-PAE/FASD to keep them socially developing together. Again, counseling experiences are different in each case. Emotions, thoughts of disappointment, feeling alone, a sense of perpetual failure, and realizing that incorrect, ineffective discipline worsened adverse consequences require psychological interventions and broader support for parents.

Validation, catharsis, cognitive realignment of beliefs, and support from peers all contribute to a more positive outlook for parents. The clinician with a nonjudgmental attitude can strengthen the familial bonds and effectively support families. Guiding parents to identify and define adequate treatment goals helps to dictate the extent and direction of the required intervention. Training in effective communication between parents is viewed as a complementary solution to the child's development and progress. Multiple adoptions, for instance, come with stressful components. Whether the

TABLE 16–4. Effective parental support programs

NAME OF PROGRAM	THEMES ADDRESSED	BENEFITS/AREAS OF IMPROVEMENT
Families Moving Forward (FMF)	Parenting attitude Parenting responses Challenging behavior Functional improvement	Caregiver self-efficacy Caregiver self-care Family needs Child problem behavior
Parent–Child Interaction Therapy (PCIT)	Parent–child relationship Child's social skills Problem behavior Positive discipline	Child behavior Parenting stress
Coaching Families (CF)	Practical parenting tips FASD education Connection to resources Advocacy	Family needs Goal attainment Caregiver stress
Breaking the Cycle	High-risk children Attachment Parent-child relationship	Child depression Attachment Family stress
Parent–Child Assistance Program (P-CAP)	Substance use Mentoring Connecting to resources Parent-child relationship	Maternal outcomes
Parenting training workshops	FASD education Managing behavior Advocacy	Parent knowledge Child behavioral functioning

adoptions were contemporaneous or occurred at separate times is also an issue. Counseling can be directed at preparing the adopting parents or resolving reactions after adoption or fostering.

Conclusion

Children and adolescents are part of the family unit, and they should be supported by that structure. PAE should be seen as a red flag that signals the need for a thorough diagnostic process and points to multiple other brain-affecting adverse factors, such as poverty and malnutrition. Biological and surrogate parents react differently to having a child affected by PAE and its consequences. Transitions are important in the future of the child and adolescent, and planning should start at the point of clinical contact, which should incorporate parents as important partners in treatment. Effective communication involving parent-child, family-professional, and interprofessional dyads should be encouraged because it is pivotal before and after the diagnostic process. Effective strategies should identify evidence-based support programs, especially those applicable to modifying deficits of executive function. The family should also be directed toward broader peer, social, and community supports.

CLINICAL PRACTICAL APPLICATIONS

- To understand adolescent behavior, clinicians should adopt the stress-diathesis model of understanding vulnerability (e.g., PAE) as foundational to the other precipitants of mental disorder (e.g., trauma).

- Comprehensive functional assessment is paramount for effective intervention, and this should involve multidisciplinary professionals, such as occupational therapists.

- Failing grades associated with externalizing behavior should prompt inquiry about neurocognitive deficit, and, if present, effective teaching strategies should be tailored to accommodate deficits and ensure success.

- To account for the wide range of neurocognitive and treatment response variables similar to and contrasting with ADHD and ND-PAE/FASD, diagnosis of ADHD should trigger screening for PAE.

- A positive history of PAE in a child and adolescent is a significant predictor of multiple family-related adverse events (e.g., poverty, poor nutrition, additional polysubstance use, domestic violence, poor access to care) that clinicians should inquire about.

- Caregivers still appreciate explanatory models of the development of disorders associated with PAE, even when scientific and professional understanding is incomplete.

References

American Psychiatric Association: Diagnostic and Statistical Manual of Mental Disorders, 5th Edition. Arlington, VA, American Psychiatric Association, 2013

Anderson T, Mela M, Rotter T, Poole N: A Qualitative investigation into barriers and enablers for the development of a clinical pathway for individuals living with FASD and mental disorder/addictions. Canadian Journal of Community Mental Health 38(3):43–60, 2020

Beckman PJ, Beckman Boyes G (eds): Deciphering the System: A Guide for Families of Young Children with Disabilities. Cambridge, MA, Brookline, 1993

Bertrand J, Interventions for Children with Fetal Alcohol Spectrum Disorders Research Consortium: Interventions for children with fetal alcohol spectrum disorders (FASDs): overview of findings for five innovative research projects. Res Dev Disabil 30(5):986–1006, 2009

Carpenter B: Pedagogically bereft! Improving learning outcomes for children with foetal alcohol spectrum disorders. British Journal of Special Education 38(1):37–43, 2011

Chasnoff IJ, Wells AM, King L: Misdiagnosis and missed diagnoses in foster and adopted children with prenatal alcohol exposure. Pediatrics 135(2):264–270, 2015

Cook JL, Green CR, Lilley C, et al: Response to "A critique for the new Canadian FASD diagnostic guidelines." J Can Acad Child Adolesc Psychiatry 27(2):83–87, 2018

Coons KD, Watson SL, Schinke RJ, Yantzi NM: Adaptation in families raising children with fetal alcohol spectrum disorder: Part I: What has helped. J Intellect Dev Disabil 41(2):150–165, 2016

Coons KD, Watson SL, Yantzi NM, Schinke RJ: Adaptation in families raising children with fetal alcohol spectrum disorder: Part II: What would help. J Intellect Dev Disabil 43(2):137–151, 2018

Dubovsky D: Co-morbidities with mental health for an individual with FASD, in Fetal Alcohol Spectrum Disorder (FASD): Across the Lifespan: Proceedings from an IHE Consensus Development Conference. Edmonton, AB, Institute of Health Economics, 2009, pp 67–71

Frankenberger DJ, Clements-Nolle K, Yang W: The association between adverse childhood experiences and alcohol use during pregnancy in a representative sample of adult women. Womens Health Issues 25(6):688–695, 2015

Fryer SL, McGee CL, Matt GE, et al: Evaluation of psychopathological conditions in children with heavy prenatal alcohol exposure. Pediatrics 119(3):e733–e741, 2007

Fuchs D, Burnside L, Marchenski S, Mudry A: Children with FASD-related disabilities receiving services from child welfare agencies in Manitoba. Int J Ment Health Addict 8(2):232–244, 2010

Georgieff MK, Tran PV, Carlson ES: Atypical fetal development: fetal alcohol syndrome, nutritional deprivation, teratogens, and risk for neurodevelopmental disorders and psychopathology. Dev Psychopathol 30(3):1063–1086, 2018

Glass L, Mattson SN: Fetal alcohol spectrum disorders: a case study. J Pediatr Neuropsychol 3(2):114–135, 2017

Hagan JF Jr, Balachova T, Bertrand J, et al: Neurobehavioral disorder associated with prenatal alcohol exposure. Pediatrics 138(4):e20151553 2016

Hellemans KG, Sliwowska JH, Verma P, Weinberg J: Prenatal alcohol exposure: fetal programming and later life vulnerability to stress, depression and anxiety disorders. Neurosci Biobehav Rev 34(6):791–807, 2010

Ipsiroglu O, Berger M, Lin T, et al: Pathways to overmedication and polypharmacy: case examples from adolescents with fetal alcohol spectrum disorders, in The Science and Ethics of Antipsychotic Use in Children. Edited by Di Pietro N, Illes J. Cambridge, MA, Academic Press, 2015, pp 125–148

Khoury JE, Milligan K: Comparing executive functioning in children and adolescents with fetal alcohol spectrum disorders and ADHD: a meta-analysis. J Atten Disord 23(14):1801–1815, 2019

Kingdon D, Cardoso C, McGrath JJ: Research review: executive function deficits in fetal alcohol spectrum disorders and attention-deficit/hyperactivity disorder—a meta-analysis. J Child Psychol Psychiatry 57(2):116–131, 2016

Lange S, Shield K, Rehm J, Popova S: Prevalence of fetal alcohol spectrum disorders in child care settings: a meta-analysis. Pediatrics 132(4):e980–995, 2013

Lange S, Probst C, Gmel G, et al: Global prevalence of fetal alcohol spectrum disorder among children and youth: a systematic review and meta-analysis. JAMA Pediatr 171(10):948–956, 2017

Lange S, Rehm J, Popova S: Implications of higher than expected prevalence of fetal alcohol spectrum disorders. JAMA 319(5):448–449, 2018

Leenaars LS, Denys K, Henneveld D, Rasmussen C: The impact of fetal alcohol spectrum disorders on families: evaluation of a family intervention program. Community Ment Health J 48(4):431–435, 2012

May PA, Chambers CD, Kalberg WO, et al: Prevalence of fetal alcohol spectrum disorders in 4 US communities. JAMA 319(5):474–482, 2018

McLennan JD, Braunberger P: A critique of the new Canadian fetal alcohol spectrum disorder guideline. J Can Acad Child Adolesc Psychiatry 26(3):179, 2017

McQuire C, Daniel R, Hurt L, et al: The causal web of foetal alcohol spectrum disorders: a review and causal diagram. Eur Child Adolesc Psychiatry 29(5):575–594, 2020

Mela M, Okpalauwaekwe U, Anderson T, et al: The utility of psychotropic drugs on patients with fetal alcohol spectrum disorder (FASD): a systematic review. Psychiatry Clin Psychopharmacol 28(4):436–445, 2018

Millar JA, Thompson J, Schwab D, et al: Educating students with FASD: linking policy, research and practice. Journal of Research in Special Educational Needs 17(1):3–17 2014

Mukherjee R, Wray E, Commers M, et al: The impact of raising a child with FASD upon carers: findings from a mixed methodology study in the UK. Adopt Foster 37(1):43–56, 2013

Murawski NJ, Moore EM, Thomas JD, Riley EP: Advances in diagnosis and treatment of fetal alcohol spectrum disorders: from animal models to human studies. Alcohol Res 37(1):97–108, 2015

O'Malley KD, Nanson JO: Clinical implications of a link between fetal alcohol spectrum disorder and attention-deficit hyperactivity disorder. Can J Psychiatry 47(4):349–354, 2002

O'Malley KD, Rich SD: Clinical implications of a link between fetal alcohol spectrum disorders (FASD) and autism or Asperger's disorder—a neurodevelopmental frame for helping understanding and management, in Recent Advances in Autism Spectrum Disorders, Vol 1. Edited by Fitzgerald M. London, IntechOpen, 2013

Popova S, Lange S, Poznyak V, et al: Population-based prevalence of fetal alcohol spectrum disorder in Canada. BMC Public Health 19(1):845, 2019

Singal D, Brownell M, Chateau D, et al: The psychiatric morbidity of women who give birth to children with fetal alcohol spectrum disorder (FASD): results of the Manitoba Mothers and FASD study. Can J Psychiatry 62(8):531–542, 2017

Streissguth AP, Bookstein FL, Barr HM, et al: Risk factors for adverse life outcomes in fetal alcohol syndrome and fetal alcohol effects. J Dev Behav Pediatr 25(4):228–238, 2004

Tsang TW, Lucas BR, Olson HC, et al: Prenatal alcohol exposure, FASD, and child behavior: a meta-analysis. Pediatrics 137(3):e20152542, 2016

Watson SL, Hayes SA, Radford-Paz E: "Diagnose me please!" A review of research about the journey and initial impact of parents seeking a diagnosis of developmental disability for their child. Int Rev Res Develop Disabil 41:31–71, 2011

Weyrauch D, Schwartz M, Hart B, et al: Comorbid mental disorders in fetal alcohol spectrum disorders: a systematic review. J Dev Behav Pediatr 38(4):283–291, 2017

Whitehurst T: Raising a child with foetal alcohol syndrome: hearing the parent voice. Br J Learn Disabil 40(3):187–193, 2012

CHAPTER 17

Special Issues in the Elderly

WHAT TO KNOW

Systematic research on subjects born after ND-PAE/FASD was clinically described is scarce. Research needs to be done in the context of the developmental origin of disease and health and to understand the lifelong perspective of PAE.

Brain changes of normal aging bear resemblance to the neurocognitive deficits of PAE and may have similar neurobiological underpinnings.

Psychosocial difficulties (e.g.,bereavement) and neurophysiological dysfunction (e.g., reduced cardiac function) compound the physical and neuronal outcomes of PAE in the elderly.

Costs and burden of care may increase when providers ignore the contribution of PAE-related cognitive deficits in elderly patients with multiple medical and mental diagnoses.

Exploitation related to increased risk of suggestibility and ease of manipulation is a real danger in elderly persons with PAE.

Most of what is known about the neurocognitive and behavioral sequelae of PAE comes from studies of the functional outcomes among children and adolescents (Moore and Riley 2015). ND-PAE/FASD has a lifelong perspective and trajectory, with age-related differences. Those in the geriatric age range today (seniors, older adults, or elderly persons—usually 65 years and older) were born almost two decades before the beginnings of the clinical description of ND-PAE/FASD. Nonetheless, although the diagnostic process has specific challenges in this population, existing guidelines do not preclude elderly patients from being diagnosed. In this chapter, I discuss the shorter life expectancy associated with PAE and cover information about brain maturation. Those with ND-PAE/FASD experience a delay in brain neuroplasticity and only benefit from full functional capacity at a later age than the general population.

Limiting the Age of Research Subjects

Most modern studies of those with PAE fix a limit on the upper age of their subjects. Studies of children and adolescents use 18 years as the maximum age; other studies by design extend to about 25 years (Ipsiroglu et al. 2015; Ozsarfati and Koren 2015). In case ascertainment studies, for example, researchers fixed a maximum of 30 years (MacPherson et al. 2011) and 40 years (McLachlan et al. 2019) of age for the invited participants. Clinical samples, however, have provided some clinical and social information on subjects older than the 40-year maximum. Still, those samples contain information on subjects below the elderly range (Astley 2010; Streissguth 1993). There is therefore a limit in research-based knowledge about the clinical presentations of and interventions for the population of elderly persons with PAE and its consequences. Challenges associated with confirming diagnosis in adults whose mothers are more likely to be deceased have also been identified in younger persons (Chudley et al. 2007). Some individuals were adopted years ago, and the chance of getting birth records and reliable collateral information about those pregnancies is slim. The records of others have been lost. That is not to say that people diagnosable with the disorder in the geriatric age range have nothing to contribute to mental health knowledge. Indeed, elderly subjects with ND-PAE/FASD are critical for understanding the developmental origins of adult health and disease (Lunde et al. 2016). PAE is recognized for its epigenetic changes in utero that influence long-term outcomes (Lussier et al. 2017).

Clinical Vignette

While examining, at the request of a lawyer, an elderly man known to be under the care of a psychiatrist, it is revealed that he was initially on probation for mischief. He committed an offense and is facing incarceration. He is diagnosed with bipolar disorder and had attempted suicide once. His cognitive decline is reported as unexpected. The man followed a female executive walking to her car. She left her briefcase to get something she forgot. He then took the briefcase and left. When he explains the theft, he insists that the woman left the briefcase in an open car, and it was too vulnerable for him to leave alone. He says he was "keeping it for her." He was in recovery at the time, having been sober for more than 35 years.

Indicators of PAE are blurred in elderly persons because of several compounding issues and diagnoses. It is difficult to access the patient's birth record and confirm maternal use of alcohol even though his father is still alive, because his father has been diagnosed with amnestic disorder. The simplistic nature of the crime, long-standing dependent living, poor employment record, and other factors suggestive of past involvement in crimes considered senseless are proposed sequelae of PAE. Diagnosis still proves difficult, and even cognitive deficits can be explained by other etiologies over the life course. Team members with expertise in managing complex cases should note the interrelated diagnoses and follow standards of treatment recommended for dysfunction in similar domains. They should also be aware that a combination of diagnoses has an augmenting effect that can linger on into old age.

Relevant Issues of PAE in Elderly Patients

Individuals involved with the care and welfare of the vulnerable sectors of the population championed the development of knowledge and services for the elderly. The roles and needs of caregivers were instrumental in conceptualizing the important aspects of holistic care. For those with ND-PAE/FASD, that care almost always intersects with several organizations and agencies. Already the justice, education, mental health, social services, and housing sectors experience overrepresentation of those with cognitive deficits related to PAE. These same agencies bear the weight of serving all elderly persons, including those without PAE and its consequences. The interface of health and social sectors in the care of elderly persons with ND-PAE/FASD calls for an intentional orientation of services. This is because the developmental and social consequences compound difficulties for these patients. Certain features indicate, depending on the age of onset, that an elderly patient could have PAE (Table 17–1).

The compounding problems have neurological and psychological correlates. The known brain changes of normal aging mirror some of the neurocognitive deficits of PAE. Reduction of white and grey matter, volume reduction in hippocampal cortices, and nerve cell loss have been reported in normal aging. In elderly persons, psychological problems of declining IQ, short-term memory deficits, and deteriorating executive function only complicate already existing deficits in those with PAE. The added social

TABLE 17–1. Age-related indicators studied as precursors to ND-PAE/FASD and supported anecdotally*

TIMING OF INDICATORS	NATURE OF INDICATORS
Prior to old age	Significant adaptive behavioral deficits in adolescents and adults
	Past mental health diagnosis or involvement
	Alcohol and drug use
	Antisocial behaviors
	Repeated pregnancy in females
	Minimal involvement in family responsibilities
During old age	Deficits in socialization and communication skills
	Dependent living and loss of residence
	Evidence of cognitive deficits
	Antisocial personality
	Repeated engagement in "non-self-serving" behavior
	Repeated risky behavior for no purpose

*Age-related indicators studied by Streissguth 1993.

problems related to aging, loss of status, bereavements, and loss of independence, complicate the neurocognitive deficits of PAE.

The interests of elderly patients with ND-PAE/FASD can be supported through the advocacy of mental health professionals who understand the compounding effects of age and cognitive deficits from PAE. Such informed clinicians are more effective when they are aware of how those special issues arise in their daily practice. Patients who present with compounding effects have preexisting problems of cognitive, physical, mental, and social relevance. Sensitivity to how these problems manifest makes it more likely that identification will occur. Education, promotion, collaboration, and innovation are among the essential strategies to support the development of special responses to the compounding challenges of the elderly affected by PAE. To be effective, strategies must address the disadvantages that elderly patients with consequences of PAE grapple with. They are usually vulnerable, easily exploited, and dependent on others.

Relevant issues such as capacity to consent to treatment, guardianship, and other decision-making abilities (e.g., regarding advance directives) are complicated by the neurocognitive deficits of ND-PAE/FASD and further complicated by the aging process and cognitive decline associated with both. Unfortunately, little is known about this area, the relationships, or outcomes. Studies of older individuals with ND-PAE/FASD reported the absence of a network of social support and different diagnostic categorization (Mela et al. 2013; Temple et al. 2015). These studies are not specific to geriatric patients. They included characteristics of the adult patient, including how to qualify for developmental assistance, issues of loss of family support, and adverse negative outcomes.

Age Limitation in Existing Studies

We can learn from adult data within longitudinal cohort studies (Astley 2010; Rangmar 2015). These studies highlight issues that may be applicable to elderly patients, many of whom are diagnosed in the social services and health sectors because they were previously unrecognized as affected by PAE (Temple et al. 2015). The current clinic-based databases contain clinical information about few geriatric patients. For instance, the Canada FASD Research Network, CanFASD, is made up of people referred to clinics in Canada and offers a good source of information with no maximum limit on age. It is, however, clear that information about the manifestations of PAE among elderly patients is still scanty. Some information can be gleaned from samples of patients reported in the literature. The long-term effects of neurodevelopmental disorders such as autism serve as potential clues of what to expect in the prospective neurodevelopmental disorders associated with PAE. Early onset of dementia in those with Down syndrome is a well-known clinical occurrence (Ballard et al. 2016), and examination of this phenomenon may shed light on the pathogenesis, clinical features, and future complications of ND-PAE/FASD. Realistic reasoning similar to that applied to neurodevelopmental disorders should contribute to knowledge of the geriatric complications of PAE, including the clinical, social, treatment, and prognostic implications to address. Such knowledge is essential to improve identification, support, and treatment of those affected. Astley (2010) reported on outcomes involving patients of about 50 years of age. The maximum age of 47 years was noted in a longitudinal population cohort study by Rangmar et al. (2015). In a study of brain morphology (Jarmasz et al. 2017), a subgroup of subjects ages 21–67 years was included. In a case series of peer mentoring and support, two individuals with FASD were more than 60 years of age (Tait et al. 2017). The issues of diagnostic identity and adequacy of community support needed for positive outcomes were described. The scarcity of information is clear in that the matters addressed in most research on adults cannot be generally or directly applied to issues concerning diagnosis and intervention in the elderly.

We are left to conjecture and are forced to extrapolate the longer-term effects of PAE in elderly persons based on findings from studies in adults (Moore and Riley 2015). For instance, the physical features of PAE appear to be somewhat moderated. In a study by Spohr and Steinhausen (2008), examining the persistence of sequelae into adulthood, differences were reported for the dysmorphic features. Short stature, microcephaly, and thin upper lips were found to be stable over the lifetime in the same person. These features are specific and thus are proposed as potential items for screening. Other features, such as height and BMI, were not that stable over the life course. In a different study across a population of those diagnosed with ND-PAE/FASD, variations in height and BMI were noted across age groups (Fuglestad et al. 2014). In that study, looking at the distribution of BMI, 85% of children diagnosed with FASD fell below the third percentile. For those over 21 years of age, only 15% fell below the third percentile. These differences indicate how challenging it is to propose unique features to be expected in geriatric patients with PAE.

Clinical Relevance of PAE-Related Issues of the Elderly

Ongoing issues of lifelong disabilities, dependent living, unemployment, and financial deprivation are common shared findings (Moore and Riley 2015; Rangmar et al. 2015). It is also possible that elderly patients with PAE may live productive lives. Better developed frontal lobe function, environmentally enriched lives, and stronger support are the important positive prognostic factors. It has been proposed that the delay in neurodevelopment may be corrected as executive function improved over time. Similar findings have been reported in those with ADHD—a form of catch-up. Although it is feasible, this argument needs to be verified by studying the longitudinal developmental trajectory of adults with PAE. Increased white matter volume, which occurs later in life, was associated with increased cognitive and executive function improvement (Gautam et al. 2014). Further research is needed to establish the specific mechanism for cognitive changes over the lifespan.

Recent theories explaining the importance of the changes that can affect elderly patients with PAE invoke the developmental origin of disease and health hypothesis. The epigenetic changes PAE caused were responsible for the adult diagnosis of ND-PAE/FASD (Lunde et al. 2016). The field of geriatrics and FASD is in its infancy, but various templates are available to facilitate the study and understanding of the relationship between geriatrics and FASD. Neurocognitive deficits are central to the consequences of PAE, and the effects on elderly patients have varying implications. Burden of care on the family and economic, social, and legal outcomes challenge existing services. Relevant to understanding is awareness of the additive effect of various factors. PAE is considered an agent of fetal programming, which exerts its influence on outcome by interacting with factors in a person's life. Childhood stress, traumatic events in later life, and biopsychosocial factors mediate or aggravate the existing damage from PAE. It will be a while yet before data accumulate to accurately define and specify relevant pressure points. There are several reasons for this. By the time an elderly person (age ≥65) is diagnosed, multiple other comorbid disorders are likely to exist as well, so much so that a separate entity of ND-PAE/FASD is difficult to fathom. In addition, given the lack of maternal confirmation of alcohol use and various contributing and complicating factors that arise throughout the trajectory of life, diagnosing older patients is challenging (Chudley et al. 2007).

Although databases that contain older individuals exposed to alcohol prenatally exist, those individuals may not have been formally and comprehensively diagnosed as recommended by existing guidelines. The data needed to compare with lifelong aspects as in case ascertainment are insufficient. It is hoped that older persons diagnosed with ND-PAE/FASD will constitute a source of important information that is needed to intervene and develop appropriate geriatric services. Given the challenge of a shorter life expectancy, maintaining a cohort for a long enough time requires deliberate efforts. However, data from these cohorts should facilitate understanding of the unique issues of elderly persons with PAE.

We can only hypothesize about PAE outcomes in elderly persons based on adult findings and trajectories reported in the literature. Loss of memory and difficulties with learning new things are common with PAE. Components of cognition present differently over time. Crystalized intelligence remains active, whereas fluid intelligence, usually affected by factors such as speed of information processing, affects learning in this population. Elderly patients with FASD are more likely than not to experience all the negative social and occupational factors related to PAE. They have an increased risk of mental disorder, unemployment, substance use disorder, and social exclusion. When these factors interact, they trigger dysfunction that compounds PAE outcomes.

Dysfunction in elderly patients manifests when clinical decisions and issues of autonomy arise. Decision-making capacity should be assessed carefully. Deficits in executive function, attention, cognition, and memory affect this capacity. Inadequate or deteriorating abilities mean that people in their older years are particularly at a disadvantage for handling the challenges of daily living. Thus, they require support, protection, and safeguards attuned to the effects of PAE to support them in making decisions. The support can be specific both to the consenting processes and to preventing exploitation. In retrospect, it may be recognized that the patient was not competent when previous decisions were made. To avoid this, clinicians must be vigilant in identifying common patterns related to neurocognitive deficits. If deficits are suspected, assessments should be requested to confirm them. Efforts to improve such assessment should employ PAE-informed approaches. For instance, the person should not be rushed to respond when interviewed. Information should be sought from reliable collateral sources to augment the patient's responses. Working with others in the patient's circle of support creates the best prospect of obtaining a patient's informed consent. Individuals with long-term knowledge of the patient develop special ways to effectively communicate with him or her. Such experience provides improved and more reliable communication, which supports the patient's autonomy.

Special Issues in the Care of Elderly Patients With ND-PAE/FASD

The preexisting challenges of ND-PAE/FASD include the common co-occurring cognitive impairments found in other mental disorders. These impairments have been indicated as cost drivers in both schizophrenia and major depressive disorder, for example, because of the recurrent rates of medical treatment and medication nonadherence. Without a good plan, elderly persons with compounding issues frequently use emergency room services, are hospitalized at a higher rate, and experience increased mental health care costs. Recognizing the causes of these cost drivers and strategically addressing them is highly valuable in caring for elderly patients with the consequences of PAE. Thus, there is a need to identify and diagnose older adults early. Interactive collaboration involving health, justice, housing, educational, and social services has the potential of offering preventive benefits to those with adverse consequences of PAE. By working synergistically and carrying out economic analysis of the outcomes, these services can fill an important gap by engaging with elderly patients with ND-PAE/FASD until enough PAE-specific research evidence becomes available. In addition to economic advantages, comprehensive initiatives will enhance appropriate care and promote the human rights of elderly persons with PAE.

Mental disorders are prevalent in old age. They are complicated by environmental and chronic organic brain conditions. The incidence of suicide, alcohol use disorder, mood disorders, and organic psychosis calls for a particular set of skills when PAE and its sequelae are part of the clinical picture. The resilience of elderly patients presenting to a mental health professional should be recognized. First, they survived the very low life expectancy associated with ND-PAE/FASD. Second, they survived the multiple complications of comorbid conditions that mostly went unrecognized. These complications require deliberate, cogent, and unified interventions. Fortunately, existing psychogeriatric services are multidisciplinary in nature. Specialists in the field are familiar with the complexities of comorbidity. They recognize the unique challenges of premorbid personality, social isolation, and access to volunteer organizations to actualizing the health goals of the individual patient. Another source of concern is the suspected high rate of dementia associated with PAE. In a cohort of more than 8,000 individuals with intellectual and developmental disorders (IDD), the prevalence of dementia (8.1%–17%) was between three and eight times the rate in those without IDD (Shooshtari et al. 2017). The cohort was made up of all cases of IDD, including FASD. It provides the only indication that dementia ought to occupy the minds of those dealing with elderly patients with a history of PAE.

When mental health care costs are high, they distract from correct and outcome-based care. Instead, the focus on blame limits care. When the manifestations of neurocognitive deficits of elderly patients are misunderstood, clinicians may characterize the manifesting features as self-inflicted. Advances in care should incorporate mental health care focused on reducing the cost burden. Service development should also involve agencies that advocate and protect elderly persons with cognitive impairment.

The challenge facing the elderly person with ND-PAE/FASD is not recognizing the risk and likelihood of exclusion from mainstream social and health services. Given the known trajectory of those with PAE, housing, criminal justice, and addiction services may inappropriately become involved. These agencies usually have a central role in providing care and organizing services for the elderly person; in turn, the individual identifies with these same services. However, to improve outcomes for elderly persons affected by PAE, services need to prepare for the unique needs of this population as they emerge. Effective responses should be informed by the awareness of the consequences of PAE. Individual plans, protection from exploitation, and flexibility of care should be high on the agenda of the service delivery and care of the mental health professional.

Individuals with ND-PAE/FASD are easily manipulated by others. Given their poor awareness of social risk, along with poor decision-making capacity, adverse consequences are common. When elderly patients diagnosed with ND-PAE/FASD interact with more competent and exploitative individuals, negative outcomes can result. Elder abuse can be problematic because of the ease of manipulation and suggestibility that distinguish individuals with PAE. These traits arise from neurocognitive limitations that are the bedrock of both aging and PAE. The mental health professional has the important role of screening for, recognizing, and interrupting elder abuse both domestically and institutionally. A comprehensive integrative-preventive approach is necessary to effectively guide the professional. Legal and government entities should proactively introduce programs that can identify and accommodate the compounding deficits of PAE, aging, and mental disorders.

Conclusion

The rate of cognitive impairment in the population is increasing. It is impossible to discount the contribution of PAE to the high prevalence of cognitive impairment. The various causes compound each other and impose a high economic cost on society. The consequences for individual patients can be reduced by alert and astute mental health professionals. Their awareness of the PAE red flags can facilitate more timely and effective intervention. However, on a larger scale, services with interactive preventive plans should be the goal. Reducing vulnerability, addressing social exclusion, and providing medical and mental health support should be the goals of such services. The economic cost of this approach can be enormous, but ultimately, it is cost-effective when older adults with PAE sequelae are identified and cared for by PAE-informed, specialized, efficient multisectoral services.

CLINICAL PRACTICAL APPLICATIONS

- Clinicians advocate better for the elderly and their caregivers when they understand the compounding effect of aging on neurocognitive deficits consequential to PAE.

- Clinical and functional variables in the elderly with PAE appear to be on a continuum, with the best outcomes associated with matured frontal lobes, enriched lives, and better support.

- Clinicians should vigilantly observe patients' decision-making ability, autonomy, and independence when treating the consequences of PAE, especially in elderly patients.

- Care of the elderly with the consequences of PAE should involve multiple services and be interdisciplinary, just, and comprehensive.

- Until PAE-specific geriatric evidence of clinical outcomes is studied, other neurodevelopmental disorders may provide a few clues about what to expect and how to address the needs of elderly persons.

References

Astley SJ: Profile of the first 1,400 patients receiving diagnostic evaluations for fetal alcohol spectrum disorder at the Washington State Fetal Alcohol Syndrome Diagnostic & Prevention Network. Can J Clin Pharmacol 17(1):e132–e164, 2010

Ballard C, Mobley W, Hardy J, et al: Dementia in Down's syndrome. Lancet Neurol 15(6):622–636, 2016

Chudley AE, Kilgour AR, Cranston M, Edwards M: Challenges of diagnosis in fetal alcohol syndrome and fetal alcohol spectrum disorder in the adult. Am J Med Genet C: Semin Med Genet 145C(3):261–272, 2007

Fuglestad AJ, Boys CJ, Chang PN, et al: Overweight and obesity among children and adolescents with fetal alcohol spectrum disorders. Alcohol Clin Exp Res 38(9):2502–2508, 2014

Gautam P, Nuñez SC, Narr KL, et al: Effects of prenatal alcohol exposure on the development of white matter volume and change in executive function. Neuroimage Clin 5:19–27, 2014

Ipsiroglu O, Berger M, Lin T, et al: Pathways to overmedication and polypharmacy: case examples from adolescents with fetal alcohol spectrum disorders, in The Science and Ethics of Antipsychotic Use in Children. Edited by Di Pietro N, Illes J. London, Academic Press, 2015, pp 125–148

Jarmasz JS, Basalah DA, Chudley AE, Del Bigio MR: Human brain abnormalities associated with prenatal alcohol exposure and fetal alcohol spectrum disorder. J Neuropathol Exp Neurol 76(9):813-833, 2017

Lunde ER, Washburn SE, Golding MC, et al: Alcohol-induced developmental origins of adult-onset diseases. Alcohol Clin Exp Res 40(7):1403–1414, 2016

Lussier AA, Weinberg J, Kobor MS: Epigenetics studies of fetal alcohol spectrum disorder: where are we now? Epigenomics 9(3) 291–311, 2017

MacPherson PH, Chudley AE, Grant BA: Fetal Alcohol Spectrum Disorder (FASD) in a Correctional Population: Prevalence, Screening and Characteristics (Research Report R-247). Ottawa, ON, Correctional Service Canada, 2011

McLachlan K, McNeil A, Pei J, et al: Prevalence and characteristics of adults with fetal alcohol spectrum disorder in corrections: a Canadian case ascertainment study. BMC Public Health 19(1):43, 2019

Mela M, McFarlane A, Sajobi TT, Rajani H: Clinical correlates of fetal alcohol spectrum disorder among diagnosed individuals in a rural diagnostic clinic. J Popul Ther Clin Pharmacol 20(3), e250–e258, 2013

Moore EM, Riley EP: What happens when children with fetal alcohol spectrum disorders become adults? Curr Dev Disord Rep 2(3):219–227, 2015

Ozsarfati J, Koren G: Medications used in the treatment of disruptive behavior in children with FASD—a guide. J Popul Ther Clin Pharmacol 22(1):e59–e67, 2015

Rangmar J, Hjern A, Vinnerljung B, et al: Psychosocial outcomes of fetal alcohol syndrome in adulthood. Pediatrics 135(1):e52–e58, 2015

Shooshtari S, Stoesz BM, Udell L, et al: Aging with intellectual and developmental disabilities and dementia in Manitoba. Adv Ment Health Intellect Disabil 11(4):134–144, 2017

Spohr HL, Steinhausen HC: Fetal alcohol spectrum disorders and their persisting sequelae in adult life. Dtsch Arztebl Int 105(41):693–698, 2008

Streissguth AP: Fetal alcohol syndrome in older patients. Alcohol Alcohol Suppl 2:209–212, 1993

Tait CL, Mela M, Boothman G, Stoops MA: The lived experience of paroled offenders with fetal alcohol spectrum disorder and comorbid psychiatric disorder. Transcult Psychiatry 54(1):107–124, 2017

Temple VK, Ives J, Lindsay A: Diagnosing FASD in adults: the development and operation of an adult FASD clinic in Ontario, Canada. J Popul Ther Clin Pharmacol 22(1):e96–e105, 2015

CHAPTER 18

Special Issues in
Forensic Mental Health

WHAT TO KNOW

The consequences of PAE readily intersect with various contact points in the criminal justice system in ways that are pervasive and expensive.

The diagnosis of ND-PAE/FASD and criminal activity share a common list of criminogenic variables.

No specific criminal activity is pathognomonic of PAE, but repeated offending, suggesting inability to learn from past experiences, is highly suspect.

Case ascertainment studies found that 15%–18% of adults in the correctional population had a diagnosis of ND-PAE/FASD, with a higher number of cases occurring in the forensic mental health system.

Current estimates are regarded as underestimates of actual rates because of the invisibility of the disorder.

Legal associations (American Bar Association, Canadian Bar Association, Truth and Reconciliation Commission of Canada) have signaled their concern about the treatment of those with PAE-associated deficits navigating the criminal justice system. Several authorities have called for the system to accommodate the deficits of ND-PAE/FASD.

It has been suggested that a substantial portion of criminal offending can be ascribed to individuals with the lifelong sequelae of PAE (Fast and Conry 2009). In one youth forensic assessment unit, the 1-year rate of FASD was 23%. These numbers indicate a high prevalence of individuals with FASD in the correctional system. The mechanism by which the deficits of PAE cause affected individuals to offend and to become and remain involved with the criminal justice system (CJS) is a matter of ongoing research and discussion. Of the total estimated cost of spending on FASD, 40% was attributable to the correctional component. Knowledge of professionals, screening to identify those with PAE consequences, diversion, and the remedy of the law are all important components of this chapter. Current case law recognizes that the consequences of PAE meet the threshold of the legal definition of mental disorder or disease of the mind. A recent systematic review and meta-analysis of PAE in the CJS called for a stronger connection between research, practice, and policy as the way forward. Considering the economic, social justice, medical, and mental health perspectives of ND-PAE/FASD, this guidance and direction is of utmost importance to public health and public safety.

Intersection of PAE Deficits and the Criminal Justice System

Forensic is a word easily replaced by "forensic science." Its origin is from the Latin word *forum*, referring to open court, public debate, or discussion. It relates to or denotes the application of scientific method or techniques in the investigation of crime. *Forensic psychiatry* is a subspecialty of medicine concerned with the application of clinical expertise at the interface of psychiatry and law. Put another way, it aims to prevent, ameliorate, and treat victimization arising from mental disorder (Gunn and Taylor 2014). It is this wider application that impacts individuals with PAE and its consequences.

The advantages of the involvement of mental health professionals who know about the deficits of PAE in the CJS are the following: caring for the patient, protecting the professionals, and, by extension, reducing victimization in society (Nelson and Trussler 2015). Without the knowledge of the sensory hypersensitivities found in those with FASD, for instance, unwarranted and unnecessary violence can occur with the police when a person who is intolerant to touch on account of sensory processing deficits is handled (Carr et al. 2010). Unrecognized diagnosis with the hidden impaired psycholegal abilities of those with FASD risks poor representation in court and diminishes the potential for diversion from court despite large numbers of PAE-affected individuals going through the courts (Chartrand

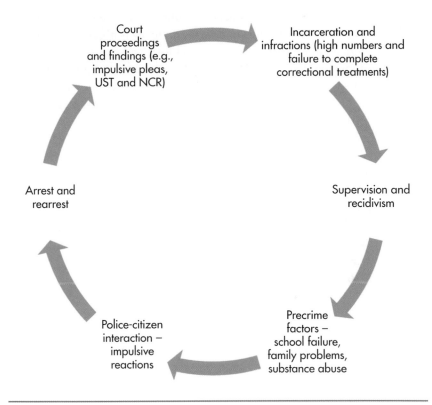

FIGURE 18–1. Intersection points of PAE-affected individuals with the criminal justice system.

NCR=not criminally responsible by reason of mental disorder; UST=unfit to stand trial.

and Forbes-Chilibeck 2003; McLachlan et al. 2014). In the custodial setting, infractions based on FASD-dependent cognitive deficits (e.g., impulse control, adaptive problems following rules, easy manipulation, unwise gang activities) are higher and result in protracted criminal involvement of affected individuals (Figure 18–1).

Lack of FASD diagnostic capacity contributes to impaired individuals falling through the cracks. Offenders with ND-PAE/FASD, by the nature of their behavioral difficulties, are classified as having a high risk to offend or be violent. This means that they will be unsuitable for early release. Release before the end of an offender's sentence guarantees a graded release plan that includes adequate support in the community, which is associated with a better chance of success. In the case of the unrecognized deficits of PAE, however, this chance is negligible. Being in the high-risk category eliminates the possibility of release with support and diversion (Brown et al. 2012). When an offender is released under supervision to a community parole officer who is not knowledgeable about the deficits associated with FASD, noncompliance with the conditions of parole is highly likely (Pei et al. 2016). Deficits in executive function, memory, and comprehension and receptive language difficulties, which may be masked by a higher-level vocabulary and seeming acquiescence to instructions—without full understanding—contribute to offenses of noncompliance (Substance Abuse and Mental Health Services Administration 2014). The revolving circle of offending continues and is likely to be uninterrupted unless mental health professionals become aware and informed about the deficits associated with ND-PAE/FASD (Fast and Conry 2009) (Figure 18–1). These deficits are better identified in comprehensive assessments completed by multidisciplinary teams (Brintnell et al. 2019).

Education and training should be enhanced in the different sections of the CJS in which clinical practice can influence outcomes, such as the following: police interactions, preadjudicatory assessments, court expert-based assessment, in-custody mental health care, and community case management (Brown et al. 2010). The large numbers of individuals with ND-PAE/FASD, who are mostly unrecognized, need FASD-informed practices. When education and training are also directed to enhancing clinicians' acumen in recognition and appropriate intervention, the benefits of screening, diagnosis, intervention, and diversion accrue to society. Mental health professionals therefore contribute to changing the negative trajectory of patients.

Diagnosis and Management in the Forensic Mental Health System

Clinical Vignette

A 25-year-old man is on probation and is referred for a psychiatric assessment. He has breached his parole condition of abstaining from alcohol, and this is his last chance before becoming homeless or incarcerated. Being of legal age, he helped purchase cigarettes and alcohol for his 16-year-old friend. The patient drank half a bottle of beer. Of the five homes he has lived in while being on probation, the current group home is the one he likes the most. He says he enjoys being with and joking with the other 10 residents and likes the food; he thinks "everybody there is nice." Reasons he lost his previous residential placements include fighting, "horseplay," making inappropriate comments to female staff, "borrowing stuff" from others, and drinking alcohol against house policy.

Adoption documents indicate that his mother drank alcohol during pregnancy and "had a low-self esteem" and that his father was "easily frustrated." His parents were accused of neglect, and he was removed from their care 4 months after birth. He was moved between several foster homes and finally adopted when he was 8 or 9 years old. He was assessed in the fifth grade and prescribed Ritalin because "I was hyper and trashed my room." Developmentally, he began antisocial behaviors at the age of 14. He struggled to read and found academic subjects very difficult, with the exception that he excelled in "gym and drama." He skipped school frequently. He readily fought in and out of school and "broke my nose eight times." In other instances, he said he tried to fight off bullies or protect others from bullies. He left a number of jobs because he was unable to wake up in the morning, follow directions, or get along with his boss.

He experiences "massive mood swings and anxiety." He complains of hearing voices, which get louder and worse when he smokes marijuana. Still, he spends money on cannabis and sometimes cannot afford food or basic necessities. He reports varied sleep patterns, sometimes sleeping until 3 P.M. and other times staying awake for days.

Red Flags: What Else Could It Be?

Red flags for this patient include early onset of behavioral problems, several foster care placements, residential instability, an adoption record suggesting PAE, stimulant prescription, and assuming people are nice. PAE is suspected with the manifestation of mood swings and impulsive and aggressive behavior related to unawareness of risk. His drama and gym skills are nonverbal and align with PAE-related abstraction difficulties of prefrontal cortical dysfunction. This manifests in challenges with concepts of time, money, math, and abstract subjects. Difficulty with school subjects and a poor work record are virtually identical in those with a diagnosis (Streissguth et al. 2004). He displays behavior suggestive of immaturity; he relates to a younger person and seems inclined to follow suggestions even from a younger person.

Possible Modifications

The vignette subject's patterns of behavior suggest initiating the assessment process for ND-PAE/FASD. The diagnosis, if present, opens up new and improved strategies for managing his case, which differ from strategies employed for neurotypical individuals. Efforts to identify his strengths and regularly commend simple positive actions and qualities reflect strength-focused interventions. To prevent exploitation and the continuing negative financial consequences resulting from his cognitive deficits, a mentor and trustee should be assigned to manage the subject's social assistance income. Diagnosis and treatment in the community can be supported by an expert diagnostic service or by the mental health system.

For managing the patient's alcohol problems, visual and pictorial representations of concepts are more effective. For instance, alcohol is represented as a cliff that he will be dragged over by negative peers and associates.

The consequences of going back to drinking and the benefits of staying away from the edge of that cliff should be clearly laid out. Arrange with the group home operator to provide a handheld notebook for the patient to record the list of house rules in his own words (or pictorially), and to review those rules periodically. Using the circle of support and fence method, the patient should be guided on how to respond to the invitations of negative peers. This takes the form of a sketch that identifies people according to their place in one of three zones: the safe zone, the avoid zone, and the interface zone. Contact with those in the interface zone must be considered based on a checklist of questions about each peer, such as the following: Does he or she care about me? What in the past supports that? What will my doctor say about associating with him or her? Approaches to true understanding and communication should be adapted to the person's level of cognitive functioning, taking into account both the person's deficits and strengths (see Chapter 21, "Future of the Interface of Prenatal Alcohol Exposure and Mental Disorder," for discussion of critical success factors).

Transition and Housing

An earlier report for transforming the correctional programs to accommodate individuals with the deficits of PAE recommended the development of better case management strategies as a first step (Boland et al. 1998). The recommendations acknowledged that the path to such management depended on comprehensive assessment, delineation of deficits, and connecting people with services that could address their deficits with flexibility. Traditional cognitive-behavioral therapy was discouraged for those diagnosed or suspected of ND-PAE/FASD because they lack the ability to develop the superior cognitive skills necessary to assimilate and to generalize or transfer the therapy concepts to daily life. It is not solely a matter of "tweaking" or making modifications to the present system to fit the needs of FASD patients; it is, rather, a rethinking of the system to fit their needs. The wrong intervention can have devastating results, as is all too apparent considering recidivism rates and the tragic stories behind these rates.

Housing for those with ND-PAE/FASD can serve as a stabilizing force, given the multiple dysfunctions that offenders must confront. The treatment team should identify the right residence based on past failures and successes, current level of dysfunction, and availability of sufficient support. During transition, special homes—those with a highly structured environment and the capability of continuing customized interventions—should be identified. If such facilities are not secured, the person is likely to be unsupported and continue the cycle of reoffending. Examples of such homes should be included in a list kept by discharge specialists. Close communication between professionals in the custodial institution and the designated home is vital. This provides the avenue for sharing information on effective strategies and discontinuing previously tried ineffective ones. The goal is to develop a framework that enables the person to generalize to improved function in a different context.

Types of Offenses Committed by Individuals With ND-PAE/FASD

In a sample of about 400 youth with FASD, the most frequently described offenses were crimes against persons (45%), which included shoplifting or theft (36%), burglary (15%), domestic violence (15%), and assault (17%) as well as drug possession or selling. Other crimes in the adolescent sample included property damage, vehicular crimes, and running away. Sexual assault, including child molestation, was identified in 18% of the sample (Streissguth et al. 2004). Another study found no difference in the types of crime committed by those affected with PAE (Flannigan et al. 2018b). Recently, however, administration of justice offenses, such as breaches (i.e., failure to attend or comply), were overrepresented among a sample of offenders diagnosed with ND-PAE/FASD in an adult prison (Brintnell et al. 2019). However, these offenders were referred for the study because correctional officers identified them as repeat offenders.

Sexually inappropriate behavior by individuals with ND-PAE/FASD has been noted as a cause of several offenses. Researchers have indicated that it is imperative to study the causes, manifestations, and interventions required to understand the relationship between PAE and sexual offending (Anderson et al. 2018; Brown et al. 2017). There is a noticeable knowledge gap in the summary of research findings and the strategies for intervention. Treatment should be FASD-informed and comprehensive. Regarding sexual offending, professionals should be capable of distinguishing the cognitive deficits associated with poor boundary awareness and the intentional malicious offending by affected persons.

Factors Contributing to Offending

The general criminogenic variables that contribute to antisocial activities and criminal behaviors also precipitate ND-PAE/FASD. Variables such as the following exert prenatal and postnatal influences that mediate the effect of prenatal alcohol exposure and criminal outcome: gender, parental social class, marital status, socioeconomic status, employment status, residential stability, parental substance use disorder, parental criminality, maternal depression, parental education level, parental IQ score, perinatal injury, use of other substances by the mother and/or the offspring, and head injury. The frequent use of cannabis, nicotine, opiates, cocaine, ecstasy, and amphetamines is known in patients with ND-PAE/FASD and also contributes to offending (Streissguth et al. 2004; Weyrauch et al. 2017). Use of alcohol and illicit substances by the male parent and poor quality of parenting are commonly shared factors in the diagnosis and criminality (Lander et al. 2013; Solis et al. 2012).

Experiences of adversity, multiple comorbidities, and varied offending histories are common in individuals with FASD. The assumptions of the CJS are often incorrectly applied to those with FASD. Having a significantly lower level of cognitive function, as reported by virtually all research studies on offenders with FASD compared with those without FASD, negatively impacts functional ability to be law abiding. Assumptions about the ability to choose right versus wrong, to consider the consequences of one's actions, and to comply with instructions are frequently fallacious. There are many reasons why the neurocognitive deficits in PAE are likely to intersect with offending behavior. For instance, with executive deficits in impulse control and deficiencies in boundary awareness, people with FASD do not grasp the social or legal significance of permanently depriving someone of property through stealing, breaking the rules, making inaccurate statements, or touching someone inappropriately. The connection between affect and situational responses is misconceived, and the inability to regulate affect can result in impulsive and aggressive behavior leading to criminal charges. Additionally, the self-regulation difficulties in youth with FASD and their tendency to be highly suggestible through peer contagion contribute to copying offenses (Dishion and Dodge 2005; Pollard et al. 2004).

Cultural Aspects of PAE in the Criminal Justice System

Clinical Vignette

A 24-year-old indigenous man comes to an outpatient clinic complaining of anger toward his father for having abandoned him and "not been there for me." He states that he was "run over by a car" when he was 5 years old and spent about 36 months (6 of these in a coma) in the hospital undergoing several corrective surgeries to repair his rib cage and fractured skull and to undergo a nephrectomy. He describes an inability to sleep without medications and a long history of significant alcohol and stimulant drug use. His mother died 2 years earlier at the age of 49 from a chronic liver disease; she had a history of chronic alcohol problems. He had been raised by his maternal grandfather, who taught him about indigenous spiritual ceremonies. However, his struggle with alcohol and substances, which began at age 11, triggered by his poor school performance, prevented him from taking part in spiritual ceremonies, which left him feeling isolated from his community. He dropped out of school in the seventh grade and became involved in socialized conduct behaviors (e.g., group theft, joint bullying, vandalism). By the time he visits the clinic, his criminal record includes over four dozen convictions, mostly breaches of parole and property offenses.

The typical unmodified pattern of managing this type of case is first to develop a case formulation. This conceptualizes a life course characterized by persistent antisocial behavior. Given the repetitive offending already manifested, the interaction between the man's criminogenic environment and his foundational neuropsychological deficits will produce a long and destructive criminal life (Snedker et al. 2017). He may be offered programs to address anger (anger management), alcohol and substances (addiction counseling, self-help, and other intensive programs), and socio-occupational dysfunction (occupational rehabilitation programs). However, predominantly considered a hopeless case, either as an intractable recidivist or a victim of unchanging social circumstances, the psychoeducational correctional programs and addiction programs are insufficient to change his life trajectory. Although some evidence exists for the value of spiritual experience in fostering prosocial behavior, the possibility of this seems negligible for the patient given his early childhood trauma, brain injury, impulsive behavior, and disqualification from spiritual engagement and activities due to ongoing alcohol use (Keightley et al. 2018).

The referral issue of anger could reveal relevant clues to the foundational problems. A carefully obtained history of chronic liver disease and death associated with the lifelong alcohol use of his mother should trigger inquiry about PAE. It is important that clinicians recognize the essential factors closely associated with PAE because current screening tools have yet to be validated in all populations. Personal history of alcohol use, family history of alcohol use, and intensive residential treatment for alcohol, drugs, and mental disorders are risk factors that can be clinically evaluated. These risk factors are positive in this man's case (Goh et al. 2008). Additional diagnostic reinforcement comes from postnatal behaviors and events. Being raised by nonbiological parents, by extended family, or in the child welfare system has been recognized as evidence for maternal dysfunction due to substance use and as a strong indicator of PAE. School failure, early onset of alcohol use, and conduct behavioral problems point to neuropsychological deficits. By extension, the accident at the age of 5 could be linked to his deficits in attention and risk awareness. These can be inquired about in a comprehensive assessment.

Health and social service systems house many individuals who are misunderstood by virtue of their disability. It behooves professionals to reexamine their approach and bias when confronted with the repeated failure of a standardized protocol and lack of success despite effort with particular patients. A different interpretation may be called for. Important to this approach, clinicians should note patterns of maladaptive behavior that align with neurocognitive deficit, and patients should be referred for a comprehensive assessment. In patients with FASD, the reported and observed behaviors form a recognizable pattern, for example, failure to remember rules of group engagement and missed appointments, which interferes with any treatment. Other individuals with FASD present with behavior suggesting slowed speed of information processing, lower level of maturity than expected for their age, inappropriateness in words or actions, and displays of inconsistent abilities. Taking unnecessary risk is anchored in risk unawareness and gullibility, a component of poor judgment from executive dysfunction (Greenspan and Driscoll 2016).

It is therefore possible that with a more informed CJS and trained professionals, the pattern of repeat offending displayed by this man will raise the following question: "What else is going on?" The strong PAE indicators that apply to him should trigger a deviation from the usual anger management recommendation. The focus should be on the essential guiding principles for effective correctional intervention (the risk-need-responsivity model). The patient's needs are articulated by the features he manifests. His level of risk for recidivism is high on account of his age, past history, failure under supervision, substance use, poor support, and mental disorders (Flannigan et al. 2018a). Responsivity represents a viable missing element in this vignette; school and correctional programs failed to respond effectively to reduce recidivism. It also hinges on a recognition of the patient's unique learning style and prompts modification of future interventions to accommodate such deficits that contribute to involvement in crime. To reduce this involvement, the risk-need-responsivity model espouses intervening to help offenders through compassionate, collaborative, and dignified human service (Bonta and Andrews 2010). Factors that predict criminal behavior should be targeted. The neuropsychological and sociocultural factors are best evaluated and identified through a comprehensive assessment of the consequences of PAE.

Although cultural factors are involved in the acceptance of alcohol use in some situations, ethnocultural background is not a defined risk for PAE. Communities with high rates of alcohol use register higher rates of PAE and its mental disorder consequences. A popularized saying is "FASD is not an Aboriginal problem, it is an alcohol problem." The man's grandfather demonstrates both the extended support system that may be available for reducing risk and the resilience in some communities despite experiencing adversity. The man's indigenous background should prompt clinicians to seek culturally appropriate interventions that support hope and resilience (Keightley et al. 2018).

Currently, few forensic mental health services exist to provide expert opinions about the mental condition of offenders and to establish whether offenders affected by PAE are competent or not (Brown et al. 2019). However, opinions on criminal responsibility (insanity), moral blameworthiness, and the appropriateness of sentencing and the death penalty have been provided by experts in the field. It is such assessments that could provide the recommendations that would lead the system to change the approach of the past (Mela and Luther 2013; Mela et al. 2019).

Comprehensive assessments for PAE and its adverse outcomes, recommended by most diagnostic guidelines, provide the impetus for a change of approach. When ND-PAE/FASD is confirmed, modified expectations and realistic communication between patient, clinician, and the mental health system are required. Central to these is the redefinition of success, which should be determined in a personal, patient-centered manner. In place of expecting the patient in the vignette to behave like everyone else, he should be provided with what he needs to successfully navigate the CJS. His repeated offending was previously understood as the result of persistent, deliberate, and willful decisions. Accepting the neurocognitive deficits identified during assessment redirects attention from blame to the root cause of the behavior difficulty: brain dysfunction. Intervention strategies should be aligned with mental rather than chronological age, deficient cause and effect thinking should be amended, and easily accomplishable tasks aimed at boosting self-esteem should be assigned. These are the beneficial aspects of assessments. Others can be invited to play a supportive role, for example, providing appointment reminders. Successful interventions derived from comprehensive assessments also contribute to public safety when criminal offending is reduced or stopped.

Modifications should be promoted because they encourage a more positive caregiving attitude, reduce caregiver stress, and improve outcomes. These improved outcomes facilitate connection with community care, which has been found to break the cycle of repeat offending. The offender is now seen as *unable* rather than *unwilling*. Rather than group interventions, which can reinforce the patient's sense of inadequacy when he is confronted with text-heavy material, individual sessions for anger management and counseling have a better chance of success. After establishing a comfortable level of patient comprehension, childhood issues can be explored. Engaging in art allows verbal communication difficulties to be bypassed; emotions can be expressed via another channel. Additional counseling should sensitively address past trauma (through a trauma-informed lens), alcohol and drug use, grief and loss, and the consequences of repeated involvement with the CJS.

Understanding the patient's level of comprehension allows for conversation that could reveal unresolved issues regarding his significant injury at the age of 5 (e.g., a sense of loss regarding his kidney and his physical vitality) as well as feelings of abandonment by his mother. Pain is complicated in ND-PAE/FASD by the hyposensitivity and hypersensitivity sensory processing difficulties. Also, sleep difficulties have multiple causes and need to be addressed systematically. Providing practical sleep hygiene techniques and evaluating and effectively managing stress, anxiety, depression, and pain create confidence in the clinician. Providing cultural and spiritual reorientation and engagement allows him to address the disconnection from his culture and to benefit from a culture-based social support system.

Case management by community correctional professionals should be enhanced by education on FASD and collaboration with clinicians with expertise in managing FASD cases. Through such collaboration, strategies to ameliorate neurocognitive deficits are shared. In the event of noncompliance by the person or treatment ineffectiveness, a clinical approach should be employed to identify the contributing factors and to strategize how best to therapeutically manage those. Successful treatment and a positive outcome in this case are possible with modified expectations, structure, support, and sensitive supervision, and the adoption of flexible strategies that recognize neurodiversity and accommodate the patient's learning style.

Therapeutic Jurisprudence (Using the Law to Help)

Once factors indicate the possibility of ND-PAE/FASD, ideally, a diagnostic assessment ensues. However, the low capacity for assessment and diagnosis makes this unlikely (Clarren et al. 2011). Nevertheless, interventions can still be provided. These interventions involve modifying existing strategies to overcome ineffective communication. Coping strategies are taught using visual and graphic representations. In some patients, noted to have early onset of problems, repeated offending, and unsupported psycholegal abilities, different legal remedies should be actively explored. Because few exist, the precedence for those cases will have to develop in the coming years.

Most jurisdictions recognize mental disorder as the pivotal condition that requires the proposal of legal solutions. Virtually all courts have accepted the neurocognitive and functional problems associated with PAE as a mental disorder. On the basis of that recognition, various decisions on capacity and competence have been rendered. Decisions of incompetence or finding an accused unfit to stand trial on account of PAE vary on a case-by-case basis. Memory problems, diminished intellectual abilities, slower speed of processing information, and severe inattention disrupt relevant abilities necessary for conducting a defense. Assessed youth overrated their abilities compared with objective assessments of true competence (McLachlan et al. 2014). Very few cases have succeeded in criminal responsibility being abrogated on account of features of PAE (Mela and Luther 2013). More commonly, the courts accept evidence about PAE with regard to diminished responsibility, mitigation, and, at times, aggravation when issuing sentences.

Not surprisingly, deficits from ND-PAE/FASD fail to meet the higher threshold of an insanity defense. ND-PAE/FASD was mentioned in the defense of diminished capacity and noted as the number one reason in 133 Canadian cases in which neuroscientific evidence was presented in court (Chandler 2015). Justice practices should be informed by an accurate estimation of the individual's ability and combined with the use of effective interventions that do not harm the individual.

Because the consequences of PAE-related deficits are not validated with respect to competency to stand trial, the legal relief associated with justice practices is limited. The courts have reasonably accepted that PAE deficits affect fitness to plead and to communicate with counsel. The majority of courts have stopped short at recognizing the neurocognitive deficits as severe enough to interrupt legal awareness of wrongdoing and consequential impact of criminal acts. More worrisome is the inconsistent manner in which FASD has been used in sentencing. The role of PAE-related deficits in mitigating moral blameworthiness is negligible compared with conclusions related to aggravation drawn in several cases.

Implications and Interpretation of Prevalence Rates of ND-PAE/FASD in the Criminal Justice System

Individuals with FASD are overrepresented in the CJS. The figures are supported by research in correctional populations. Research ranges from studies in the community among youth under correctional supervision to youth in correctional and psychiatric facilities. Other studies reported rates of FASD in adult correctional facilities and adult outpatient forensic psychiatric clinics. However, these published data paint an uncertain picture of the extent of the problem. The reported rates range from 0.008% to 36% of the studied populations (Flannigan et al. 2018b). The most reasonable explanation is the use of different methods of calculating the rates of individuals in the system diagnosed with ND-PAE/FASD. In one set of studies with rates as low as fractions of a percentage, the data were obtained from prison directors and policy makers, who relied on diagnosed cases contained in official documents (Burd et al. 2003, 2010). By counting the officially diagnosed individuals in the institutional records available to them, the reliability of their figures cannot be questioned because they report what is actually recorded. If the lower figures are credible, it insinuates the middle and higher rates are exaggerated.

However, if the very low rates are discounted on account of the misguided research method applied, the other rates can be assumed to be correct and not overinflated. The most sophisticated method of estimating the rate of FASD in the correctional population depends on a study type: active case ascertainment study. It involves inviting virtually all potential candidates in the population to allow themselves to be ascertained as having or not having the diagnosis in question. During the study, those who agree to participate will undergo a complete and comprehensive assessment. These long assessments adhere to an accepted process defined by the Canadian diagnostic guidelines (Cook et al. 2016). This is a published account that combines current research evidence with the agreement of experts on how diagnosis should be performed. Rates determined through this method employ the rigor required to achieve credibility. Policy proposals should use the rates derived from these studies.

Correctional Services of Canada researchers conducted an incidence study among 92 new admissions to the federal penitentiary system. In the analysis, the confirmed incidence was 10%, and the possible incidence, given the challenge of confirming maternal alcohol consumption, was 18% (MacPherson et al. 2014). A systematic review found youth with FASD were 19 times more likely to be incarcerated than those without FASD (Popova et al. 2011). Little is known about mentally disordered offenders with FASD, for example, how well they are supported in the community and what works in their forensic rehabilitation.

Identification of neurocognitive deficits in patients in forensic outpatient clinics lags behind because of a lack of neurobehavioral assessment. The importance of this assessment for diagnostic and treatment planning purposes cannot be overemphasized (Woods et al. 2012).

The accepted figures from case ascertainment include youth and adults (Table 18–1). The rates from the prospective case ascertainment studies are more reliable than those obtained through retrospective chart reviews. In case ascertainment studies, researchers interested in getting good numbers in support of their hypothesis of the significant overrepresentation of FASD

TABLE 18–1. Existing studies on rates of ND-PAE/FASD in different criminal justice system settings

STUDY CITATION	POPULATION	METHOD	RATE OF ND-PAE/FASD, %	COMMENTS
Rojas and Gretton 2007	230 youth (12–18 years)	Retrospective file review	10.9	Sexual offender community program
Murphy and McCreary Centre Society 2005	137 youth (14–19 years)	Adolescent health questionnaire survey	11.7	In custody and only 14% females
Fast et al. 1999	287 youth (12–18 years)	Active case ascertainment (diagnostic)	22.3	In forensic psychiatric facility
MacPherson et al. 2014	91 adults (19–30 years)	Active case ascertainment (diagnostic)	10–18	Only those <30 years
Stinson and Robbins 2014	Secure forensic psychiatric hospital, N=235, Midwestern United States	Diagnostic survey	8	Only FAS and not FASD
McLachlan et al. 2019	90 adults in prison	Active case ascertainment (diagnostic)	17	<50 years, PAE confirmed in 50%
Bower et al. 2018	Youth prison	Active case ascertainment (diagnostic)	36	Latest Australian study
Mela et al. 2019	Outpatient forensic clinic	Active case ascertainment	27	No age limit and community based

in the offender population can make their diagnostic criteria less robust so that it is easier to establish a diagnosis. For instance, reducing the age of those who are included in the study can have a double effect (increase or decrease) rates in the calculated final numbers. By including individuals whose mothers are likely to be alive, such researchers increase the chances of confirming diagnosis over researchers who include older subjects with less likelihood of PAE confirmation, a vital criterion for diagnosis.

Be that as it may, the reported rates of ND-PAE/FASD are considered an underestimation of the actual rates because the disorder is not easily recognizable and is thus invisible compared with perceptible intellectual disability. Except in a formal case ascertainment or a clinical query, individuals with ND-PAE/FASD in the CJS remain undetected. Adult diagnosis suffers from a lack of confirmation of maternal drinking during pregnancy. The older the person being assessed, the less likely such information is available. Circumstances such as the mother being deceased, mother and offspring not being in contact, or the mother being reluctant to admit to alcohol use because of guilt and shame are more prevalent. This age-related phenomenon led to common reports that misdiagnosis and underdiagnosis are the norm in populations with a high risk of vulnerability to PAE. Misattribution of FASD to other disorders contributes to a negative outcome. Also, people who are not identified early are not able to access timely appropriate care. Their trajectory through the health and social care sectors can involve or end in the CJS. Invisibility delays diagnosis and perpetuates the adverse consequences of mistreatment or no treatment. This invisibility affects individuals with PAE more than those with other disorders and disabilities.

What is known about the overrepresentation of FASD in the CJS is similar to what is known about FASD in vulnerable populations. There is a lack of knowledge of the disorder in those affected, their families, and the clinicians or caregivers looking after them. Virtually all studies in adolescents and children or high-risk populations (fostered, adopted, and correctional) consistently find high rates of subjects who have no knowledge of their diagnosis among the people they subsequently diagnose in their research studies. Those who calculated this lack of awareness reported that between 30% and 85% of subjects did not know they had a diagnosis of FASD until participating in the study (Chasnoff et al. 2015; Fast et al. 1999). Although the rates of diagnostic unawareness vary widely, it is hard to argue that such unawareness is uncommon. The implications are broad and important, especially when most individuals have another mental health diagnosis also. When labeled with a disorder other than FASD, people become "attached" to those labels and identify more strongly with them (Tait et al. 2017). This self-identity provides a potential explanation for their prolonged difficulties. The incomplete diagnostic labels persist and become entrenched when the individuals experience some level of success in the management advanced by the treatment team. This may be coincidental because patients are treated with shared approaches and methods. FASD and other mental disorders have common interventional strategies: supportive therapy, stable residential conditions, and biological treatment. Yet treating the other disorder almost always takes precedence over FASD-targeted intervention. It is likely that advances in treatment of other disorders, especially with guidelines accepted in the field, encourages clinicians to focus on the non-FASD condition. When those treatments are insufficient for effective outcomes, missed opportunities to correct PAE-related damage and gravitation toward the CJS can occur.

By the time legal practitioners are consulting, representing, and advocating for older youth and adult offenders, the burden of missed opportunities and undertreatment of those with FASD are almost universal. This should prompt lawyers to obtain good background information about those pressure points that stymied diagnosis (see Figure 18–1). Legal and medical representatives may need to advocate for processes that will guarantee cost-effective and readily available assessments. The assessments should be comprehensive and functionally oriented. Assessments not only identify weaknesses, they also outline strengths that can be used to fashion the correct strength-based treatment modality. Treatment planning that is FASD informed and based on evidence depends on such comprehensive assessments.

The implications of a good relationship with the patient cannot be overemphasized. Affected individuals develop means of coping with their disability, and these adaptations may help conceal their deficits. Even with adaptation, however, the deficits may still contribute to offending and negative outcomes, especially because stress interacts with cognitive deficits and actually increases the risk of dysfunction. During an event such as loss of support or failure in a job, there is no buffering or moderation of the impact of the stress. The "true" unbuffered condition may lead to poor judgments, impaired decision making, and impulsivity, which can result in offending behavior and its associated difficulties.

Making the Criminal Justice System FASD Informed

FASD is based on a deficit model, so its link to correctional and forensic populations is easy to make. Given the overrepresentation of FASD in criminal and populations of mentally disordered individuals in contact with the law, understanding the reasons for the high rates is an important area of inquiry and research. The implications are clinical, correctional, and public in nature. To stem the tide of the ever-increasing numbers of those with FASD in the CJS, adequate clinical identification and intervention are necessary. Only through such active management, can the risk to the public by those individuals who are involved with the system be checked and reduced.

Current approaches to managing people with FASD include strength-based strategies alongside accepted evidence-based treatments. The attention paid since 2010 by the public and nongovernmental organizations to the issues involving PAE has influenced the current level of treatment for FASD. Examining the various aspects of FASD and how they relate to the CJS is part of this progression of interest.

Examples of Initiatives Over a Decade (2010–2020)

The Canadian Bar Association was astute in recognizing the hitherto unattended high rates of CJS involvement among those with FASD. They accurately observed the disparity between the normative assumptions about deterrence and consequential thinking and the deficits in these abilities found in many with FASD. Given the negative outcomes of lack of recognition in services and public policy, the association passed a resolution in 2010 to address these issues. The resolution called for alternative approaches to sentencing and the administration of justice, as well as policies to accommodate the deficits inherent in those with the disability. In 2012, the American Bar Association followed suit by passing a resolution recognizing the seriousness of the problem of FASD, its relationship to disability benefits, and the importance of considering mitigating circumstances in sentencing those with the disorder. The American Bar Association resolution cites the impact of the *Atkins v. Virginia* (2002) case, which involved imposition of the death penalty on an individual with intellectual disability.

The Canadian Bar Association was clearly well informed when it passed a more specific and action-oriented resolution in 2013. Included in this resolution were how to legally define FASD, options to order a comprehensive assessment, recognition of FASD as a mitigating factor, and the need to accommodate offenders with FASD in the correctional system. In the same year, the Institute of Health Economics in Alberta, Canada, organized a conference of experts to develop a consensus statement on FASD and the CJS (Flannigan et al. 2018b). These recommendations, many of which were based on scientific findings, have been brought together in a document that has served in many settings as a reference document for FASD planning within the CJS.

The strategy required to impact the CJS should include the words *understand* and *support*. There are serious implications for individuals with

FASD navigating the CJS. They can be misunderstood in court, victimized in jails, and mismanaged in the transition back to the community, unless the people working with them are aware of FASD and its implications (Fast and Conry 2009). Failing that, the tide of increasing numbers of individuals with FASD entering the CJS will not be stemmed. The risk to the public is also likely to continue unchecked because of missed diagnosis and under-treatment. Diversion of these individuals to the mental health system is a viable recommendation and option.

In Canada, as in other countries, the overrepresentation of indigenous persons in the CJS has been a source of distress for the government. The trajectory of many remains almost predictable, abetted by misguided child welfare policies and a broken and inadequate foster care system that produces troubled youth who begin offending early and invariably enter the CJS. Once involved with the system, return to normal life is tough; circling endlessly in the proverbial revolving door is easier and, unfortunately, a too common outcome. The Truth and Reconciliation Commission of Canada assumed a broad perspective and released calls to action heralded as a useful framework through which corrective measures can help redress inequities affecting indigenous people. It is hoped that these calls to action will be put into practice throughout society (Truth and Reconciliation Commission of Canada 2015). One of the calls to action concerns the many people diagnosed or who should be diagnosed with FASD who are caught in the web of the CJS. In addition to diversion, the commission calls for understanding of FASD in order to deliver justice and create resources that will facilitate community care as a standard. The effect of these calls to action will foster a larger discussion on indigenous people in general and those with FASD within indigenous society specifically.

Over the decade from 2010 to 2020, knowledge of FASD among court protagonists and police has been steadily increasing (Cox et al. 2008; Gagnier et al. 2011). Research among court officials supports this, but calls for more justice require that workers be conversant with FASD. Diversion through the structure of the mental health court with a prominent indigenous focus was reported as both unique and successful. There were benefits for the perpetrators, victims, legal professionals, and the community at large (Flannigan et al. 2018a).

Management in Residential or Custodial Settings

In addition to focusing on how individuals' characteristic neurocognitive deficits affect their interaction with the CJS, the deficits present an enduring risk for patients. People with the kind of limited cognition characteristic of ND-

PAE/FASD are more susceptible to modeling, almost exactly, behaviors they observe. The risk is obvious when those with FASD are incarcerated and left to the "mentoring" of convicted peers. The social deficits of PAE lead offenders to mimic the popular youth and adults in these settings. To manage these unfortunate reactions and outcomes, mental health specialists in the correctional, justice, and forensic mental health systems have paramount roles as agents of change. They should help to steer impressionistic offenders from obvious revictimization and halt their learning by observation and imitation (Bandura et al. 1963; Baumbach 2002). Imitative learning can be an advantage, however, if the patient is assigned to a prosocial mentor. Skills for handling stressful events and managing peer interaction are sorely needed. Mentors can model these skills, and the staff within the correctional system are better practical models as well. Refusing to do what the more experienced offenders ask them to do can result in physical and/or sexual assault. Patients require empowerment and education about safe sex and negotiating safe sex. Given the volatile situations of unsafe sex and exploitation that occur in the CJS, case workers and front-line staff should strive to engage vulnerable patients and roleplay how they can navigate tense conversations with predators and potentially violent situations. Equally important is support in consensual peer-to-peer sexual involvement from professionals and case managers attached to the cases of those with neurocognitive deficits (Brown and Singh 2016).

Behavior therapy using preplanned staff responses of both reinforcement and loss of reward is the mainstay of treatment in correctional programs. Unfortunately, the literal nature of, inappropriate application by, and slow cognitive processing in those with ND-PAE/FASD limit the utility of these approaches. Within the context of the general custodial environment, however, protection and structure are beneficial for the affected person (Brown et al. 2012). Predictability and simplified supervision and structure not only help to control stress but, at times, support learning (Mela 2016). Self-regulation techniques are much-needed approaches to handling the aggression common in the CJS environment. Individual treatment plans make it impossible to adhere to inter-individual consistency, but they should support consistent intrapersonal strategies. Behavioral modification with clear and consistent expectations in the prison milieu should link to individually tailored treatment plans and services as well as a behavioral reinforcement program (Brown et al. 2015).

Before release, discharge planning that identifies what the person has learned and will miss from the experience and what the person fears about reentry into the community should form the basis for transitional planning. Transition to the community and the generalization and maintenance of new skills become top priorities. For this reason, caregivers must be closely and regularly involved in inpatient treatment to the extent possible and trained on how to duplicate successful strategies employed while the person was incarcerated (Brown et al. 2012). Information about any aspects of behavioral modification techniques that appear beneficial should be communicated to the new community caregiver and case manager.

Role of Diversion

Therapeutic jurisprudence includes as one of its tenets the use of psychological means to support the social justice principles and practices dictated by the rules of the CJS. The mental health court is an ideal type of therapeutic jurisprudence in which many offenders are spared intolerable prison sentences by diversion that incorporates components of community treatment programs. A number of diversion programs specifically for FASD have begun to be evaluated. These innovations are, however, being hampered by the economic cost of establishing new systems within the CJS. Encouraging positive outcomes, including recognition, decreased adverse outcomes, meaningful sentencing, community collaboration, and reduced familial burden, have been observed in preliminary evaluations (Longstaffe et al. 2018; Mela et al. 2019). In another innovative, culturally based court, focus group interviews of participants (i.e., judge, lawyers, police, clerks) identified important themes. The respondents suggested that building capacity, humanizing the offender, creating bridges, and moving forward formed the gestalt of care relevant to good outcomes (Flannigan et al. 2018a). The following vignette depicts an example of how diversion from the correctional centers may be crucial to altering a person's outcome.

Clinical Vignette

A 24-year-old offender is assessed in the weekly correctional center psychiatric clinic. He complains of feeling overwhelmed with others asking him for his lisdexamfetamine, the medication he takes to help with focus in the psychoeducational program classes. He reveals hopelessness and suicidal ideation, anxiety, and inability to sleep and says he was diagnosed with "panic disorder, anxiety disorder, depression, FASD, intellectual deficiency, and memory problems." He reports that he tried multiple psychotropic medications in the past but experienced bad side effects with many of them. Lorazepam is the only medication that helps his severe panic attacks and anxiety.

His past contact with psychiatric services included dozens of emergency room visits to various hospitals. He was admitted six times because of prolonged anxiety and panic. Smoking marijuana worsens his panic attacks, and the only drug he abused before coming to the correctional center was alcohol. His parents were said to have abandoned him at the age of 5. He went through the foster care system and obtains support from his older sister who is currently completing a course to become a police officer. He has more than 50 convictions on his criminal record, mainly property offenses and system-generated offenses (e.g., breaches of parole, failures to comply). When facing stress, he demonstrates suicidal behaviors, including taking overdoses of medications, risking his life by jumping in front of oncoming traffic, and running to the top of a building and threatening to jump off.

His index offense of mischief, robbery, and avoiding police reveals a pattern of behavior. He visited his son in the hospital who was on life support. Hospital staff prevented him from seeing his son because of a legal restraining order prohibiting contact with his partner and son because of past violence. Immediately, he ran out of the hospital, broke a large glass window, and asked someone to call the police. He waited in the hospital parking lot for the police to arrive. When they arrived, he professed that he had a gun. He said he wanted the police to shoot him. He was disappointed when they came and talked with him and left, only charging him for destroying hospital property. He hotwired a car in the parking lot, stole it, and drove to another part of the city. He went into a convenience store there and again acted as if he had a gun, asked for cash, and then asked to have the police called. He stated to the police he had a gun and that he was going to shoot. He hoped they would shoot him, but they arrested him. He received a reduced sentence when he argued he really did not have a gun but wanted the police to shoot him because he feared his son would die without him having an opportunity to see him.

He reports that a particular source of anxiety is that members of his family have begun to cut him off because of "this suicide thing." The only family members who still support him are feeling worn out by his incessant demands, suicidal behaviors, and complaints of anxiety.

Red Flags: What Else Could It Be?

This young man revealed, rightly or wrongly, that he had multiple diagnoses, including FASD. His behaviors—suicide attempts, risky behaviors, and repeated offending with no evidence of learning from the past—are indicative of some of the well-known behavioral issues in offenders with FASD (Brintnell et al. 2019). He was involved with the foster care system, demonstrated poor coping skills relating to the stress of not seeing his son, and was prescribed a stimulant. He also reports what appears to be hypersensitivity to certain medications. His prison-based behavior (e.g., disobeying unit rules and codes of dressing, possessing contraband and "wheeling and dealing") and use of substances are not unique to PAE but support the suspicion. To clarify the diagnosis, information about any cognitive tests, access to birth records, and additional details about his development is needed.

Modifications of Care

Because he was convicted more than 50 times, it is safe to assume, and can be confirmed, that this individual was previously involved with and participated in treatment programs such as correctional programs and substance use programs. It is evident that none of these has changed his outcomes. His behaviors may have necessitated the use of behavior modification but to no avail. His medications and their benefit should be reviewed. The full psychological assessment, if accurately done in the context of a multidisciplinary team assessment, should outline his strengths and deficits and will form the basis for building a strong relationship with his clinician. Together they should formulate an individualized plan with new strategies. The neuropsychological assessment evaluates cognitive functioning and learning styles; knowing this also facilitates individual treatment planning (Sparrow et al. 2013). A discharge plan with the goal of connecting him with mental health services and FASD informed services should be initiated early. This allows a postsentence type of diversion from the criminal justice system to the mental health system before his release into the community.

Using visual communication and checking true understanding are necessary to ensure absorption of program material. He should benefit from simple and concrete instruction and support regarding the losses in his life: parental, relational, and social. Depending on the social support in the community and the level of FASD education among case managers, a mentor with knowledge of PAE and its deficits, financial assistance, housing stability, and structure in his day are foundational interventions following his release from prison. During the transition from prison to the community, he should identify successful interventional strategies, and these should be transferred to his new living environment. Case managers who adopt a modified approach, using flexible, regular, short-duration check-in and appointment reminders, are likely to positively influence the response to case management. This fits the risk-need-responsivity model of correctional treatment.

This form of postsentence treatment should include ongoing reviews with case managers and case presentations of challenges along the treatment trajectory. Patients who are prescribed stimulants should be supported by team members with experience in managing issues that arise, such as medication diversion and misuse, memory-related loss of medication, and correct administration of the medications. The role of alcohol and substances in perpetuating the offending behavior is real and should be a focus of ongoing intervention. The patient should be guided in identifying those in the circle of support with positive attitudes who actively champion him. Those who derail his progress should be pointed out, and the patient should roleplay a strategy of how he will respond to the next invitation to be involved in criminal activities by those acquaintances and peers.

Conclusion

FASD is overrepresented in the CJS. Current estimates of high rates of FASD and corresponding neurocognitive deficits in all offenders call for new approaches in identification and systemic support for individuals whose awareness of wrongfulness is compromised. The point has been made that an urgent response and strategy is required to address the missed opportunities related to PAE. Some have considered PAE to be a path to adapted interventions. To be relevant to public safety, the CJS should accommodate and respond to the deficits identified in those with ND-PAE/FASD. By using effective prevention and intervention management techniques, the potential to reduce crime and victimization is real and can be transformative to the system. It brings the forensic mental health system and CJS closer together to solve the age-old problem of crime and its consequences.

CLINICAL PRACTICAL APPLICATIONS

- For offenders with ND-PAE/FASD, stable housing is critical for any intervention to be successful.
- Clinicians should elicit from neurocognitively impaired patients whether sexual offenses arose from poor awareness of boundaries or intentional self-serving behavior.
- In assessing impaired psycholegal abilities, those with ND-PAE/FASD are at higher risk of being misclassified as capable.
- Early onset of alcohol and drug use, offending behavior, and school failure should prompt a search for PAE in an offender.
- Case managers should be aware of and search for significant neurocognitive deficits and multiple diagnoses comorbid with PAE in individuals in the criminal justice system and the forensic mental health system.
- Best practice by mental health professionals should involve repeated attempts to divert those with ND-PAE/FASD from the criminal justice system to the mental health system.

References

Anderson T, Harding KD, Reid D, Peia J: FASD and Inappropriate Sexual Behaviour. CanFASD, 2018. Available at: https://canfasd.ca/wp-content/uploads/2018/07/CanFASD-Issue-Paper-Inappropriate-Sexual-Behaviour-Final.pdf. Accessed November 6, 2019.

Atkins v. Virginia, 536 U.S. 304 (2002)

Bandura A, Ross D, Ross SA: Vicarious reinforcement and imitative learning. J Abnorm Psychol 67(6):601–607, 1963

Baumbach J: Some implications of prenatal alcohol exposure for the treatment of adolescents with sexual offending behaviors. Sex Abuse 14(4):313–327, 2002

Boland FJ, Burrill R, Duwyn M, Karp J: Fetal Alcohol Syndrome: Implications for Correctional Service. Ottawa, ON, Canada Correctional Service, 1998

Bonta J, Andrews DA: Viewing offender assessment and rehabilitation through the lens of the risk-need-responsivity model, in Offender Supervision: New Directions in Theory, Research and Practice. Edited by McNeill F, Raynor P, Trotter C. Oxon, UK, Willan Publishing, 2010, pp 19–40

Bower C, Watkins RE, Mutch RC, et al: Fetal alcohol spectrum disorder and youth justice: a prevalence study among young people sentenced to detention in Western Australia. BMJ Open 8(2):e019605, 2018

Brintnell ES, Sawhney AS, Bailey PG, et al: Corrections and connection to the community: a diagnostic and service program for incarcerated adult men with FASD. Int J Law Psychiatry 64:8–17, 2019

Brown J, Singh JP: Perceptions of FASD by civil commitment professionals: a pilot survey. Sexual Offender Treatment 11(1):1–6, 2016

Brown J, Hesse ML, Wartnik A, et al: Fetal alcohol spectrum disorder in confinement settings: a review for correctional professionals. Journal of Law Enforcement 4(4), 2015

Brown J, Cooney-Koss L, Harr D, et al: Fetal alcohol spectrum disorder and sexually inappropriate behaviors: a call on sex offender treatment clinicians to become informed. The Journal of Special Populations 2(1):1–8, 2017

Brown J, Carter MN, Haun J, et al: Fetal alcohol spectrum disorder (FASD) and competency to stand trial (CST): a call on forensic evaluators to become informed. J Forensic Psychol Res Pract 19(4):315–340, 2019

Brown NN, Wartnik AP, Connor PD, Adler RS: A proposed model standard for forensic assessment of fetal alcohol spectrum disorders. J Psychiatry Law 38(4):383–418, 2010

Brown NN, Connor PD, Adler RS: Conduct-disordered adolescents with fetal alcohol spectrum disorder: intervention in secure treatment settings. Crim Just Behav 39(6):770–793, 2012

Burd L, Selfridge RH, Klug MG, Juelson T: Fetal alcohol syndrome in the Canadian corrections system. Journal of FAS International 1:e14, 2003

Burd L, Fast DK, Conry J, Williams AD: Fetal alcohol spectrum disorder as a marker for increased risk of involvement with correction systems. J Psychiatry Law 38(4):559–584, 2010

Carr JL, Agnihotri S, Keightley M: Sensory processing and adaptive behavior deficits of children across the fetal alcohol spectrum disorder continuum. Alcohol Clin Exp Res 34(6):1022–1032, 2010

Chandler JA: The use of neuroscientific evidence in Canadian criminal proceedings. J Law Biosci 2(3):550–579, 2015

Chartrand LN, Forbes-Chilibeck EM: The sentencing of offenders with fetal alcohol syndrome. Health Law J 11:35–70, 2003

Chasnoff IJ, Wells AM, King L: Misdiagnosis and missed diagnoses in foster and adopted children with prenatal alcohol exposure. Pediatrics 135(2):264–270, 2015

Clarren SK, Lutke J, Sherbuck M: The Canadian guidelines and the interdisciplinary clinical capacity of Canada to diagnose fetal alcohol spectrum disorder. J Popul Ther Clin Pharmacol 18(3):e494–e499, 2011

Cook JL, Green CR, Lilley CM, et al: Fetal alcohol spectrum disorder: a guideline for diagnosis across the lifespan. CMAJ 188(3):191–197, 2016

Cox LV, Clairmont D, Cox SC: Knowledge and attitudes of criminal justice professionals in relation to fetal alcohol spectrum disorder. Can J Clin Pharmacol 15(2):e306–e13, 2008

Dishion TJ, Dodge KA: Peer contagion in interventions for children and adolescents: moving towards an understanding of the ecology and dynamics of change. J Abnorm Child Psychol 33(3):395–400, 2005

Fast DK, Conry J: Fetal alcohol spectrum disorders and the criminal justice system. Dev Disabil Res Rev 15(3):250–257, 2009

Fast DK, Conry J, Loock CA: Identifying fetal alcohol syndrome among youth in the criminal justice system. J Dev Behav Pediatr 20(5):370–372, 1999

Flannigan K, Pei J, Rasmussen C, et al: A unique response to offenders with fetal alcohol spectrum disorder: perceptions of the Alexis FASD Justice Program. Can J Criminol Crim Just 60(1):1–33, 2018a

Flannigan K, Pei J, Stewart M, Johnson A: Fetal alcohol spectrum disorder and the criminal justice system: a systematic literature review. Int J Law Psychiatry 57:42–52, 2018b

Gagnier KR, Moore TE, Green JM: A need for closer examination of FASD by the criminal justice system: has the call been answered? J Popul Ther Clin Pharmacol 18(3):e426–e439, 2011

Goh YI, Chudley AE, Clarren SK, et al: Development of Canadian screening tools for fetal alcohol spectrum disorder. Can J Clin Pharmacol 15(2):e344–e366, 2008

Greenspan S, Driscoll JH: Why people with FASD fall for manipulative ploys: ethical limits of interrogators' use of lies, in Fetal Alcohol Spectrum Disorders in Adults: Ethical and Legal Perspectives: An Overview on FASD for Professionals (International Library of Ethics, Law, and the New Medicine, Vol 63). Edited by Nelson M, Trussler M. Cham, Switzerland, Springer, 2016, pp 23–38

Gunn JC, Taylor PJ (eds): Forensic Psychiatry: Clinical, Legal and Ethical Issues, 2nd Edition. Boca Raton, FL, CRC Press, 2014

Keightley M, Agnihotri S, Subramaniapillai S, et al: Investigating a theatre-based intervention for indigenous youth with fetal alcohol spectrum disorder: Exploration d'une intervention basée sur le théâtre auprès de jeunes autochtones atteints du syndrome d'alcoolisme fœtal. Can J Occup Ther 85(2):128–136, 2018

Lander L, Howsare J, Byrne M: The impact of substance use disorders on families and children: from theory to practice. Soc Work Public Health 28(3–4):194–205, 2013

Longstaffe S, Chudley AE, Harvie MK, et al: The Manitoba Youth Justice Program: empowering and supporting youth with FASD in conflict with the law. Biochem Cell Biol 96(2):260–266, 2018

MacPherson PH, Chudley AE, Grant BA: Fetal Alcohol Spectrum Disorder (FASD) in a Correctional Population: Prevalence, Screening and Diagnosis (Research Report R-247). Ottawa, ON, Correctional Service Canada, 2014

McLachlan K, Roesch R, Viljoen JL, Douglas KS: Evaluating the psycholegal abilities of young offenders with fetal alcohol spectrum disorder. Law Hum Behav 38(1):10–22, 2014

McLachlan K, McNeil A, Pei J, et al: Prevalence and characteristics of adults with fetal alcohol spectrum disorder in corrections: a Canadian case ascertainment study. BMC Public Health 19(1):1–10, 2019

Mela M: Medico-legal interventions in management of offenders with fetal alcohol spectrum disorders (FASD), in Fetal Alcohol Spectrum Disorders in Adults: Ethical and Legal Perspectives: An Overview on FASD for Professionals (International Library of Ethics, Law, and the New Medicine, Vol. 63). Edited by Nelson M, Trussler M. Cham, Switzerland, Springer, 2016, pp 121–138

Mela M, Luther G: Fetal alcohol spectrum disorder: can diminished responsibility diminish criminal behaviour? Int J Law Psychiatry 36(1):46–54, 2013

Mela M, Coons-Harding KD, Anderson T: Recent advances in fetal alcohol spectrum disorder for mental health professionals. Curr Opin Psychiatry 32(4):328–335, 2019

Murphy A; McCreary Centre Society: Time Out II: A Profile of BC Youth in Custody. Vancouver, BC, McCreary Centre Society, 2005

Nelson M, Trussler M: (eds.): Fetal Alcohol Spectrum Disorders in Adults: Ethical and Legal Perspectives: An Overview on FASD for Professionals (International Library of Ethics, Law, and the New Medicine, Vol 63). Cham, Switzerland, Springer, 2015

Pei J, Leung WSW, Jampolsky F, Alsbury B: Experiences in the Canadian criminal justice system for individuals with fetal alcohol spectrum disorders: double jeopardy? Canadian Journal of Criminology and Criminal Justice 58(1):56–86, 2016

Pollard R, Trowbridge B, Slade PD, et al: Interrogative suggestibility in a US context: some preliminary data on normal subjects. Pers Individ Diff 37(5):1101–1108, 2004

Popova S, Lange S, Bekmuradov D, et al: Fetal alcohol spectrum disorder prevalence estimates in correctional systems: a systematic literature review. Can J Public Health 102(5):336–340, 2011

Rojas EY, Gretton HM: Background, offence characteristics, and criminal outcomes of Aboriginal youth who sexually offend: a closer look at Aboriginal youth intervention needs. Sex Abuse 19(3):257–283, 2007

Snedker KA, Beach LR, Corcoran KE: Beyond the "revolving door?": incentives and criminal recidivism in a mental health court. Crim Just Behav 44(9):1141–1162, 2017

Solis JM, Shadur JM, Burns AR, Hussong AK: Understanding the diverse needs of children whose parents abuse substances. Curr Drug Abuse Rev 5(2):135–147, 2012

Sparrow J, Grant T, Connor P, Whitney N: The value of the neuropsychological assessment for adults with fetal alcohol spectrum disorders: a case study. Int J Alcohol Drug Res 2(3):79–86, 2013

Stinson JD, Robbins SB: Characteristics of people with intellectual disabilities in a secure U.S. forensic hospital. J Ment Health Res Intellect Disabil 7(4):337–358, 2014

Streissguth AP, Bookstein FL, Barr HM, et al: Risk factors for adverse life outcomes in fetal alcohol syndrome and fetal alcohol effects. J Dev Behav Pediatr 25(4):228–238, 2004

Substance Abuse and Mental Health Services Administration: Addressing Fetal Alcohol Spectrum Disorders (FASD). Treatment Improvement Protocol (TIP) Series 58. HHS Publication No (SMA) 13-4803. Rockville, MD, Substance Abuse and Mental Health Services Administration, 2014

Tait CL, Mela M, Boothman G, Stoops MA: The lived experience of paroled offenders with fetal alcohol spectrum disorder and comorbid psychiatric disorder. Transcult Psychiatry 54(1):107–124, 2017

Truth and Reconciliation Commission of Canada: Truth and Reconciliation Commission of Canada: Calls to Action. Winnipeg, MB, Truth and Reconciliation Commission of Canada, 2015. Available from: http://trc.ca/assets/pdf/Calls_to_Action_English2.pdf. Accessed October 5, 2020.

Weyrauch D, Schwartz M, Hart B, et al: Comorbid mental disorders in fetal alcohol spectrum disorders: a systematic review. J Dev Behav Pediatr 38(4):283–291, 2017

Woods GW, Freedman D, Greenspan S: Neurobehavioral assessment in forensic practice. Int J Law Psychiatry 35(5–6):432–439, 2012

CHAPTER 19

The Emergency Room

WHAT TO KNOW

Patients with ND-PAE/FASD come to the emergency room (ER) frequently. Sensitivity to the needs of these patients is crucial for improving outcomes.

The ER environment can present barriers to care unless those who screen, triage, and refer patients are aware of the distinct, yet frequently appearing, deficits of PAE and how atypically the deficits can manifest.

PAE deficits portend an increase of health-interfering behaviors, such as risky acts with medications; thus, linking patients with support persons is important.

Although fast-paced, the ER presents a good environment to properly intervene in the multiple manifestations of PAE and provide needed diversion for those affected.

Not recognizing PAE contributes to the exorbitant direct and indirect cost of health care.

In the emergency room (ER), or the accident and emergency (A&E) department as it is called in other medical centers, many professionals intersect with patients, albeit temporarily. Although ER specialists manage and triage incoming patients, virtually all specializations are connected with and represented in the ER. Because of the consequences of PAE, a large number of patients diagnosed with ND-PAE/FASD require ER services. Those with PAE are disproportionately misdiagnosed and experience adverse outcomes consistent with the results of treatment resistance. Statistically, they are frequently diagnosed with multiple pathologies, simultaneously or in combination, and are at risk of noncompliance to treatment. Unfortunately, surveys of different professions that interact with patients in the ER (e.g., psychiatric residents, nurses, occupational therapists, pediatricians, paramedical first responders) depict a lack of knowledge and insufficient skills for managing the outcomes of PAE when manifested (Johnson et al. 2010; Mukherjee et al. 2015; Tough et al. 2005). PAE has the potential to damage multiple organs. Medical professionals need training and skill to first identify those affected by consequences of PAE, mentally and physically, and then modify their approaches to be effective with these patients.

Knowledge Gap of Professionals

As noted, surveys of professionals tasked with identifying, classifying, and intervening with individuals with ND-PAE/FASD in the ER indicate a concerning inadequacy (Mukherjee et al. 2015). Survey results point to knowledge gaps in those who work in or take referrals from the ER (Johnson et al. 2010). Incorrectly identifying patients with ND-PAE/FASD carries the risk of increasing stigma by perpetuating negative secondary issues such as unnecessary side effects and inappropriate treatment plans. The education of professionals in the ER does not cover the requisite details of presentation and strategies for disposition to support successful assessment of and intervention with patients with the lifelong deficits associated with PAE. Recognizing how inadequate their training in FASD is, almost 90% of psychiatric residents surveyed wanted more education on FASD (Eyal and O'Connor 2011). Pediatricians were knowledgeable about PAE, but only 34% of more than 800 surveyed felt ready to manage and coordinate services for children with ND-PAE/FASD (Gahagan et al. 2006). Training is no better for first responders and other subspecialists (e.g., anesthesiology, internal medicine, surgery). Sufficient knowledge and expertise in treatment professionals is critical for the many patients seeking help in the ER (Tough et al. 2005).

Factors That Increase Morbidity in ND-PAE/FASD in the Emergency Room

The way professionals provide services for the clinical and social needs of patients with substance- and alcohol-related disorders or problems is structured differently in the ER. *Triage*, prioritizing levels of severity, and referral for those who require additional specialist care are the essential components of the standard of emergency care. There are a plethora of individual, professional, and system-relevant factors that guide referral and, ultimately, care. Optimum emergency care is achieved by an all-around service of specialists and their support trainees and staff. Services include ordering laboratory tests, completing brief and focused physical examinations, referring to specialists, and monitoring patients. If these component services are not adequate or available, patients are misclassified, and the potential for negative outcomes arises. In ND-PAE/FASD, the respective neurocognitive deficits arguably interfere with the delivery of such optimum care.

The patient whose PAE-induced impaired neurocognitive ability (i.e., executive function, memory, impulse control, and organization skills) is significant may fail to recognize symptom-based sensations, fail to adhere to advice to seek help for particular problems because the patient is unable to sense and correctly interpret the sensation, and fail to communicate distress adequately to the ER clinician. In that event, the information gathering of essential clinical material will likely and unintentionally be incorrect and insufficient. In some instances, the patient with ND-PAE/FASD lacks understanding due to poor comprehension, which is characteristic of neurocognitive deficit and contributes to the patient's failure to comply with instructions. This interferes with consequent care and is compounded over time and during repeated visits to the ER. Symptom misinterpretation can occur from the other direction as well; ER clinicians, including mental health specialists, may fail to recognize the unusual presentation (or impaired communication of clinical symptoms and signs) of an individual with ND-PAE/FASD or to detect presentations consistent with PAE and its consequences.

Conditions Manifesting in the ER

Findings of high rates of medical comorbidities and a shortened lifespan in patients with ND-PAE/FASD suggest that individuals with the consequences of PAE frequently visit the ER. These consequences involve a number of medical diagnoses. As a whole-body disorder, no organ is spared from the teratogenic effect of PAE (Shelton et al. 2018). In a study of the ICD diagnostic categories affecting those with a diagnosis of FAS, researchers found an alarming rate of 428 separate comorbid conditions in the diagnosed patients (coming from 18 out of 22 chapters in ICD-10) (Popova et al. 2016). The most common disorders found in the study appear to be those also likely to manifest in ERs, including congenital malformations, deformities, chromosomal abnormalities, and mental and behavioral disorders (Popova et al. 2016). These categories correlate with disorders presenting acutely and affecting the eye, ear, skin and circulatory, respiratory, digestive, or musculoskeletal systems. Through these acute presentations, a profile can be formulated that serves as a pattern of warning signs for PAE. Medical complications associated with behavioral deficits and compliance issues contributed to a shortened life expectancy in a mortality study on FAS. Death resulted from medical diseases of the nervous (8%), respiratory (8%), and digestive (7%) systems and congenital malformations (7%). These death rates are much higher than in those without the diagnosis of ND-PAE/FASD (Thanh and Jonsson 2016).

In a study by Himmelreich et al. (2017), acute and chronic infections (chest, sinus, and middle ear) in subjects with FASD were reported twofold or threefold the rate in the general population. Rates of chronic otitis media were estimated in 77%. Asthma was also highly prevalent. Patients presenting with medical and mental disorders are at risk of having no attention paid to the impact of PAE on their presentation and behavior. Multiple disorders with odds in the hundreds were reported by those diagnosed with ND-PAE/FASD surveyed online (Himmelreich et al. 2017). Renal abnormalities (pyelonephritis, painless hematuria, and renal failure) and hepatic disorders are more common in those with consequences of PAE (Assadi 2014). Shortened lifespans were also evident in siblings of those with PAE and its consequences, which indicates that relatives of those exposed are at increased risk and should either be screened or closely evaluated, keeping PAE warning signs in mind.

The overrepresentation of mental disorders from all sections of DSM-5 (American Psychiatric Association 2013) suggests that individuals with ND-PAE/FASD comorbid with mental disorder traverse the ER on a frequent basis. The incidence and effect of neurocognitive impairment add to the risk of frequent ER visits, inappropriate care, possible exclusion (e.g., "frequent flyers"), and negative outcomes (Mela et al. 2019). Some of the negative outcomes relate to the effect of stigma and misinformation about PAE among health professionals (Choate and Badry 2019). Stigma constitutes an important clinical risk factor because treatment is sought late. Cumulatively, stigma was found to worsen course and outcome, reduce compliance, and increase the risk of relapse (Shrivastava et al. 2013). Mood, anxiety, and personality disorders and risk-elevating behaviors are common in ND-PAE/FASD and so are self-harm and suicidal gestures (Lange et al. 2017; O'Connor et al. 2019). These problems present as acute difficulties that require the expertise of ER physicians and specialists.

Mental and physical disorders compound each other in patients requiring the services of specialists in the ER (Shelton et al. 2018). Services should be in tune with patient needs. Lack of recognition of PAE was exemplified by a 6-year study looking at the rates of alcohol and drug testing in the ER

TABLE 19–1. Indices of PAE in the emergency room

Frequent discharge against medical advice

Receptive verbal language problems

Altered sensation manifestations

Unreasonable refusal of care

Heightened sensitivity during brief physical examination

Unfounded lack of coping

among pregnant women compared with nonpregnant women. Pregnant women were 75% less likely to be tested for drug and alcohol use (Moyer et al. 2018). Without attention to indicators (obvious in relatives of those with PAE who accompany the patient), appropriate services and interventions will not be provided. ER clinicians should exercise a high level of suspicion with regard to those who come frequently, appear to not learn from the past, conduct their lives in a way suggestive of impaired judgment, and have a family history of alcohol and substance use disorder. If some criminal justice systems indict mothers for PAE, how will clinicians who do not screen pregnant women be viewed? The ER offers an environment for screening and aligning services for those with the consequences of PAE or at risk of exposing their offspring to alcohol.

Support for individuals with neurocognitive deficits, especially before diagnosis, is inadequate and places them at significant disadvantage. Patients' lack of impulse control can contribute to impatience and discharge against medical advice. Medical advice verbally communicated to a patient with a receptive language problem in the context of higher expressive abilities is regularly misunderstood. The deficit reduces the comprehension of instructions and leads to seemingly deliberate noncompliance. Deficits involving sensory processing are also a source of misidentification. High pain threshold can mask serious and significant problems, and excessive sensitivity to touch or phobic reactions (common comorbid conditions) will contribute to refusal of care. Patients may decline to have a physical examination or to have blood drawn in the ER (see Table 19–1 for ER risk factors). The busy nature of the departments and the speed of medical activities, lifesaving and directing care, take attention away from those vulnerable patients, who are made more vulnerable because of neurocognitive deficits.

Family Practice Environment

Although the family practice environment is not typically organized like an ER, patients with PAE have reported similar levels of frustration and intimidation in their family physicians' offices. Impersonal encounters, communication problems, and culture-specific issues must be addressed to facilitate uptake of services in both emergency and family practice settings. Knowledge of the impairing cognitive abilities should propel services to identify high-risk patients and assess behaviors construed to be part of a spectrum of warning signs to identify service links for those suspected of PAE and its consequences. Culturally sensitive care should be offered to groups not frequently recognized in the ER.

Focusing on Red Flags

Clinical Vignette

A 23-year-old man is referred from the emergency service center of the university hospital for admission to the psychiatric inpatient unit. He yelled at, threatened, and cursed at his father. After punching a hole on the living room wall in the family house, he shot at his father's car. He was violent and verbally threatening when police arrived. This is his third psychiatric hospital admission through the ER in 16 months. His persistent complaint is of "hearing voices, seeing things, and feeling paranoid." He reports a history of snorting cocaine and crystal methamphetamine and states that he quit about 2 weeks earlier. He acknowledges smoking unknown quantities of marijuana daily and drinking alcohol to reduce his feelings of anger. His adoptive father, a religious minister, is frustrated with him and cannot tolerate his son's use of cannabis because of his own religious beliefs. This is a source of ongoing family conflict.

After the patient's last admission, he was prescribed injectable antipsychotics and a medication (benztropine) for any extrapyramidal side effects (stiffness, tremors, and rigidity). He is only minimally compliant, stating he does not like the reactions he is having from the injection and has lost the medication for side effects. He attempted to work in a grocery store where he stocked the shelves but felt overwhelmed because the manager gave him more work than he could handle. He felt exploited and made many mistakes and was dismissed a week before the current hospital admission. He expresses irritation and is upset that he is not able to see his 3-year-old daughter, who is living with his partner. His partner has no interest in a relationship with him, and he repeatedly fails to comply with a civil court order to provide child support.

When the patient was 7 years old, because of his biological parents' extensive use of alcohol and drugs, he was taken from the home. He lived in several different foster homes. He started using alcohol and drugs at the age of 12 and dropped out of school in the ninth grade. He was angry with classmates and was not able to focus in class. He was involved in bullying both as a perpetrator and a victim.

The issues raised by patients with neurocognitive deficits who come to the ER are diverse. As in this vignette, more visits will occur if the underlying causes of relapse and noncompliance are not addressed. Data about the number of visits and hours in the ER were factored into the estimation of the cost of health care calculated for those with a history of PAE. In one such study, 15- to 29-year-old patients with FAS accounted for the highest utilization rate for acute care, psychiatric care, and ER visits (Popova et al. 2012). Calculated costs for those with FAS, which included acute care, psychiatric care, day surgery, and ER services, were twice that of the general population. Ignoring certain factors in this case means that the patient's outcome will be worse because the presentation in the ER is likely to continue the pattern of the last three visits. Rethinking the case to determine what is perpetuating these problems is a search for red flags.

School failure may arise from difficulty with attention, impaired cognition, hyperactivity, home-based stresses (parental alcohol use), and early substance use (e.g., beginning at age 12). Stresses associated with residential instability or specific childhood adverse events such as abuse are common in patients in the mental health system. Adult women with alcohol use problems also report high rates of traumatic events. Research found that the average number of foster care homes for those with PAE was between three and four, and those with PAE had a fourfold higher rate of adverse childhood events (Choate and Badry 2019; Frankenberger et al. 2015). The patient in the vignette is said to have been in different foster homes when his parents could not manage him. The higher the number of placements and associated emotional dysregulation (e.g., anger, aggression, bullying behavior), the more PAE is suspected. Having a poor estimation and awareness of risk can occur in those with alcohol and substance use disorder; however, this occurs frequently in those with PAE. If the reported psychotic-like symptoms are a result of perceptual disturbance from alcohol withdrawal or drug withdrawal, one can suspect heritable factors in substance use disorder in the patient.

Neurocognitive deficits of poor memory, planning, generalization, and communication correlate with failed employment. Suspecting PAE will become more reasonable if additional factors are demonstrated from his replies to questions such as the following: Is he more likely to experience side effects? Is the loss of medication a product of poor memory and executive dysfunction, and is there a history of pervasive noncompliance to treatment? Does he get easily overwhelmed and show no cognitive ability to problem solve and resolve conflict? What explanation is there for failing to provide child support while still expressing a strong desire to connect with his daughter? Is alcohol and substance use purely a diversion or an attempt to self-medicate? Could disorganization be a consequence of the neurocognitive deficits of PAE? Is he capable of learning from past experience, and is he flexible to change? How much insight does he have about his problems?

What is his ability to estimate the risk of harm when in possession of a gun? Does he show a pattern of poor cause and effect reasoning?

Clinical Reasoning Applied to the Vignette

The patient's responses to clinical inquiries may indicate a drug-induced psychotic disorder. However, investigating the possibility of PAE and its negative outcomes is astute and relevant if his repeated hospital admissions are to be managed better. Responsivity dictates that learning styles and deficits be remediated with community support that addresses the level of dysfunction or cognitive performance specific to the patient.

To apply practice-informed steps capable of improving the quality of care for the patient, a screening tool would be helpful. In the absence of a specific tool, the Life History Screen, applied in cases of addiction treatment, can be used (Grant et al. 2013). The best strategy is to pose a number of inquiries that could elicit answers that support a reasonable suspicion of PAE. To confirm the diagnosis, referral to a specialty team or additional assessment (psychological, social, educational, and genetic) is called for. The assessment can thus support or exclude PAE as a contributing factor in the patient's presentation.

Collateral information may be available from foster parents. With the patient's permission, one or all of his foster parents may be interviewed if they are available. They may have information about his developmental history that would help to situate the occurrence of certain behaviors. If his biological mother is alive and willing to be interviewed, a sensitive and non-guilt-inducing inquiry may help determine quantity, timing, and frequency of alcohol use if it did occur. Given the association of PAE with guilt and self-blame, this patient and his mother need to be prepared individually if PAE is confirmed. In situations in which PAE is confirmed, having an empowering relationship with a patient's mother and making home visits rather than questioning them in the office led to more positive outcomes (Parkes et al. 2008). In addition, taking steps to obtain support for rather than castigating women is therapeutic. There are many reasons a woman drinks alcohol during pregnancy; deliberate desire to harm her baby is not one of them. Helping the patient comprehend this fact is as important as engaging in efforts with the mother to access help and support.

Special diagnostic teams usually develop processes for obtaining diagnostic information. Questions are designed to identify abnormal functioning in daily living, social responsibility, and the practical and social adaptive domains. Certain questionnaires have been suggested for use at this juncture. The Independent Living Scale measures cognitive skills necessary for independent living. Scores on this scale can indicate the level of supervision needed for an individual. The Vineland Adaptive Behavior Scales measure adaptive function in individuals with cognitive abnormalities. Their scores provide estimates of capacity in spheres such as communication, socialization, and adaptive function.

Treatment depends on the primacy of the PAE in the patient's overall presentation. Strategies of engagement should especially include mentoring support by a case manager with knowledge of the neurocognitive deficits. If it is determined that PAE has little impact and substance use is the likely problem, intervention will focus on drug detoxification, psychoeducation, rehabilitation, use of self-help tactics, and day or residential programs. Alternatively, and with a diagnosis of ND-PAE/FASD as in the vignette, intervention and strategies for managing neurocognitive deficits are germane (see Chapter 13, "Pharmacological Intervention," and section "Specific Treatment for Neurocognitive Deficits" in Chapter 14, "Psychological Treatment").

Monitoring Treatment

Laboratory, electrophysiological, and neuroimaging studies provide comprehensive assessments and assistance in finding or excluding other disorders. The medical disorders frequently associated with ND-PAE/FASD, if detected, require specific treatment appropriately different from that of a purely mental disorder.

Knowledge of psychopharmacology is essential for the treating clinician both to ensure a choice of medications backed by evidence (limited as it may be) of effectiveness and to differentiate side effects of medication from symptoms of the disorder (Mela et al. 2018).

The involvement of mental health professionals in monitoring children and adolescents becomes important when they present with subthreshold symptoms. Longitudinal follow-up of those whose symptoms transitioned to severe treatable symptoms in adulthood identified certain features as risk elevating: female sex, family history of and severity of depression, presence of medical symptoms at baseline, history of anxiety, and suicidal ideation (Astley et al. 2000; Larcher and Brierley 2014; Petrenko et al. 2014). Because of the medical symptoms associated with FASD, additional risk-elevating features, and the role of subthreshold symptoms in potently increasing risk, patients with FASD require specialist follow-up. A system of identification for these risk-amplifying factors can be adequately incorporated into health care service for those with FASD.

Consideration of Policy Affecting Emergency Care

Referral systems are composed of different processes by which assessments are initiated, completed, and evaluated. Referral sources are guided by clinic and government policies; some policies insist on using a screening tool, confirming maternal exposure from history or from medical records (Cook et al. 2016). With that approach, one of the diagnostic criteria (proposed Criterion A for ND-PAE in DSM-5) is being used to determine appropriateness of the referral. Although this simplifies the process by eliminating the task of comprehensively assessing that criterion, it is fraught with other problems. Other criteria should be examined thoroughly and their endorsement rigorously debated by the multidisciplinary team members. Confirming PAE is difficult to do in the ER, and insisting on confirmation before diagnostic assessment still does not guarantee the veracity of the account of PAE. Moreover, many individuals cannot provide information about their prenatal exposure, and their imminent exclusion will need to be examined through a social justice lens.

As services evolve, innovation should be the guiding principle in managing the growing waiting list for diagnosis. Services that accommodate deficits are flexible and responsive to unique needs. Policies that guide such service development should also be informed by current evidence. Various referral pathways are possible. Behavioral problems, social dysfunction, employment failures, and homelessness are more pragmatic indices and offer relevant reasons for referral, rather than just diagnosis. These reasons sensitize the system, making it more comprehensive and allowing accessibility to other service options and thus reducing the exclusion of those who need the services (Bakhireva et al. 2018). Among the challenging issues in the literature is the lack of and challenges to adult diagnosis. Beware that patients with multiple problems coming to the ER may experience revictimization on account of inadequate policies affecting identification and intervention.

Conclusion

Because PAE contributes to multiple compounding mental and medical disorders, the ER, which serves as the gateway to most medical systems and services, is frequented by patients with ND-PAE/FASD. The operations and procedures of the ER can serve as a barrier to meeting the needs of those whose neurocognitive deficits interfere with care pathways. The ER environment and FASD-informed professionals can transform those interferences and enable access to relevant care. Patients who appear to be misusing the ER and yet receive the least effective help require a modified approach that understands the reasons for past failure. When these reasons are addressed and resolved rationally and appropriately, clinical, economic, and health outcomes can be improved.

CLINICAL PRACTICAL APPLICATIONS

- All professionals in the emergency room should be aware that many of their patients have experienced PAE and its consequences.

- More careful examination from an FASD perspective of those with PAE is essential because PAE could complicate presentation, treatment adherence, and clinical outcome.

- Mental and medical disorders compound each other and are highly prevalent in those with PAE who come to the emergency room.

- Lack of recognition of the consequences of PAE and stigma create a resistant patient group with a revolving-door relationship with the emergency room.

- Clinicians should share information with emergency room colleagues about patients who may present with diverse symptoms and be ineffective in communicating them.

References

American Psychiatric Association: Diagnostic and Statistical Manual of Mental Disorders, 5th Edition. Arlington, VA, American Psychiatric Association, 2013

Assadi F: Renal dysfunction in fetal alcohol syndrome: a potential contributor on developmental disabilities of offspring. J Renal Inj Prev 3(4):83–86, 2014

Astley SJ, Bailey D, Talbot C, Clarren SK: Fetal alcohol syndrome (FAS) primary prevention through FAS diagnosis: II: A comprehensive profile of 80 birth mothers of children with FAS. Alcohol Alcohol 35(5):509–519, 2000

Bakhireva LN, Garrison L, Shrestha S, et al: Challenges of diagnosing fetal alcohol spectrum disorders in foster and adopted children. Alcohol 67:37–43, 2018

Choate P, Badry D: Stigma as a dominant discourse in fetal alcohol spectrum disorder. Adv Dual Diag 12(1/2):36–52, 2019

Cook JL, Green CR, Lilley CM, et al: Fetal alcohol spectrum disorder: a guideline for diagnosis across the lifespan. CMAJ 188(3):191–197, 2016

Eyal R, O'Connor MJ: Psychiatry trainees' training and experience in fetal alcohol spectrum disorders. Acad Psychiatry 35(4):238–240, 2011

Frankenberger DJ, Clements-Nolle K, Yang W: The association between adverse childhood experiences and alcohol use during pregnancy in a representative sample of adult women. Womens Health Issues 25(6):688–695, 2015

Gahagan S, Sharpe TT, Brimacombe M, et al: Pediatricians' knowledge, training, and experience in the care of children with fetal alcohol syndrome. Pediatrics 118(3):e657–668, 2006

Grant TM, Brown NN, Graham JC, et al: Screening in treatment programs for fetal alcohol spectrum disorders that could affect therapeutic progress. Int J Alcohol Drug Res 2(3):37–49, 2013

Himmelreich M, Lutke CJ, Travis E: The lay of the land: final results of a health survey of 500+ adults with diagnosed FASD. Plenary panel at the 7th International Conference on FASD, Vancouver, BC, University of British Columbia, March 4, 2017

Johnson ME, Robinson RV, Corey S, et al: Knowledge, attitudes, and behaviors of health, education, and service professionals as related to fetal alcohol spectrum disorders. Int J Public Health 55(6):627–635, 2010

Lange S, Probst C, Gmel G, et al: Global prevalence of fetal alcohol spectrum disorder among children and youth: a systematic review and meta-analysis. JAMA Pediatr 171(10):948–956, 2017

Larcher V, Brierley J: Fetal alcohol syndrome (FAS) and fetal alcohol spectrum disorder (FASD)—diagnosis and moral policing; an ethical dilemma for paediatricians. Arch Dis Child 99(11):969–970, 2014

Mela M, Okpalauwaekwe U, Anderson T, et al: The utility of psychotropic drugs on patients with fetal alcohol spectrum disorder (FASD): a systematic review. Psychiatry Clin Psychopharmacol 28(4):436–445, 2018

Mela M, Coons-Harding KD, Anderson T: Recent advances in fetal alcohol spectrum disorder for mental health professionals. Curr Opin Psychiatry 32(4):328–335, 2019

Moyer CL, Johnson S, Klug MG, Burd L: Substance use in pregnant women using the emergency department: undertested and overlooked? West J Emerg Med 19(3):579–584, 2018

Mukherjee R, Wray E, Curfs L, Hollins S: Knowledge and opinions of professional groups concerning FASD in the UK. Adopt Foster 39(3):212–224, 2015

O'Connor MJ, Portnoff LC, Lebsack-Coleman M, Dipple KM: Suicide risk in adolescents with fetal alcohol spectrum disorders. Birth Defects Research 111(12):822–828, 2019

Parkes T, Poole N, Salmon A, et al: Double Exposure: A Better Practices Review on Alcohol Interventions During Pregnancy. Vancouver, BC, British Columbia Centre of Excellence for Women's Health, 2008

Petrenko CL, Tahir N, Mahoney EC, Chin NP: Prevention of secondary conditions in fetal alcohol spectrum disorders: identification of systems-level barriers. Matern Child Health J 18(6):1496–1505, 2014

Popova S, Lange S, Burd L, Rehm J: Health care burden and cost associated with fetal alcohol syndrome: based on official Canadian data. PLoS One 7(8):e43024, 2012

Popova S, Lange S, Shield K, et al: Comorbidity of fetal alcohol spectrum disorder: a systematic review and meta-analysis. Lancet 387(10022):978–987, 2016

Shelton D, Reid N, Till H, et al: Responding to fetal alcohol spectrum disorder in Australia. J Paediatr Child Health 54(10):1121–1126, 2018

Shrivastava A, Bureau Y, Rewari N, Johnston M: Clinical risk of stigma and discrimination of mental illnesses: need for objective assessment and quantification. Indian J Psychiatry 55(2):178–182, 2013

Thanh NX, Jonsson E: Life expectancy of people with fetal alcohol syndrome. J Popul Ther Clin Pharmacol 23(1):e53–e59, 2016

Tough SC, Clarke M, Hicks M, Clarren S: Attitudes and approaches of Canadian providers to preconception counselling and the prevention of fetal alcohol spectrum disorders. J FAS Int 3:e3, 2005

Wedding D, Kohout J, Mengel MB, et al: Psychologists' knowledge and attitudes about fetal alcohol syndrome, fetal alcohol spectrum disorders, and alcohol use during pregnancy. Prof Psychol Res Pract 38(2):208–213, 2007

PART VII

Systems of Care

PART VII

Systems of Care

CHAPTER 20

Clinical Relevance of Fetal Alcohol Spectrum Disorder in the Mental Health System

<u>WHAT TO KNOW</u>

Expert interest in PAE should be developed rather than a new alternative service/system to cater to those with ND-PAE/FASD.

Clinicians should be aware that reasons for referral of a patient may be diametrically different from the clinical picture that unfolds.

Multiple diagnoses in an individual labeled as noncompliant may be a red flag for the consequences of PAE.

Residential instability arising from the failure of multiple placements and adverse childhood experiences reported for a patient are associated with a history of PAE.

Labeling patients as uncooperative, noncompliant, resistant, and unmotivated, without fully exploring and excluding neurocognitive deficits puts them at increased risk of exclusion from mainstream services.

Screening tools should only be used with the goal of providing modified intervention by the mental health professional.

On the whole, the system of care and clinical pathway for those primarily diagnosed with FASD currently looks entirely different from that of those diagnosed with other mental disorders. Even though individuals mostly experience symptoms at the interface of mental disorder and FASD, the referral criteria and level of evidence for intervention are different. The consequences of PAE that coexist with mental disorders frequently present a challenge to the mental health system (Chudley et al. 2007; Clarke and Gibbard 2003). The factors relevant in producing positive or negative outcomes across the lifespan with respect to the comorbid conditions need to be more fully explored. These prognostic factors could be considered separately with each disorder or together but in the context of the mental health system. Special FASD diagnostic clinics employ different referral reasons and processes. A high suspicion or confirmed history of PAE and a history of maladaptation or dysfunction are the most common reasons for referral. Dysfunction in school, work, relationships, and social responsibility triggers the requisite comprehensive diagnostic assessment. Consequences of PAE and mental disorder share clinical and social features. People who are potentially diagnosable with either mental disorder or ND-PAE/FASD enter the health and social service sectors with a high probability of crisscrossing multiple systems and services within those sectors.

As a result, patients exhibiting dysfunction in various life demands are sometimes inappropriately referred to mental health systems. In some situations, male parents have reported inaccurate histories of PAE when engaged in child custody battles. Desire for social support can lead some to offer unconfirmed/inaccurate histories of PAE. Some parents have claimed PAE to obtain neurocognitive assessment for their child even when there was no exposure. The starting point for these referrals falls somewhere on the pathway navigated for accessing clinical services (Hoyme et al. 2016). In this chapter, I discuss the different avenues in the system that accommodate those with neurocognitive deficits and detail the role and insufficiency of the mental health system in supporting those with primarily neurocognitive deficits resulting from PAE. I recommend how clinicians and service providers can flexibly respond no matter where along the clinical pathway they encounter these deficits in patients.

Desirable Clinician-Led Changes in the Mental Health System

Clinicians function well when they can identify patients in need of care or patients whose illness is not responsive to treatment. To correct the lack of clinical response, and following a full case review, a more specialized assessment and intervention is required. This service-related gap applies poignantly to those with neurodevelopmental disorders, those with mental disorder associated with medical conditions, and those with comorbid conditions. To appreciate the extent and importance of the neurodevelopmental disorder category, under which those with ND-PAE/FASD and those with genetic disorders and intellectual disability fall, clinicians should adopt a lifetime perspective. Upon referral, such patients should undergo a complete review, comprehensive assessment, and application of effective treatment strategies. They should then be provided with supports to address the medical condition and the identified neurocognitive deficits, preferably support that is not compartmentalized. The appropriate treatments for the conditions identified or for new and emerging disorders diagnosed should be incorporated into the overall management plans.

Referring patients who "fall between the cracks" for a comprehensive assessment should be considered for when clinical patterns indicate neurocognitive deficits. These are best recognized when patients are viewed from a lifelong perspective. Hence, a high index of suspicion should be cast on those who repeatedly and senselessly miss clinical appointments, those who are usually described as patients who "just don't get it," and those who invariably become frustrated with the process when they participate in group sessions. These patterns are typically associated with failure on the part of the patient and, for the most part, with irritability and feelings of being overwhelmed in caregivers, and clinical frustration in the treatment team.

By adopting an FASD lens (recognizing the lifelong neurocognitive developmental deficits) in approach and practice, the mental health clinician enables effective care by limiting the obstacle of ignorance in treatment (Anderson et al. 2017; Rutman 2013). Misdiagnosis leads to more negative outcomes (Chasnoff et al. 2015). Additional barriers to effective care arise when traditional approaches are used without considering the unique difficulties of individuals with neurocognitive deficits. Clinical assumptions by mental health professionals have immediate treatment implications. For instance, a cognitively impaired patient assumed to be fully and cognitively competent, and treated as such, could be erroneously expected to act and behave beyond the limits of their abilities. It is not hard to imagine where obvious failures could be misinterpreted and negative responses directed at the patient. Such countertransference reactions can be subtle or overt, but if unrecognized and left unprocessed, they contribute to the failure of mental health treatment. Patients will be regarded as choosing negative behavior, as being unmotivated and obstructionist to treatment planning.

Clinicians and researchers interested in the interface of ND-PAE/FASD and the mental health system describe unfortunate conclusions when the abilities of patients with neurocognitive deficits are overestimated. At first, these patients appear truly competent, especially because of the superior verbal skills and expressive language they commonly possess. The perspective regularly taken, albeit without recognition of the need to accommodate those with deficits, leads to a negative interpretation and view of the respective patients. (Substance Abuse and Mental Health Services Administration 2014). Consequently, the patient is viewed as noncompliant, uncooperative, resistant, manipulative, and unmotivated, which creates more social stigma and additional treatment barriers (Choate and Badry 2019; Dubovsky 2005). Changes in brain structure and function should first be carefully considered and targeted so that the patient is not blamed for the treatment failure. This modification of the treatment approach is part of the patient-oriented or patient-centered care advocated by most professional groups. Such care is responsive first and foremost to the patient's deficits; treatment is individualized and thus associated with more positive outcomes (Gelb and Rutman 2011).

There is sufficient evidence that those with FASD and the consequences of PAE form a sizable proportion of those involved with mental health and addiction services. To meet patients' needs and goals, the mental health system must plan and execute an overhaul that involves professional development. Clinicians must learn innovative interventions and focus on prevention of negative outcomes to enhance functional outcomes (Mela et al. 2019; Pei et al. 2017). The resulting efficient system made possible by protocols in the mental health system to respond to deficits is a side benefit. Clinicians pursue optimum care by minimizing misunderstanding and maximizing flexibility to support attendance and compliance with recommended services. To accomplish such care, clinicians first must direct their efforts to understanding patients' behavior and how that behavior arises from their neurocognitive deficits. Next, they must recognize the specific disabilities associated with brain-based behaviors; this is a hallmark of understanding. These primary deficits are the basis for developing highly targeted interventions. An FASD-informed approach becomes particularly useful as successes influence the mental health system to change the paradigm applied to certain behaviors. Instead of being labeled "noncompliant," the patient's limited abilities and intellectual problems provide a well-founded explanation for such behaviors.

Clinical Vignette

A 21-year-old adopted African American man is referred to inpatient treatment for drug and alcohol abuse. He is described as homeless, unemployed, and anxious and depressed. He reveals having been diagnosed with "bipolar, schizophrenia, attachment, and antisocial personality disorders and PTSD." He reports that he started drinking alcohol at the age of 6 and using illicit substances at the age of 8. He is also involved in petty crimes and will usually stick up for the people he commits crimes with. He engages poorly in intervention programs. He is known to disrupt psychoeducational classes, divert his stimulant medications, and fail to attend appointments with therapists. He is currently not taking any medications despite his persistent cognitive distortions. His regular medications include haloperidol injections, amitriptyline, buspirone, carbamazepine, and venlafaxine. He was previously treated with methadone but was uncooperative.

Considering treatment resistance, interference, and deadlocks, clinicians are better off if they consider each of the following contributors. A patient classified as uncooperative and difficult to engage is not always the easiest to help. Some of the unstable and seemingly noncompliant behaviors in the vignette will likely exclude the patient from accessing services or at least serve as an obstacle to care. The behaviors result from a combination and interaction of his social condition and mental disorders. As indicated in Figure 20–1, a patient with these features, known to be noncompliant and with multiple diagnoses and medications should trigger the need to take a closer look at the existent deficits. The described presentations and historical information (childhood adversity, residential instability, and maternal risk factors) call for specific tailor-made interventions. These consider functional improvement, reduction of trauma effect, and provision of the needed structure and support. Once the historical information leads to corrective measures, the focus shifts to detection of and intervention for impairments. These are usually related and flow out of neurocognitive deficits. The deficits can then attract care in the form of correcting the indices of affect, attention, and impulse regulation.

Understanding the Interaction and Development of FASD and Associated Mental Disorders

Patients with the neurocognitive deficits of PAE experience and manifest many symptoms of mental disorder; individuals with mental disorder also experience and exhibit cognitive deficits. The source of cognitive deficits varies with obvious etiologies associated with medical conditions, such as traumatic brain injury, Down syndrome, and tertiary syphilis. Cognitive features identified in patients with severe and persistent mental disorder such as schizophrenia include deficits in attention and spatial memory (Carter et al. 2010). Occurring at both the early and later stage of schizophrenia, deficits in psychomotor speed, pattern recognition memory, and executive function have been described (Bozikas et al. 2006; Riley et al. 2000). Similar neurocognitive deficits arising in those with PAE encountered in the men-

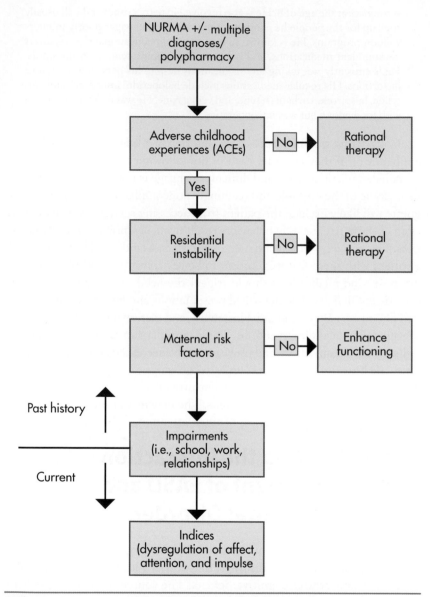

FIGURE 20–1.   Turning the disadvantage of negative perception about complex patients into an interpretative and productive exercise.

NURMU=noncompliant, uncooperative, resistant, manipulative, unmotivated.

tal health system can be subtle, unrecognized, or invisible and, unfortunately, linked to negative outcomes.

Relevant to the mental health system, the role and significance of PAE in the broader categories of mental disorders are still being studied. From the perspective of phenomenology, behavioral manifestations of FASD-related deficits closely resemble presentations of externalizing disorders such as conduct disorders, ADHD, and personality disorders. Deficits in neurocognitive functions found in chronic mental disorders like schizophrenia, mood disorders, and learning disorders also occur in individuals diagnosed with FASD. Family histories of substance and alcohol use among those with FASD is similar to familial accounts found in those with a primary substance use disorder, suggesting both disorders have possible etiological correlations. Apart from some minor variations, the treatment responses of patients with ND-PAE/FASD to stimulants and adrenergic, atypical neuroleptic, and mood stabilizing agents are not distinctly different from those of patients being treated for other mental disorders (Figure 20–2). So, it is important to understand the underlying mechanisms by which PAE relates to both manifestations of neurocognitive deficits and features of comorbid mental disorders. From clinical and therapeutic perspectives, such knowledge is vital to informing appropriate patient care.

Role of PAE in the Mental Health System

As a response to the hand-in-glove relationship between FASD and mental disorder, a diverse system of health and mental health services has been proposed and created. One example is learning disability (LD) services; usually national in scope and embedded within psychiatry and mental health services, LD services have been the default system for those with FASD and mental disorder (Lyon 1996; Sheehan et al. 2016). Intellectually disabled patients in LD services in substantial numbers can be identified by physical characteristics. Only 15% of those with FASD have physically and facially identifiable features (Astley 2010; Nash et al. 2006). As a consequence of a general failure to meet the unique mental health challenges of those with the hidden disorder of FASD, the literature has focused on the description of specialist clinics (Coles et al. 2018; Mukherjee et al. 2019). These rare specialist services have mostly been clinician led, research heavy, and cutting-edge in approach. They are more resource intensive and have not been widely available for the multitude of patients who need that level of expert service.

To accommodate the need for and limitations of these separate services, teams with an interest in the interface between FASD and mental disorder have become a new service focus. At a basic level, these newer clinics serve a particular targeted need. Among young offenders and adult forensic patients, needs-driven services focus on assessment and violence prevention (Fast et al. 1999; Flannigan et al. 2018; Mela et al. 2019). Some services were established as part of research projects, whereas others are part of ex-

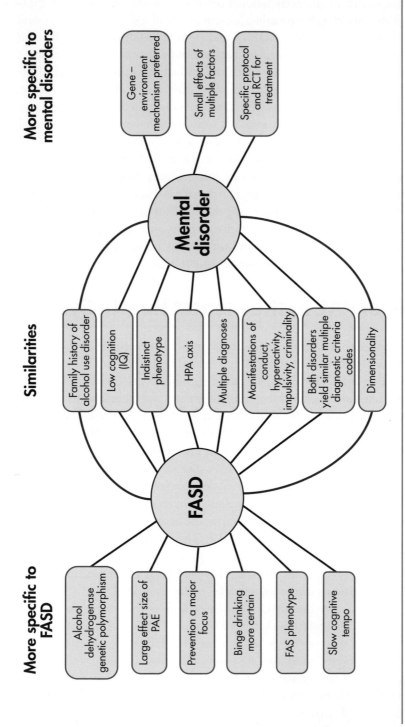

FIGURE 20–2. Understanding the mechanisms of the relationship between PAE and mental disorder.

HPA = hypothalamic-pituitary-adrenal axis; RCT = randomized controlled trial.

isting child and youth rural and urban health systems (Bower et al. 2018; McFarlane 2011). Another service example consists of a special expert forensic team providing services for those on death row who have a neurocognitive disorder associated with PAE (Brown 2017). Similar to this model are individual clinicians who provide assessments and unique recommendations either through consultancy or interdisciplinary contribution to a team.

Recognizing that significant monetary, philosophical, and monumental changes are required to affect the relevant system in adjusting to the "emerging" population of those with both FASD and mental disorder, different approaches have informed the new wave of collaboration. Intense training for those in the mental health and addiction services sector is called for. The training helps mental health specialists with no knowledge of or skills pertinent to FASD to identify and modify their approaches to match individuals' unique deficits. These strategies create in mental health professionals innovative expert interest that guides their practice in caring for those with PAE. Initial anecdotal evidence reported at a recent conference indicated positive individual outcomes in the patients of the trained staff (Fitzpatrick 2019). Existing training uses the Treatment Improvement Protocol (TIP) rolled out by the Substance Abuse and Mental Health Services Administration in 2014. A number of these initiatives have sprung up and need to be evaluated as potential effective methods within existing services.

The reasons why patients with ND-PAE/FASD require specialized systems vary depending on their age and location. Certain countries and communities require a diagnosis based on a set of criteria in order to access services. Services that depend and insist on diagnosis also rely on the biological model in which the joint expression of signs and symptoms is recognized diagnostically. According to this model, deficiencies in neural migration, direct cell death, and neurotransmitter abnormalities associated with genetic inheritance are common to mental disorder and the consequences of PAE. To adequately align clinical features with the diagnostic criteria intended by the classification system, a diagnostic formulation that accounts for all essential factors in the presentation should be made. Lack of recognition and inadequate service response led to a sizable number of patients falling through the cracks. Their treatment has been complicated by a monolithic mental health approach devoid of an FASD lens. Mental health expertise incorporates the skill set needed for recognizing complexity, accepting uncertainty, and differentiating comorbidity to provide the most effective interventions.

The results of training programs focused on modifying and enhancing the skills of mental health professionals in adapting to the unique needs of patients with FASD are encouraging. Outcomes such as the recognition of patients' strengths and deficits (Petrenko et al. 2014), completion of addiction therapy (Grant et al. 2013), improved metal health symptoms (Mela et al. 2019), and increased professional confidence (Reid et al. 2020) are positive and encouraging. Services directed at training clinicians to accurately identify and effectively intervene with those with FASD intersecting the mental health system should be encouraged. Such training opportunities should be evaluated and globally implemented. It is important to evaluate on a continuing basis how well the goals and foci of patients, the care team, and economic and public policy are being met.

Professional Apathy in Recognizing PAE and Mental Disorder Outcomes

A distinctive finding related to FASD is the frequent assertion of parents and caregivers that health professionals, including those in the mental health fields, are less knowledgeable and less willing to listen to their concerns (Petrenko et al. 2019; Whitehurst 2012), particularly professionals who gravitate toward minimizing the severity of the deficits associated with PAE. The disconnect between the anticipated validation and level of therapeutic attention and what is actually offered by mental health professionals adds to the already heavy burden of care for families and caregivers. These overburdened families report that professionals who discount the impact of the mental health consequences of PAE opine that PAE is similar to other minor risk factors in mental health challenges (Coons et al. 2018). These professionals downplay the contributions of PAE and the constellation of FASD-associated deficits as both insignificant to management and of no added complication in those with established mental disorders. In one study, clinicians were quick to evaluate the presence and rates of ADHD among children and adolescents exposed to alcohol prenatally. This practice was heralded as prudent and comprehensive because comorbidity was accounted for in the management of those patients. In the same study, clinicians were asked why they did not consider it prudent to evaluate histories of PAE among patients already diagnosed with ADHD. The answers they gave were instructive. Clinicians and professionals with expertise in diagnosing and treating ADHD who did not inquire about PAE said doing so was just stigmatizing and unnecessary for treatment purposes (Howlett et al. 2019; Peadon and Elliott 2010).

Engaging Mental Health Professionals

PAE leads to many and varied symptoms that patients may present to the mental health professional. To be informed and helpful to patients, clinicians should know something about the mechanism that produces these symptoms. Similar to the effect of biopsychosocial factors in developing mental disorders, cell death, abnormal neuronal migration, hormonal insufficiency, and inhibited neurotransmission all contribute to ND-PAE/FASD. Along with biological determinants in the stress-diathesis model of affect, precipitants such as problems with employment, relationships, and other psychosocial issues play active etiological roles. Unresolved issues and stressful events precipitate clinical symptoms. Such knowledge is helpful for understanding ND-PAE/FASD as well as recognizing similarities in the comorbid states common with the diagnosis. Clinicians should be aware of the range of diagnosable mental disorders (virtually all classifiable categories) comorbid with the consequences of PAE (Lange et al. 2017; Weyrauch et al. 2017). The consequences of PAE are encountered along the continuum of care from outpatient to secure inpatient care (Brown et al. 2018).

Mental health professionals may only be introduced to the clinical outcomes of PAE later in their careers. By which time, they have developed particular approaches and models of care strictly guided by acquired assessment and diagnostic practices. The practices may contradict the modifiable approaches used to effectively manage those with ND-PAE/FASD. Behaviors observed and labeled noncompliant in a person with major depressive disorder will have a different connotation if viewed through the lens of neurocognitive deficits. Impaired adherence to medications and repeated behaviors suggestive of risk unawareness also require a different interpretation for those affected by PAE. An advantage that the mental health professional has in dealing with ND-PAE/FASD is in the interpretation of what purposes diagnosis serves. Similar purposes have been expounded for mental disorders: informing specific intervention, ensuring adequate interprofessional communication, supporting access to disability-related financial support, and preventing secondary disability. Specific to PAE and its consequences, additional benefits from diagnosis include linking mothers to support, providing transitional care for affected persons, and reducing negative outcomes associated with misdiagnosis. These are within the purview of the mental health professional.

It is important for mental health professionals to note that the diagnostic process required to identify alcohol-exposed patients is not as onerous and complicated as it may appear. Having to collaborate with a multidisciplinary team and conduct screening and psychological assessment, including physical measurements, could be considered a deterrent, especially when these added steps are incorporated into the diagnostic process. Yet, a closer look reveals that these are essentially what clinicians are likely already doing. In the assessment of a person suspected of having autism spectrum disorder, for instance, the clinician sets in motion a process of referrals to obtain psychological, laboratory, electrophysiological, and medical examinations. This requires referrals to multidisciplinary members of a team, and it may take a while for the process to be completed. To be true to our calling as professionals and to provide comprehensive care, nothing less is expected when assessing patients with complications from PAE. The rigor of the diagnostic process should not be compromised. Moreover, complete information about the deficits is a crucial component of treatment and appropriate care and, ultimately, of ensuring good quality of life for the patient.

As prescribed by most diagnostic guidelines, the path to a diagnosis involves a multidisciplinary team. In the event that members of the team do not assemble in one location to deliberate the diagnostic considerations, an alternate process should involve them sequentially or virtually, as resources permit (Figure 20–3).

Whether the DSM-5 ND-PAE features and consequences are refined or allowed to serve as diagnostic criteria will depend on the utility and ease of use of the research criteria (American Psychiatric Association 2013). The mental health professional who is aware that a diagnostic criterion allows for brain domain–based behaviors to be identified is at an advantage in supporting patients with neurocognitive impairment. These clinicians already have experience in examining features delineating behavioral clusters that align with the neurocognitive, adaptive, and self-regulation superdomains and their deficits. Aware that their clinical subjects are made up of the more than 90% of those with PAE recognized as having additional mental diagnosis, clinicians need only be vigilant about identifying the neurocognitive deficits in patients they assess and manage (Brown et al. 2018). Research indicates that alcohol and substance use occurs five times more often in those with PAE than in those without. Although involved with mental health and addiction services, more than a quarter of those with PAE are misdiagnosed or misclassified (Weyrauch et al. 2017). Thus, these patients regularly encounter clinicians who lack the insight and advanced skills to detect and appropriately intervene with them.

Given that initiating and developing new services is a difficult undertaking for policy makers, notwithstanding its advantages, training and enhancing the skills of mental health professionals offers the best option for introducing positive interventions into the mental health and addiction systems. Key indicators of the direct expression of neurocognitive deficits (impairment in language, memory, executive function, and attention) will help clinicians identify red flags. The consequences of these features, such as poor educational achievement and reduced social, law-abiding, and relational function, could be integrated into a framework to help clinicians recognize and manage patients under their care with the consequences of PAE. Mental health professionals could rely on the most common diagnoses (ADHD and intellectual, substance use, alcohol use, mood, and anxiety disorders) or most reported combinations of disorders occurring in those with

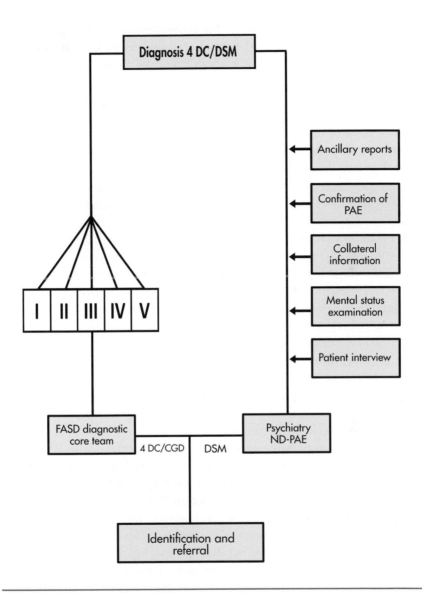

FIGURE 20–3. Diagnostic guidelines for ND-PAE/FASD may require a variety of professionals and processes.

CGD=Canadian diagnostic guidelines; 4 DC=four-digit code.

PAE as red flags (Weyrauch et al. 2017). In the case of ADHD, for instance, experts reported that a specific type of attention deficit, type of treatment response, and additional social factors screen well for ND-PAE/FASD (Young et al. 2016). These insights and approaches can transform service delivery in the mental health system for those with ND-PAE/FASD.

Knowledge that appears attainable should improve the engagement of mental health professionals with their alcohol-exposed patients. Physical features of facial dysmorphia occur in about a tenth of those exposed, and these features may be more difficult to recognize in older patients. To appreciate the extent of neurocognitive deficits, clinicians with mental health expertise should focus less on intelligence tests to identify PAE-affected patients. The average range of IQ in studies of those with PAE is 65–85 (Streissguth et al. 2004), and only about a quarter of those exposed will fall below the 2 standard deviation deficit margin of IQ of 70 (Greenspan et al. 2016). Genetic factors contribute to IQ levels even among those with PAE (Lewis et al. 2012). Clinicians should recognize the importance of deficits in executive, attention, adaptive, and self-regulatory function because these are more relevant features to consider for identification (Greenspan et al. 2015). Those who care for older patients are at an advantage if they focus on individuals in their care whose behaviors are suggestive of inability to regulate attention, affect, and impulse. A greater level of detection of ND-PAE/FASD could be achieved in the history-taking part of the evaluation interview if awareness of those behaviors is combined with daily dysfunction known to suggest PAE. Mental health professionals can easily deduce the risk of PAE when they combine maternal risk factors associated with PAE and the patient's school, employment, and relationship problems (Astley et al. 2000). These rather than direct PAE confirmation in the adult lend confidence to an FASD diagnosis in the mental health system. Substantiating this diagnostic process requires rigorous clinical judgment.

A rather counterintuitive method of detecting patients with PAE in the mental health system is recognizing the intolerable behaviors they display. Although these behaviors are viewed negatively in general mental health patients, they can imply the consequences of PAE. These patients are easily overwhelmed because of poor internal resources for managing discomfort and distress. Executive function deficits lead to difficulties in problem solving, poor judgment, and impaired decision making. Impaired patients are more likely to engage in behaviors they were advised against, report losing their medications more frequently, and perform or repeat actions with negative consequences because they do not learn from past mistakes. Taking part in risky behaviors involving manipulation by others or a desire for companionship demonstrates an unawareness of risk and impulse control problems. As a result of executive function problems, these patients are more disorganized and, thus, are often late for appointments or fail to arrive at all. When asked about missing appointments, most appear to be genuinely surprised that they forgot. Learning difficulties from PAE memory deficits are responsible but superficially not detectable. Additional long-term consequences, which again could be red flags, include exclusion from services and countertransference reactions from clinicians.

In clinical settings, patient histories of dependent living, school difficulties, and residential instability, especially in the context of adverse childhood experiences, are quite common. Inadequate skills for meeting the daily demands of self-care, social responsibility, and independence will be displayed. Immaturity will be exhibited as impaired socialization; friendships are usually with others younger than the chronological age of the individual with PAE. A patient's poor social skills, due to an inability to perceive social cues, manifest as lack of tact, inappropriate boundary violations, and inappropriate comments and behaviors. However, there is usually a wide variation of skill displayed by the affected person. This is described as *dysmaturity*; some cognitive functions are well advanced whereas others are underdeveloped.

Effective intervention begins with mental health professionals becoming well informed about these characteristics and adopting modified treatment approaches to accommodate the patients' deficits and provide the relevant support within the mental health system. The development of an alternative and parallel system, such as an addiction or LD service, is unlikely. Maintaining the status quo will perpetuate the negative outcomes associated with nonrecognition, misdiagnosis, and inappropriate intervention. These, along with stigma, are the significant obstacles in the clinical pathways of those with ND-PAE/FASD seeking help in the mental health system (Anderson et al. 2017).

Solutions for enabling adequate care in mental health and addiction services have been advanced from research that involved surveys and focus group discussion among individuals who attempted to navigate the mental health system. Respondents indicated that what was most needed to remove barriers and facilitate evidence-based practice was the inclusion of professionals with an interest in and knowledge of PAE complications within the system (Anderson et al. 2017). Those experts should be knowledgeable navigators, and they should advocate that each service accommodate, rather than exclude, individuals with common PAE-related deficits who need services and support.

Addiction Services and Response of the System

The traditional approach of group psychoeducational classes and language-rich material couched in metacognitive principles fails to address and meet the needs of patients with FASD. Innovative treatment applications within the mental health and addiction systems are needed to accommodate those with PAE who desire change. Group processes are intimidating, distracting, and, at times, confusing for the individual with ND-PAE/FASD. Program content was devised to solve complex needs, using abstract concepts and language. Individuals with FASD, especially those with deficits in comprehension, receptive language, and attention, are known to struggle when taught using such approaches (Grant et al. 2014). As a result, they terminate involvement too soon. Even with adequate motivation, patients find the expectations and inflexibility of the mental health and addiction programs too great, and they are therefore excluded. The problem is exacerbated if staff is not knowledgeable about FASD and not willing to accommodate these patients' deficits (Anderson et al. 2017). For mental health and addiction services to be relevant, they must examine these pitfalls and introduce corrective and innovative approaches.

Functional communication is generally impaired in those with FASD. Because communication is dependent on language and executive function indices, such as inhibition, abstract thinking, working memory, and attention, a person with these deficits is not likely to express concepts well. Those with ND-PAE/FASD do not grasp abstract content easily unless it is modified, which is not possible in a group setting. When they are asked in the group context if they understand the material presented, they will acquiesce and nod in the affirmative out of fear of looking stupid. Patients who do not exhibit neurodevelopmental disorders are at increased risk of attrition if clinicians do not accommodate their slow processing speed or deficient receptive language. Using plain, concrete language to explain concepts and tactfully asking these patients to restate the information in their own words is an example of a modified approach that the mental health professional can use to effectively accommodate those deficits. Content should be broken down into the simplest understandable units, and enough time should be allowed for patients to think without being pressured, thus accommodating the slow speed of information processing. Approaches that support memory include jotting down information and using text messages and journaling as reminders. Group settings make these strategies difficult, but even individual interactions need modification. For instance, school or homework assignments for students with ND-PAE/FASD can be presented in visual rather than written form. Clinicians function in a psychoeducational role by helping teachers understand this unique strategy. Also, they should adopt an active supervisory role in supporting classroom practices that enhance group safety and ensure an atmosphere conducive to learning, one free of bullying and accepting of those with neurocognitive impairment.

Participating in Perinatal Care

Clinical Vignette

While browsing the website of the national medical association for a conference that supports a continuing medical education credit, a specialist in obstetrics chooses and attends a meeting workshop session of an obstetrical society titled "The Role of the Obstetrician in Eliminating Teratogens in Pregnancy." Subsequently, in the outpatient antenatal clinic, the obstetrician assesses a 37-year-old patient who is 12 weeks pregnant and has been diagnosed with substance use disorder, major depressive disorder, a history of postnatal depression, PTSD, and alcohol use disorder. She is taking 225 mg of venlafaxine daily, 2 mg of clonazepam, and 150 mg of quetiapine at night. Sensitized by the conference discussion about clinical needs during pregnancy, the specialist smells alcohol during one consultation with the patient and makes an effort to secure access to residential addiction rehabilitation services for her. The policy of the addiction services in that catchment area requires an addict to be sober for minimum of 7 days before entering a residential program. The two rehabilitation centers in that jurisdiction also restrict the use of benzodiazepines.

Adopting an active advocacy, the specialist asks the family doctor to refer the patient to a psychiatrist working in the mental health system. On assessment, the woman reports she has been pregnant nine times, suffered domestic violence in the hands of several partners, was previously homeless for a total period of 3 years, and is currently in a temporary shelter with her 3-year-old son. The boy's informal foster placement fell apart because of his significant behavioral problems, including disturbed sleep, violent behavior, and oppositional tendencies toward the foster parents (the patient's older sister and her common-law partner). The patient has attempted three rehabilitation programs over the past year but left each before completing the program. She was expelled from one program when, on three consecutive occasions, she refused to attend the compulsory morning walk expected of residents. In another situation, she was disruptive in the group. In her most recent program, she left the center, smoked marijuana with two other residents, had three beers, and returned inebriated.

The psychiatric assessment further reveals chronic anxiety, depression, and nightmares about sexual abuse and the domestic violence she suffered at the hands of two partners. Both partners were addicted to drugs and alcohol and had violent tempers. She experienced three miscarriages; four of her live births culminated in adoption, each within the first year of life, because of her inability to care for the babies and her unstable lifestyle. Her 3-year-old son was fostered by her sister because she expressed a desire to "stay clean and be a mom for him." She reports using drugs and drinking alcohol during all of her pregnancies, "just like my mum."

Red Flags: What Else Could It Be?

Although this patient's maternal instincts and desire to care for children may explain her many pregnancies, they occurred in patterns highly suggestive of poor planning, inability to learn from past experience, risk unawareness, and thoughtless recapitulation of family life. Her risk unawareness, poor judgment, and possible impulsivity are ingredients contributing to poor decision making in partner choice, which may factor into the repeated domestic violence she experiences. Although sexual abuse is pervasive, especially

TABLE 20–1. Suggested red flags prompting mental health professionals to suspect PAE

History of abuse and maltreatment
Family history, especially maternal, of alcohol use problems
History of residential instability
Indices of neurocognitive deficits (comprehension, verbal, memory)
PAE-related sleep problems
Signs of gullibility and easy exploitation
Repeated cycles of ineffective intervention
Evidence of ineffective group participation

among females seeking mental health support, the rates of maltreatment in those with ND-PAE/FASD is almost four times that of the general population (Totten 2010). Considering her poor judgment, patterns of behavior, and unstable living arrangements, the possibility of cognitive problems in this patient is high (Table 20–1) (Streissguth et al. 1998).

Helpful in detecting neurocognitive deficits is the red flag of repeated failed attempts at rehabilitation. The patient's renewed and expressed desire to have children may be taken as a reasonable internal motivation to quit drugs and alcohol. Attending rehabilitation programs more than once points to some level of commitment. It is therefore difficult to justify a lack of motivation as the cause for treatment termination. Her behavior reveals a person with some challenges that, in spite of intentions to change, make adherence to the expectations of program regimens impossible. The vignette illustrates a situation in which the patient is obliged to fit the demands of the system (e.g., sobriety before admission, early morning waking to walk with everyone despite variations in circadian rhythm). For individuals with FASD and those affected by PAE, obstacles within mental health and addiction systems are a recurring theme (Petrenko et al. 2014).

Entering three rehabilitation programs with inflexible admission criteria (i.e., satisfying a 7-day sobriety requirement) demonstrates the patient's higher level of commitment. Patients who disrupt group or class sessions, as in the vignette, are viewed as oppositional and unmotivated. Fear of being viewed as dumb or foolish because of a lack of understanding can be displayed as antagonistic behavior. Certain patients, in situations similar to that described here, show behavior that combines impulsive and distractible acts ensuing from undiagnosed ADHD or FASD. Aggravated by poor understanding of group content, they may act deliberately to conceal their lack of comprehension. Morning walks are important components of therapy. They promote the benefits of physical activity: better attention and bonding with staff and other clients before group sessions. Unrecognized sleep problems (usually related to PTSD and depression or consequences of PAE) can manifest as a sleep-reversal pattern; patients known to be sleepier in the morning are noted to have circadian challenges (Chen and Olson 2008). The chances of continuing in a program that insists on morning walks are diminished when the patient's lack of participation is viewed as disobedience rather than the result of a specific sleep difficulty that needs accommodation.

If this patient also has deficits related to ND-PAE/FASD that make her easily suggestible and gullible (Greenspan and Driscoll 2016), the negative influence of peers can have a strong effect. Such patients have been known to become the group scapegoat and are often the only one to get caught when the group engages in rule breaking (Grant et al. 2014). The act of breaching the rehabilitation center policy on using alcohol and substances during treatment should be taken seriously. This policy must be upheld to protect the integrity of the program and maintain safety in a nondistracting way for all those who desire to complete the program and lead a sober life. In the case of those with neurocognitive deficits, efforts should be made to address and accommodate those deficits that directly or indirectly work against the tenets of the program and the trajectory of well-being of the patients in the center.

Inquiry should focus on learning styles and type and level of educational achievement. Previous assessment of inattention and distractibility and early onset of alcohol and substance use are telltale signs of PAE. Forensic history, psychiatric hospitalization if any, and level of compliance with treatment should be evaluated. Attempts should be made to identify factors that previously contributed to poor performance. These could be limited to individual factors such as poor verbal learning or include system-based barriers contributing to adverse outcomes (Anderson et al. 2020; Petrenko et al. 2014). Equal attention should be given to factors that foster accomplishment of any task. To support completion of the next program, factors associated with success should be encouraged to enhance the patient's potential for rehabilitation.

The role of neurocognitive deficits as responsible for this pregnant woman's lack of success is, up until this stage, still just suspected. Confirmation one way or another will require a formal and comprehensive assessment. Following the existing diagnostic guidelines, the DSM-5 criteria require clinical assessment to elicit evidence for neurocognitive deficits affecting the intellectual, executive function, adaptive, and affect regulation domains. These deficits are to align with the finding, in the patient, of confirmed "more than minimal exposure to alcohol" (American Psychiatric Association 2013). Clinical evaluation should establish if the woman's mother is alive, and if so, permission to gather collateral information through sensitive questioning about PAE should be obtained to determine if the patient's mother used alcohol outside the period of pregnancy and if she was ever admitted to a treatment program. Maternal risk factors of depression, poverty, childhood adversity, and psychiatric treatment are also relevant, especially if the confirmation of PAE is impossible on account of parental death or social pressures limiting the admission.

Telltale signs of neurocognitive deficits and a neurological examination embedded in the mental state examination can support features of ND-PAE/FASD. The Luria three-step motor test, word fluency tests, abstract testing using proverbs, and test of similarities allow basic screening for executive dysfunction. The patient's fund of knowledge, trajectory of school life, and evidence of affect dysregulation are helpful in the process to confirm PAE and its effects. In a clinical setting and in the absence of a multidisciplinary diagnostic team, the options available to the psychiatrist include individual assessment or referral to an occupational therapist or psychologist in the mental health system. The following tests have been recommended, even in situations with minimal resources: the Mini-Mental State Examination (MMSE), the Montreal Cognitive Assessment (MoCA), the Executive Interview (EXIT 25), and the INECO frontal screening (IFS) test (Moreira et al. 2017). Occupational therapists are also able to administer and interpret these scales and suggest the level of deficit, including recommendation of strategies to accommodate those deficits (Baez et al. 2014; Coons-Harding et al. 2019).

Modification and Adaptation of Interventions

Before any adaptation can be made in the approach to support the patient in the vignette, a baseline level of function should be determined. This is one of the advantages of completing assessment scales. The scores are monitored over time and can be used to guide any adjustment to recommended interventions. Strategies devised on the basis of test results help modify the identified deficit, even when the diagnosis of FASD is not confirmed. Specific findings prompt new actions from clinicians. For instance, the patient's poor ability to tell time leads the clinician to advise about types of reminders and cues (e.g., via smartphone) that can be implemented for her to increase the chances of success.

Ideally, a team approach with a comprehensive assessment using a battery of psychological tests is the standard of care (Chudley et al. 2005).

Where no teams exist, clinicians with an interest develop the skills to perform these tests because they help with devising effective accommodation. Such clinician engagement makes sense, especially when the population served is a high-risk group, such as patients with dual diagnoses or those with complex needs. Women who have multiple diagnoses and who use alcohol and substances, such as the patient in this vignette, clearly meet the threshold for neurocognitive assessment. Alternatively, a multidisciplinary team can perform a complete deficit assessment and make informed recommendations based on the identified impairments. Another option is to refer the patient to a psychologist who can complete the battery of tests necessary to identify and address the neurocognitive deficits suspected. The results can be used to plan a more successful treatment (Olson 2015). Once an accurate diagnosis is made, differential diagnoses should also be listed to maintain a broader perspective of possibilities, which guarantees access to care. Treatment should be informed by protocols and guidelines that have been shaped by advanced evidence (Substance Abuse and Mental Health Services Administration 2014).

Modifications Based on Knowledge of Neurocognitive Deficits

The clinician's perception of this patient's behavior as a manifestation of inability and disability rather than as willful defiance better serves the patient's clinical needs. The previous use of nonaccommodating and inefficient approaches was costly and wasteful. Even when this woman's deficits are hidden or not specifically PAE related, her presentation demonstrates a clear need for support, which a modified approach guarantees. Rather than punishing failure, the level of expectation should be modified to be realistic and in keeping with her impairment. Modified approaches, applicable in a clinical context, use the patient's strengths so she can flourish and reminds everyone involved in her care of those strengths. Professionals should support interventions that encourage hope, resilience, and the expectation of success in the long run (Pei et al. 2016). Training professionals to use adapted interventional methods based on the severity of the difficulties displayed is a priority (Olson 2015). The next time this patient is in a treatment program, staff should communicate with her in simple, clear, and concrete sentences and present one idea at a time. Following orientation, she should be asked to explain in her own words what the unit rules say and mean.

Additional modification involves decluttering classrooms and program rooms in the treatment settings. The patient could be encouraged to stand up and pace during group sessions or use a fidget if it aids attention, with the hope of prolonging her participation in the group and promoting success and ensuring completion (Rutman 2016). To encourage self-advocacy, she could share with the group members how each can help her. In some situations, she will need to be in a smaller group (with three to five members), preferably followed by one-on-one individual psychoeducational sessions. Programs in tune with cognitive deficits readily provide patients like this pregnant woman with journals and technology that enables recording of lessons, homework, and reminders of commitments and schedule tracking.

This patient should be encouraged to attend appointments and programs. A thorough review of her sleep pattern should be undertaken, specifically to find agents to reduce nightmares, improve mood, and reduce anxiety. Exercises and information about improved diet and nutrition should be introduced. Strength-based approaches that select interesting ideas and games that facilitate learning about addictions should be identified (Substance Abuse and Mental Health Services Administration 2014).

To complete the required intervention, the essential components for this patient, in and out of residential treatment, are structure and mentoring supervision, which will help to protect her from the negative influences of others. Negative pressures usually come in the form of suggestions to go against treatment policies, such as leaving the unit to drink alcohol. Coaching should include ways to establish and maintain boundaries; these are best demonstrated visually and pictorially (Rutman 2016). Positive verbal reinforcement works well as a response to the successful baby steps of days without relapse, and linking these successes with the patient's ultimate goal of being able to care for her child is likely to maintain her motivation.

Instead of a "three strikes and out" strategy, occasions of noncompliance, slips, or relapses should be a time to reflect on what did not work and provide an opportunity to identify factors related to neurocognitive deficits that contributed to the failures so that different behavioral plans can be activated in the future. An accurate estimation of the patient's deficits may be what is needed to apply for and obtain guaranteed governmental social and financial support. Benefits from these social safety nets enhance stability and can also reduce some of her risky behavior. With the availability of adequate financial means, she may now be able to afford a designated mentor with expertise in neurocognitive deficits. Recognition and understanding of the patient's neurocognitive deficits form the core of successful treatment outcome.

A systematic transitional program that ensures the patient's new skills are transferable and generalized beyond the residential setting to her new residence should be implemented. Aftercare should include the regular practice of successful strategies; the patient should display her goals visually as a reminder. The clinician should furnish a referral to a parent–child assistance program and strongly recommend continued obstetrical care. Reassurance should be provided that by quitting alcohol, the patient stands a better chance of giving birth to an unaffected child (although later children are more affected [Parent-Child Assistance Program 2018]). At the time of delivery, referral to a neonatal infant psychiatrist should be facilitated (Friedman et al. 2011).

The appropriate care for comorbid symptoms of PTSD and mood, anxiety, and other substance use disorders should focus on stress management at the level of the patient's cognitive ability. Known FASD-informed strategies include flexibility, support, simple steps, supervision, and structure, which apply in both inpatient and community settings. In the community, care within self-help groups should monitor and interrupt negative suggestions to a vulnerable person like the patient in this vignette. Parents of children affected with PAE experience high levels of parenting stress, higher than with other neurodevelopmental disorders, and predictors of high stress should be managed (Paley et al. 2006).

It is important to involve the child welfare system in the new approach, so a plan should include parenting classes, parent and child therapy with the 3-year-old, and parenting support. A special FASD-informed training oriented toward increased FASD knowledge, acquisition of strategies, advocacy, and peer support has been associated with beneficial parenting in a case similar to that of the woman in the vignette (Gibbs 2019). Awareness and recognition of the symptoms of FASD by professionals are beneficial to and supportive of parents raising children with FASD (Coons et al. 2018).

Effective Screening for ND-PAE/FASD in the Mental Health System

A set of facial features that characterizes the syndrome associated with PAE is specific enough to indicate screening of patients. These features arise as a result of PAE during the specific developmental period when the formation of the face occurs, about the third week of gestation (Moore et al. 2007). Using these distinctive facial features to identify patients affected by PAE, notwithstanding their specificity, is a limited approach; only about one-tenth of those affected will have the characteristic features (Astley and Clarren 2000). Growth delays and organ defects are also linked to PAE and could serve as another means of screening (Astley et al. 2016), but these conditions are also not specific enough. It can be argued that measuring these physical deficits is more cumbersome for the mental health clinician. Because these physical features only screen positive in a small percentage of those suffering the sequelae of PAE, they have not been used in the mental health system as screening tools.

Screening can be limited to clinical settings or applied to a large population. Current screening methods target the birth mother or the individual with the diagnosis of ND-PAE/FASD; each has different implications. The reason for screening women who drink during pregnancy and women who have had children with FASD is prevention of the behavior during future pregnancies. Such screening also contributes to understanding the various facets of and mechanisms in the development of ND-PAE/FASD. Research has found that mothers of children with FASD are themselves more likely to be affected or to have more than one affected child. For example, the psychosocial context of these findings included the following: up to 40% of mothers in a study received inadequate or no prenatal care. Poverty, single parenthood, and mental health disorders were prominent in these mothers (Singal et al. 2017). Screening using such common prominent social features is highly recommended. However, the study still found a large number of mothers who gave birth to a child with FASD who also received adequate prenatal care.

The socioeconomic and medical costs of ND-PAE/FASD are vast. In order for a screening program to be successful, a set of criteria is required. For a screening tool to be ethical and the diagnostic process to be effective, the following are needed: knowledge of the process leading to the disorder, assessment availability, cost-effectiveness, and acceptable and effective interventions.

Some diagnostic clinics have adopted confirmation of PAE as a screening method for FASD. However, absence of the mother, stigma, and social pressures make it impossible to confidently and accurately confirm PAE in many cases in the mental health system, especially in adults. Multiple brain regions are affected adversely by PAE setting off several detectable functional abnormalities; these detectable abnormalities are potential candidates for developing screening tools. Batteries of neuropsychological tests are too elaborate, cumbersome, and costly to be useful as screening tools. The Child Behavior Checklist (CBCL) was modified into a screening tool, the Neurobehavioral Screening Tool (NST); it is based on identifying behavioral and functional problems arising from PAE-induced CNS damage. This parent-report questionnaire focuses on immature actions, restlessness, and lying. Findings in validating studies include better psychometric properties for older children, good sensitivity (62%–70%), and excellent specificity (100%) (LaFrance et al. 2014). NST was part of a tool kit developed by the Public Health Agency of Canada (Koren et al. 2014).

Several other screening tools are in use. The Asante Centre for Fetal Alcohol Syndrome Probation Officer Screening and Referral Tool was developed to assist community corrections case managers in detecting cases of young offenders in the community likely to be diagnosed with FASD (Koren et al. 2014). Meconium testing of fatty acid ethyl esters (FAEE) was also included in the Public Health Agency of Canada tool kit because it offers the possibility of postnatal detection of those exposed to alcohol during the last 6 months of gestation. High levels of FAEE suggest a risk for FASD. The Medicine Wheel screening tool was developed as a culturally specific screening tool for use in the indigenous community. These tools received various degrees of validation but are not universal. They require results from more population-wide studies to be certified as reliable and valid screens. In addition, the population risk varies with the degree of alcohol use and differences in vulnerability to ND-PAE/FASD. It remains to be seen how these helpful tools can be transferred and used in the general and specialist mental health system.

One advance relevant to the mental health practitioner is that the neurocognitive deficits are aligned with the common screening tools. These deficits are the same targets for adaptation and modification of intervention approaches. Although the level of dysfunction can be established by estimating the measures of neurocognitive performance, indicators in daily living allow for ease of screening, with applicability to the mental health system. Indicators include outcomes of brain dysfunction such as poor school record, social exclusion, socioeconomic disruption, and mental instability. Populations differ, however, and until a universal set of criteria is developed, population-based modifications to the adaptive dysfunction screening are likely.

To develop a globally universal scale that recognizes the brain dysfunction, screening by mental health clinicians should consider three major screening tools. The Fetal Alcohol Behavior Scale (FABS) used common features among 472 individuals diagnosed with FASD to develop a screening scale. FABS is unaffected by common variables such as diagnosis and IQ, shows high item-to-scale reliability, and predicts dependent living. The FASD 4-Digit Code Caregiver Interview Checklist is designed to identify at-risk individuals. It collates the caregiver's observation of the presence or absence of indicators of problems with planning, mood regulation, memory, and other brain dysfunction. This tool was adopted by the Substance Abuse and Mental Health Services Administration (2014) TIP initiative. The third approach includes a list of brain dysfunctions jointly considered to be more indicative of those with FASD. The acronym ALARMMERS (representing adaptation, learning, attention, reasoning, memory, motor, executive function, regulation of affect, and speech and language) and a shortened form, ALARM, refer to abnormal function detectable for screening. These require more in-depth knowledge of the abnormal function and of the person being assessed. The available evidence for the screening tools is separating those likely to have the diagnosis from people without the disorder. It is too early to adopt these tests in the mental health system, where ND-PAE/FASD needs to be separated from other brain-based disorders.

In mental health treatment, active screening is needed. Those with maladaptive problems and with a history of or indicators suggesting a risk of PAE should be referred for a comprehensive assessment. At this stage, it is better to cast the net wider rather than not wide enough. The risk of false positive screens is real. However, those so identified face no real disadvantage for having a comprehensive neurocognitive assessment. This is routinely requested in those with documented neurological disorders. Testing is a quality-improvement activity because it isolates the patient's functional limitations and residual cognitive strengths. Specific tools for mental health clinicians may require a two-stage screening approach. Patient-based criteria are evaluated first and then informant-based features are evaluated, similar to what occurs in assessment for dementia. Mothers as informants in the screening process should be evaluated for elevated rates of low IQ, maltreatment, and multiple mental diagnoses; they are more likely to have few friends, be socially isolated, and have a history of trauma.

How to Assess for the ND-PAE Criteria

The designation ND-PAE was introduced to assist mental health professionals in conducting diagnostic assessment of those with the lifelong neurodevelopmental disabilities arising from PAE. These are very common, manifest frequently in the mental health system, and go unrecognized or misclassified as other mental disorders (Chasnoff et al. 2015). FASD was the umbrella term accepted by consensus in 2004 to represent a spectrum of various clinical presentations of the teratogenic effects of PAE. Absent any obvious signs of facial dysmorphia and growth deficiency, alcohol-related neurodevelopmental disorder is not easily identified along the spectrum of PAE-related disability. ND-PAE correlates very closely (95%–100%) with alcohol-related neurodevelopmental disorder (Chasnoff et al. 2015; Johnson et al. 2018). Insisting on a multidisciplinary team approach allows for rigor and comprehensiveness of diagnosis. Diagnostic systems, however, serve more than these purposes. To combat the low capacity and uneven distribution of specialty diagnostic teams that focus more on children, the ND-PAE category offers an opportunity to improve access to treatment (Clarren and Lutke 2008; Ryan et al. 2006). Such changes in classification will help reduce the societal impact of the rather high prevalence of those affected and not diagnosed (Olson 2015). Superordinate or superdomains refer to the most closely and uniquely shared presentations of those living with the consequences of PAE. These superdomains—neurocognitive functioning, behavioral or self-regulatory functioning, and adaptive functioning—were adopted as the criteria for ND-PAE, and they can be instructive as red flags in a clinical screening process.

Screening for PAE in the Mental Health System

The Substance Abuse and Mental Health Services Administration (SAM-HSA) proposed screening populations of mental health patients to detect patients with PAE. The TIP was developed to provide care for those who screened positive for PAE. This model is now being applied in the training of mental health and addiction specialists. To identify the many with PAE and its negative outcomes who pass through the mental health and addiction services, intake staff receive training on how to apply FASD-informed practices (screening and modification of treatment approaches). They train in the administration of a particular screening tool. They then learn communication approaches that facilitate the introduction of appropriate interventions to those identified as likely to have a diagnosis. The program recognizes the gap between screening and diagnosis. When no diagnostic service exists and in the event patients screen positive, a modification of approaches is included for the interventional aspect of the process.

The Life History Screen (LHS) contains items from the Addiction Severity Index modified to screen those likely to have been exposed to alcohol prenatally. Components of the screening tool include, for example, number of mental disorder diagnoses, type of residential resources, and history of maternal alcohol and substance use at different points in time. The tool also lists modifiable strategies that can be used by the staff when items on the scale are positively present. This approach translates adequately to the needs in the mental health system, which does not yet have the full diagnostic capacity required for those screened. The mental health system is frequently navigated by patients who screen positive for addiction, with or without PAE. More relevantly, the modified approaches can be directly applied to patients with addiction issues and can be universally efficacious. Evidence to evaluate the benefit of the LHS is required from the staff, patient, and service perspective to make it the standard of care and practice.

Modifications in communication guide staff on how to go beyond superficial acceptance of information to a reasonable level of comprehension. The combination of screening and adapted intervention supports the ethical mandate of screening: to undertake action as the result of a positive screen. Modifications ensure that screening questions arise from a place of individuality. They ensure respect for the person and the self-determination that guides just practices. Comprehensive and collaborative FASD-informed services are such that the harm of screening without intervention is avoided, and thus the beneficence of the process is maintained.

Conclusion

Given the socioeconomic and public health costs related to the consequences of PAE, understanding the pathophysiological, diagnostic, and treatment implications for patients at the interface of mental disorder and the consequences of PAE is important for mental health professionals. The field is now a subject of increasing public health attention and research exploration. Clinicians care for patients affected by the coexistence of both conditions across the lifespan. The neurocognitive deficits of ND-PAE/FASD are common in those with multiple comorbid mental conditions and those involved with the criminal justice system; this offers an opportunity for identification and diversion. Because of the unique medical and mental health needs of the patient population at the interface of PAE and mental disorder, mental health professionals must correctly identify them. Screening tools are being developed for the fields dealing with PAE and mental disorders. Only when validated and reliable screening tools exist can effective approaches be globally adapted to improve quality of care. For advanced quality of care, every patient opening and entering the proverbial service "door" should be served by those who are well informed and knowledgeable about the multiple coexisting mental and developmental disorders the patient may have.

CLINICAL PRACTICAL APPLICATIONS

- Rather than focusing on IQ to identify those with PAE, regulation of affect, impulse control, and attention are simpler and more effective targets.
- Countertransference reactions to a risk unaware patient should prompt a neurocognitive review using an FASD lens.
- Managing those with PAE requires flexibility of existing structures and processes, as well as adoption of a lifelong perspective to care.
- Management of patients with PAE requires recognition of deficits, a strong positive relationship, readjustment of expectations, and adoption of realistic strength-based strategies.
- Unique deficits found through assessment should lead to individualized and targeted interventions with varying levels of support, supervision, and structure.

- To reduce their burden, attention should be paid to caregivers because they have felt their needs have been ignored.

References

American Psychiatric Association: Diagnostic and Statistical Manual of Mental Disorders, 5th Edition. Arlington, VA, American Psychiatric Association, 2013

Anderson T, Mela M, Stewart M: The implementation of the 2012 Mental Health Strategy for Canada through the lens of FASD. Canadian Journal of Community Mental Health, 36(special issue):69–81, 2017

Anderson T, Mela MA, Rotter T, Poole N: A qualitative investigation into barriers and enablers for the development of a clinical pathway for individuals living with FASD and mental disorder/addictions. Canadian Journal of Community Mental Health 38(3):43–60, 2020

Astley SJ: Profile of the first 1,400 patients receiving diagnostic evaluations for fetal alcohol spectrum disorder at the Washington State Fetal Alcohol Syndrome Diagnostic and Prevention Network. J Popul Ther Clin Pharmacol 17(1):e132–e164, 2010

Astley SJ, Clarren SK: Diagnosing the full spectrum of fetal alcohol-exposed individuals: introducing the 4-digit diagnostic code. Alcohol Alcohol 35(4):400–410, 2000

Astley SJ, Bailey D, Talbot T, Clarren SK: Fetal alcohol syndrome (FAS) primary prevention through FAS diagnosis: II: a comprehensive profile of 80 birth mothers of children with FAS. Alcohol Alcohol 35(5):509–519, 2000

Astley SJ, Bledsoe JM, Davies JK: The essential role of growth deficiency in the diagnosis of fetal alcohol spectrum disorder. Adv Pediatr Res 3(3):9, 2016

Baez S, Ibanez A, Gleichgerrcht E, et al: The utility of IFS (INECO Frontal Screening) for the detection of executive dysfunction in adults with bipolar disorder and ADHD. Psychiatry Res 216(2):269–276, 2014

Bower C, Watkins RE, Mutch RC, et al: Fetal alcohol spectrum disorder and youth justice: a prevalence study among young people sentenced to detention in Western Australia. BMJ Open 8(2):e019605, 2018

Bozikas VP, Kosmidis MH, Kiosseoglou G, Karavatos A: Neuropsychological profile of cognitively impaired patients with schizophrenia. Compr Psychiatry 47(2):136–143, 2006

Brown JM, Trnka A, Harr D, et al: Fetal alcohol spectrum disorder (FASD): a beginner's guide for mental health professionals. Journal of Neurology and Clinical Neuroscience 2(1):13–19, 2018

Brown NN: FASD in the capital context. Paper presented at the Capital Habeas Seminar, Chattanooga, TN, May 2017

Carter JD, Bizzell J, Kim C, et al: Attention deficits in schizophrenia—preliminary evidence of dissociable transient and sustained deficits. Schizophr Res 122(1-3):104–112, 2010

Chasnoff IJ, Wells AM, King L: Misdiagnosis and missed diagnoses in foster and adopted children with prenatal alcohol exposure. Pediatrics 135(2):264–270, 2015

Chen ML, Olson CH: Caregiver report of sleep problems in children with fetal alcohol spectrum disorders. Am J Respir Crit Care Med 177:A707, 2008

Choate P, Badry D: Stigma as a dominant discourse in fetal alcohol spectrum disorder. Advances in Dual Diagnosis 12(1/2):36–52, 2019

Chudley AE, Conry J, Cook JL, et al: Fetal alcohol spectrum disorder: Canadian guidelines for diagnosis. CMAJ 172 (5 suppl):S1–S21 2005

Chudley AE, Kilgour AR, Cranston M, Edwards M: Challenges of diagnosis in fetal alcohol syndrome and fetal alcohol spectrum disorder in the adult. Am J Med Genet C Semin Med Genet 145C(3):261–272, 2007

Clarke ME, Gibbard WB: Overview of fetal alcohol spectrum disorders for mental health professionals. Can Child Adolesc Psychiatr Rev 12(3):57–63, 2003

Clarren SK, Lutke J: Building clinical capacity for fetal alcohol spectrum disorder diagnoses in western and northern Canada. Can J Clin Pharmacol 15(2):e223–e237, 2008

Coles CD, Kable JA, Taddeo E, Strickland D: GoFAR: improving attention, behavior and adaptive functioning in children with fetal alcohol spectrum disorders: brief report. Dev Neurorehabil 21(5):345–349, 2018

Coons KD, Watson SL, Yantzi NM, Schinke RJ: Adaptation in families raising children with fetal alcohol spectrum disorder: part II: what would help. J Intellect Dev Disabil 43(2):137–151, 2018

Coons-Harding KD, Flannigan K, Burns C, et al: Assessing for fetal alcohol spectrum disorder. J Popul Ther Clin Pharmacol 26(1):e39–e55, 2019

Dubovsky D: Addressing child welfare and mental health issues for people with an FASD and their families. Presented at the Building State Systems Meetings, San Antonio, TX, 2005

Fast DK, Conry J, Loock CA: Identifying fetal alcohol syndrome among youth in the criminal justice system. J Dev Behav Pediatr 20(5):370–372, 1999

Fitzpatrick K: Building an FASD System of Care within Michigan's Community Mental Health System. Paper presented at 8th International Conference on Fetal Alcohol Spectrum Disorder (FASD), Vancouver, BC, March 2019

Flannigan K, Pei J, Stewart M, Johnson A: Fetal alcohol spectrum disorder and the criminal justice system: a systematic literature review. Int J Law Psychiatry 57:42–52, 2018

Friedman SH, Yang SN, Parsons S, Amin J: Maternal mental health in the neonatal intensive care unit. NeoReviews 12(2):e85–e93, 2011

Gelb K, Rutman D: Substance Using Women with FASD and FASD Prevention: A Literature Review on Promising Approaches in Substance Use Treatment and Care for Women with FASD. Victoria, BC, University of Victoria School of Social Work, 2011

Gibbs A: An evidence-based training and support course for caregivers of children with foetal alcohol spectrum disorder (FASD) in New Zealand. Adv Dual Diag 2(1/2):73–84, 2019

Grant TM, Brown NN, Graham JC, et al: Screening in treatment programs for fetal alcohol spectrum disorders that could affect therapeutic progress. Int J Alcohol Drug Res 2(3):37–49, 2013

Grant TM, Brown NN, Graham JC, Ernst CC: Substance abuse treatment outcomes in women with fetal alcohol spectrum disorder. Int J Alcohol Drug Res 3(1):43–49, 2014

Greenspan S, Driscoll JH: Why people with FASD fall for manipulative ploys: ethical limits of interrogators' use of lies, in Fetal Alcohol Spectrum Disorders in Adults: Ethical and Legal Perspectives. Cham, Springer, 2016, pp 23–38

Greenspan S, Harris JC, Woods GW: Intellectual disability is "a condition, not a number": Ethics of IQ cut-offs in psychiatry, human services and law. Ethics Med Public Health 1(3):312–324, 2015

Greenspan S, Brown NN, Edwards W: FASD and the concept of "intellectual disability equivalence," in Fetal Alcohol Spectrum Disorders in Adults: Ethical and Legal Perspectives. Cham, Switzerland, Springer, 2016, pp 241–266

Howlett H, Mackenzie S, Strehle EM, et al: A Survey of Health Care Professionals' Knowledge and Experience of Foetal Alcohol Spectrum Disorder and Alcohol Use in Pregnancy. Clin Med Insights Reprod Health 13:1179558119838872, 2019

Hoyme HE, Kalberg WO, Elliott AJ, et al: Updated clinical guidelines for diagnosing fetal alcohol spectrum disorders. Pediatrics 138(2):e20154256, 2016

Johnson S, Moyer CL, Klug MG, Burd L: Comparison of alcohol-related neurodevelopmental disorders and neurodevelopmental disorders associated with prenatal alcohol exposure diagnostic criteria. J Dev Behav Pediatr 39(2):163–167, 2018

Koren G, Chudley A, Loock C, et al: Screening and referral to identify children at risk for FASD: search for new methods 2006–2013. J Popul Ther Clin Pharmacol 21(2):e260–265, 2014

LaFrance MA, McLachlan K, Nash K, et al: Evaluation of the neurobehavioral screening tool in children with fetal alcohol spectrum disorders (FASD). J Popul Ther Clin Pharmacol 21(2):e197–e210, 2014

Lange S, Probst C, Gmel G, et al: Global prevalence of fetal alcohol spectrum disorder among children and youth: a systematic review and meta-analysis. JAMA Pediatr 171(10):948–956, 2017

Lewis SJ, Zuccolo L, Davey Smith GD, et al: Fetal alcohol exposure and IQ at age 8: evidence from a population-based birth-cohort study. PloS One 7(11):e49407, 2012

Lyon GR: Learning disabilities. Future Child 6(1):54–76, 1996

McFarlane A: Fetal alcohol spectrum disorder in adults: diagnosis and assessment by a multidisciplinary team in a rural area. Can J Rural Med 16(1):25–30, 2011

Mela M, Coons-Harding KD, Anderson T: Recent advances in fetal alcohol spectrum disorder for mental health professionals. Curr Opin Psychiatry 32(4):328–335, 2019

Moore ES, Ward RE, Wetherill LF, et al: Unique facial features distinguish fetal alcohol syndrome patients and controls in diverse ethnic populations. Alcohol Clin Exp Res 31(10):1707–1713, 2007

Moreira HS, Costa AS, Castro SL, et al: Assessing executive dysfunction in neuro-degenerative disorders: a critical review of brief neuropsychological tools. Front Aging Neurosci 9:369, 2017

Mukherjee RAS, Cook PA, Norgate SH, Price AD: Neurodevelopmental outcomes in individuals with fetal alcohol spectrum disorder (FASD) with and without exposure to neglect: clinical cohort data from a national FASD diagnostic clinic. Alcohol 76:23–28, 2019

Nash K, Rovet J, Greenbaum R, et al: Identifying the behavioural phenotype in fetal alcohol spectrum disorder: sensitivity, specificity and screening potential. Arch Womens Ment Health 9(4):181–186, 2006

Olson HC: Advancing recognition of fetal alcohol spectrum disorders: the proposed DSM-5 diagnosis of "neurobehavioral disorder associated with prenatal alcohol exposure (ND-PAE)." Curr Dev Disord Rep 2:187, 2015

Paley B, O'Connor MJ, Frankel F, Marquardt R: Predictors of stress in parents of children with fetal alcohol spectrum disorders. J Dev Behav Pediatr 27(5):396–404, 2006

Parent-Child Assistance Program: Prevention & Intervention With High-Risk Mothers and Their Children. Seattle, University of Washington Alcohol and Drug Abuse Institute, 2018. Available at: http://depts.washington.edu/pcapuw/inhouse/PCAP_Summary_of_Evidence.pdf. Accessed October 2, 2020.

Peadon E, Elliott EJ: Distinguishing between attention-deficit hyperactivity and fetal alcohol spectrum disorders in children: clinical guidelines. Neuropsychiatr Dis Treat 6:509, 2010

Pei J, Leung WSW, Jampolsky F, Alsbury B: Experiences in the Canadian criminal justice system for individuals with fetal alcohol spectrum disorders: double jeopardy? Canadian Journal of Criminology and Criminal Justice 58(1):56–86, 2016

Pei J, Baugh L, Andrew G, Rasmussen C: Intervention recommendations and subsequent access to services following clinical assessment for fetal alcohol spectrum disorders. Res Dev Disabil 60:176–186, 2017

Petrenko CL, Tahir N, Mahoney EC, Chin NP: Prevention of secondary conditions in fetal alcohol spectrum disorders: identification of systems-level barriers. Matern Child Health J 18(6):1496–1505, 2014

Petrenko CL, Alto ME, Hart AR, et al: "I'm doing my part, I just need help from the community": intervention implications of foster and adoptive parents' experiences raising children and young adults with FASD. J Fam Nurs 25(2):314–347, 2019

Reid N, White C, Hawkins E, et al: Outcomes and needs of health and education professionals following fetal alcohol spectrum disorder-specific training. J Paediatr Child Health 56(2):317–323, 2020

Riley EM, McGovern D, Mockler D, et al: Neuropsychological functioning in first-episode psychosis—evidence of specific deficits. Schizophr Res 43(1):47–55, 2000

Rutman D: Voices of women living with FASD: perspectives on promising approaches in substance use treatment, programs and care. First Peoples Child Fam Rev 8(1):107–121, 2013

Rutman D: Becoming FASD informed: strengthening practice and programs working with women with FASD. Subst Abuse 10 (suppl 1):13–20, 2016

Ryan DM, Bonnett DM, Gass CB: Sobering thoughts: town hall meetings on fetal alcohol spectrum disorders. Am J Public Health 96(12):2098–2101, 2006

Sheehan R, Gandesha A, Hassiotis A, et al: An audit of the quality of inpatient care for adults with learning disability in the UK. BMJ Open 6(4):e010480, 2016

Singal D, Brownell M, Chateau D, et al: The psychiatric morbidity of women who give birth to children with fetal alcohol spectrum disorder (FASD): results of the Manitoba Mothers and FASD Study. Can J Psychiatry 62(8):531–542, 2017

Streissguth AP, Bookstein FL, Barr HM, et al: A fetal alcohol behavior scale. Alcohol Clin Exp Res 22(2):325–333, 1998

Streissguth AP, Bookstein FL, Barr HM, et al: Risk factors for adverse life outcomes in fetal alcohol syndrome and fetal alcohol effects. J Dev Behav Pediatr 25(4):228–238, 2004

Substance Abuse and Mental Health Services Administration: Addressing Fetal Alcohol Spectrum Disorders (FASD) (Treatment Improvement Protocol [TIP] Series 58, HHS Publ No SMA 13-4803). Rockville, MD, Substance Abuse and Mental Health Services Administration, 2014

Totten M: Investigating the linkages between FASD, gangs, sexual exploitation and woman abuse in the Canadian Aboriginal population: a preliminary study. First Peoples Child Fam Rev 5(2):9–22, 2010

Weyrauch D, Schwartz M, Hart B, et al: Comorbid mental disorders in fetal alcohol spectrum disorders: a systematic review. J Dev Behav Pediatr 38(4):283–291, 2017

Whitehurst T: Raising a child with foetal alcohol syndrome: hearing the parent voice. British Journal of Learning Disabilities, 40(3):187–193, 2012

Young S, Absoud M, Blackburn C, et al: Guidelines for identification and treatment of individuals with attention deficit/hyperactivity disorder and associated fetal alcohol spectrum disorders based upon expert consensus. BMC Psychiatry 16(1):324, 2016

CHAPTER 21

Future of the Interface of Prenatal Alcohol Exposure and Mental Disorder

WHAT TO KNOW

Future screening approaches should embrace new genetic findings and combine the assessment of these with the existing clinical and environmental factors.

Recognizing the biomarkers of PAE will improve access to care.

Artificial intelligence using data on patients with PAE has the potential to guide future strategies of identification and intervention.

Progress is being made in understanding the underlying mechanisms of mental disorders and the outcomes of PAE. That interface is attracting new approaches and offers a great opportunity to innovate treatment and service development. The biological underpinnings of PAE damage remain a foundational reality for aligning the social and psychological risk factors with the disciplines of prevention, identification, and intervention in individuals with PAE and its negative outcomes. Although stigma threatens the trajectory of success, current evidence applied liberally to formulate policy on PAE has the potential to stimulate cutting-edge service development. Examining the interface of mental disorder and the outcomes of PAE affords a new way to think about multiple diagnoses and to conceptualize the contributions of multidisciplinary professionals involved in caring for those affected by PAE.

Imagining the Future

The future of ND-PAE/FASD treatment should involve innovative biopsychosocial approaches to identify and intervene with affected persons. Distinct DNA methylation patterns have been identified and continue to be characterized in those affected by PAE and its outcomes. The genetic analytic methods, highly valuable and necessary for future advancement in neurodevelopmental disorders, should sufficiently overcome the limitations of screening, diagnosis, and access to effective interventions. Current clinical and laboratory approaches to screening of those with PAE and mental disorder continue to employ knowledge closely related to findings from epigenetic research. Certain genetic compositions found in particular alcohol-exposed persons were more predictive of threshold dysfunction (de la Morena-Barrio et al. 2018; Lussier et al. 2018; Zuccolo et al. 2013). When fully developed, the screening approaches with the most clinical and public health utility will likely derive from combined biological, neurocognitive, and psychosocial variables (Chudley 2018). These variables should be applied to standardized instruments to test populations for the accurate identification of potential patients. The more objective the tests are, the wider their applications are. In clinical and public health settings, it will be important that screening methods target and accurately identify individuals with complicated overlapping clinical symptoms with other mental disorders and in need of early intervention yet without the observable physical features, such as facial dysmorphia. With growing evidence supporting the etiological role of epigenetic factors, epigenetic markers should emerge as potential biomarkers and mediators of environmental exposures.

Reducing Stigma

Clinical Vignette

A 30-year-old woman with alcohol use disorder relapses and for 3 weeks is binge drinking. Her alcohol use occurs after her 16-year-old son contacts her and accuses her of causing his disabilities. While searching for his biological parents, he found out that his mental disorders and difficulties (school dropout, conduct problems, and self-harm behaviors) are related to the alcohol his mother drank when she was pregnant with him. He was taken from her after birth and had not seen or been in contact with her since then. He was initially diagnosed with conduct disorder and recently charged with theft of a car. The court assessment concludes that his repeated car thefts since the age of 14 are related to the role PAE plays in his inability to understand consequences and manage his impulsivity. His mother is guilt stricken. She was sober for 18 months before he confronted her. She was diagnosed with postnatal depression after the birth of her second son 5 years earlier.

Interface of Risk Factors and Management

In managing the treatment of this patient, consider if she has cognitive deficits and determine her level of dysfunction due to mood problems (exclude hypomania and mania). Establish the level of drinking during the time since the relapse, length of time and quantity of alcohol she is drinking, and consequences such as neurological and cognitive problems. Check her hormonal levels, especially thyroid (include electrolyte and liver function tests and complete blood count as well), and history of seizures. Ascertain what withdrawal effects she displays and determine the level of impairment to decide whether to initiate home or hospital detoxification. If she can be managed at home, find out what level of support and stress the patient has at home (e.g., partner drinking, caring for her 5-year-old, relationship pressures, work-related stresses). Her level of commitment and use of support through addiction services will be guided by her motivation and readiness to change (Miller and Tonigan 1997). These management steps are part of routine care in dealing with relapse in the context of alcohol use disorder (Soyka et al. 2017).

Vital information can be gleaned from current studies on the characteristics of mothers of those with FASD. These features include a high rate of self-harm, depression, sexual victimization, and other risk factors associated with mental and substance use disorders (Singal et al. 2016). The vulnerability displayed by this mother is typical and can be understood from the background trauma she was likely to have endured. A sensitive approach is required to help her handle the guilt and shame involved and to understand what her son's diagnosis entails. The next step is to develop a plan and strategies to address the impact of her actions on her well-being, her son, and the wider society. Recognizing she can be a support person, if her son later chooses, and accepting that her current parenting arrangement limits access to her son should be explained and stressed, respectively. Accepting these circumstances and managing her guilt are instrumental to instilling hope and motivating her desire for change. In preparation for engagement with addiction services, she should be counseled about the advantages and disadvantages of sobriety. During her individual sessions, the role of guilt should be closely monitored. Potential vulnerability factors and mood changes associated with relapses should be identified and specifically addressed. There may be a time when discussions between the mother's and son's teams can take place, and if indicated and reasonable, mother-son face-to-face meetings should be considered. The goals developed by the youth should guide this process. It is perfectly possible that such a meeting may not be possible without a court order changing prior parental restrictions.

Management of guilt is foundational to patient-centered positive outcomes and an antistigma, empowering strategy. In the mother, guilt can arise from the experience of depressive thoughts or can be directly linked to the accusatory actions of her son. The suddenness and unexpected manner of the verbal attack likely precipitated the feelings of guilt and thus the relapse. Guilt-driven relapse is managed by isolating the issue in question, examining the pros and cons of her responses against the background of her knowledge about the danger of alcohol use during pregnancy. To reduce self-blame, it is necessary to examine the factors that contributed to her being vulnerable to drinking alcohol 16 years earlier. The link between the vulnerability factors and the eventual reasons that contributed to her drinking during pregnancy (e.g., unawareness of actual risk or misinformation) should be pointed out. Individual patterns of relapse can be cyclical, and the patient needs to know that. An emotional stress wears out an individual's strength and resistance and can become a starting point in the relapse trajectory. When the protective factors against drinking alcohol are overwhelmed, resilience may be equally insufficient to maintain sobriety. A pattern for a mood-related induced relapse can develop. This requires the full management of the clinical features of depression.

In such a negative cognitive atmosphere, the patient should be encouraged to relish her current successes, appreciate her improvement, and adopt a self-advocacy mindset. Sobriety for 18 months, apparent involvement with mental health services, caring for a 5-year-old, and other positive functioning should be acknowledged and validated. This should be communicated in ways she can understand and assimilate. Strength-focused therapy has been shown to ignite a patient's desire and motivation for change (Corrigan et al. 2018, 2019; Manthey et al. 2011). The patient should be referred to groups set up to manage guilt or other vulnerabilities (e.g., her experience of child abuse) if such factors are present and assessed to be relevant. The current existence of support in her life should be emphasized. It should be stressed with the patient that in the early stages most women do not know they are pregnant, and a significant amount of drinking may have already occurred. That knowledge puts into context the alcohol-related harm that may have affected the fetus even before the mother is aware of her pregnancy status. Although knowing this does not excuse drinking, it draws attention to future prevention options and can reduce the weight of guilt, the guilt that she intended to hurt her baby (Helgesson et al. 2018). The saying that "no pregnant woman deliberately wants to harm her baby" stems from this state of maternal unknowing. Information about the mechanisms of inheriting an alcohol use disorder (from genetic to environmental perspective) should be outlined to help her accept her diagnosis and reduce self-imposed responsibility. Groups that help reinforce these therapeutic themes should be identified, and counseling to explore responses to her son's accusations should be continued. The patient should consider apologizing to her son; this act might put to rest future accusations.

There are unique additional considerations for managing the mother–son relationship even though two distinct clinical teams have joint responsibility for their care. The son's age, available mental health services for youth offenders, and diversionary services provide opportunities for intervention. At 16 years of age, confirming maternal alcohol and substance use during pregnancy is more reliable. For the most part, services supporting the individual's mental conditions and behavioral problems exist, and quality care is easier to achieve if those services are correlated. Several jurisdictions, recognizing the link between neurocognitive deficits and offending, have initiated court diversion schemes. These provide diagnostic services for those with PAE and its mental disorder outcomes. Individuals identified are directed to services that are well informed about neurocognitive deficits to develop individual strength-based interventions that are likely to prevent re-involvement with the criminal justice system (Longstaffe et al. 2018). The 16-year-old son should be involved in long-term supportive psychotherapy, or if he has limited cognitive capacity, individual counseling and mentoring should be employed.

Therapies such as multimodal therapy, family system interventions, and problem-solving therapies involve support persons to improve functioning. Patients are then assisted by case managers capable of exerting firm and yet flexible supervision to ensure successful community care. Inpatient care was studied among a group of youth with conduct disorder and with FASD (Brown et al. 2012). The authors proposed guidelines that recognize the contribution of neurocognitive deficits to self-regulation and affect regulation. Intentional strategies for such deficits, awareness of boundaries, and protection from exploitation form the essential components of care, and these tactics should be suggested to this patient by his team of specialists. When managing the transition into the community, the full spectrum of deficits should be taken into account, and attempts should be made to match interventions with identified deficits to correct them. By so doing, patients are more equipped to modulate those features that contribute to impulsivity and behavior dysregulation. The "circle and fence" system offers the youth an opportunity to identify positive role models and support persons to associate with and lean on in times of need and to identify those he needs to avoid, such as negative peers and exploitative associates and acquaintances. Establishing this system before conditions are set for community care is preferable in cases in which care was initially residential or custodial.

These informed practices name PAE directly, acknowledge the danger, and leave no one in doubt. They provide a measured approach to education, support, and prevention, which are essential if stigma about PAE and alcohol is to be addressed.

Future of Diagnosis

The weights ascribed to PAE in current diagnostic schemes vary and influence the available criteria applied in clinical practice. Standardizing diagnostic approaches is likely to introduce more consistency in the process and outcome of ND-PAE/FASD diagnosis. These efforts are championed by international consortiums such as the Collaborative Initiative on Fetal Alcohol Spectrum Disorders and made possible through innovative surveys conducted among conference attendees (Brown et al. 2019; Mattson et al. 2010). Multifaceted views and patients' engagement are needed to achieve a practical diagnostic process with real-world application. In the meantime, advances in genetics, imaging, and electrophysiology should be incorporated into the future development of valid and highly reliable diagnostic schemes. By improving the psychometric qualities of screening, assessment, and diagnosis, therapeutic innovation is likely, which will then change practice among mental health professionals in the future.

In addition, future endeavors to improve diagnosis need to recognize some of the criticisms levied at current diagnostic practices. One of the contentious issues in ND-PAE/FASD—the interface of PAE with mental disorder—is the very reason for writing this book. Understanding and support for patients with different contributing factors is crucial. Efforts to represent the shared features at the interface were addressed by a small step in the Canadian guidelines for diagnosing the consequences of PAE. The guidelines were recently revised and incorporated the affect regulation domain as one of the 10 neurocognitive domains assessed with functional maladaptive outcomes (Chudley et al. 2005; Cook et al. 2016). It is one of the domains that, combined with two other criteria, can fulfill the requisite number of domains (minimum of three) used to diagnose ND-PAE/FASD. Another approach was the identification of the superdomains (self-regulation, neurocognition, and adaptive function), identical to all maladaptive dysfunction, by DSM-5.

These proposals were criticized as being too hasty and ahead of scientific evidence. When the proposals are measured against the understanding of pathophysiology of PAE effect, the critique is right. It, however, misses the point about the purposes of diagnosis, especially when proposing advances for the future. To achieve the future ideal of a patient-focused diagnosis framework, it is necessary to ensure that the rigor of diagnosis does not overshadow the need to increase access or satisfy the understanding of the mechanisms of pathophysiology. Still, the clinical uniqueness of PAE, given that comorbidity is the norm and not the exception, needs to be analyzed and understood. Depending on how soon a rigorous process of diagnosis develops, a widely applicable system of diagnosis will necessarily remain, at least until systems adopt and accommodate impairment-based, not diagnostic, services.

Sophisticated Facial Measurements

Efforts are now directed at proficiently distinguishing patients with inconclusive facial features but characteristic deficits for the purpose of diagnosis-driven intervention. Innovative approaches with promising evidence for accurate representation of facial measurements include computerized anthropometry and computer algorithms of three-dimensional laser-scanned facial images (Fang et al. 2008; Moore et al. 2007). The field is advancing in bringing together various contributing components of diagnosis, for instance, combining neurocognitive, neuroimaging, and facial measurements to establish more accurate predictors of PAE. Recently, researchers demonstrated the value of this approach by combining dense surface models of facial features and surface shape of the corpus callosum and caudate nucleus. Asymmetry of the caudate nucleus was reduced for those with heavy PAE compared with control subjects, and this is strongly associated with deficits in general cognitive ability, verbal learning, and recall in those with PAE (Suttie et al. 2018). Combined with neurocognitive correlates, this type of research will potentially revolutionize diagnosis of ND-PAE/FASD.

Approaches and Benefits of Innovative Screening

Clinicians trained in screening and early detection of those with ND-PAE/FASD in the health and social sectors should also be proficient in adopting appropriate responsive strategies. These strategies apply across the neurodiversity displayed in individuals they encounter in clinical settings. These individuals present in those settings on account of PAE and related causes of neurodevelopmental disorders. Using the Life History Screen (LHS), researchers incorporate interventionist approaches to complement the screening. Training now categorizes the specific domain that the intervention should focus on. Using the LHS, those identified as screening positive for the consequences of PAE are classified based on the specific neurocognitive deficit (Grant et al. 2013). For instance, screening can identify an individual who demonstrates difficulties with managing change. The next step of the training is to equip the clinician to intervene even when a diagnosis of ND-PAE/FASD is not fully confirmed or, as is more common, cannot be obtained. This means guiding the individual on prechange planning and involving caregivers in announcing, predicting, and adequately preparing for the outcomes of any potential change. Changes in clinic staff, school mates, living circumstances, and sports friends are a few of the natural and expected changes in life. They may have no consequences in the unaffected person, but those with hypersensitivity to stress due to PAE damage of the hypothalamic-pituitary-adrenal axis, for example, do not do well with the increased stress associated with even minor changes in routine. This screen and manage or modify approach is a future innovation that can revolutionize large mental health systems. Patients do not have to have the diagnosis but only show impairment in the domain, which will trigger the specific modification to remediate the deficits in the affected domain(s). The screen and manage approach recognizes the enormous gravity of the deficits and the insufficient resources to screen and diagnose all those with ND-PAE/FASD. Once the neurocognitive impairment is recognized, approaches are modified in line with the deficits.

Eye Tracking and Screening

New and advanced means of screening are being tested using the abnormalities of eye tracking. Current methods proved to be easy and cheap but require technical expertise because computer mapping is the applied approach. Using new deep machine learning to develop neurodevelopmental profiles, researchers combined eye-tracking measures, neurocognitive assessments, and neuroimaging data (Zhang et al. 2019). Using a cost-benefit analysis, the researchers derived a subset of eye movement and psychometric tests predictive of FASD. They recommend an annual process of screening children and youth as an economically viable strategy. In the future, a refined eye-tracking approach can be applied in adult mental health, correctional, and other social sectors to identify those with PAE. This has direct applicability for professionals with no prior curriculum-based training and practice.

Mental Health Professionals' Embrace of PAE

As the vignette illustrates, obtaining a psychiatric history can reveal occurrences of alcohol and substance use in the patient's family. Family history of alcohol and substance use has genetic, clinical, and preventive implications for the patient. Given PAE's significant etiological and pathophysiological contribution to mental disorder, a more in-depth inquiry and consideration is required if the future mental health clinician intends to appropriate PAE for the clinical benefit of the patient. Education and application form the dual components available to the mental health professional to impact the clinical future of PAE in the mental health system. Training, expertise, and special application of knowledge by the professional on recognition of PAE and its consequences ensure the public health goal of intervening at the individual as well as the societal level. Different levels of education and specialization were identified as affecting the quality of data obtained from clinicians about publicly recorded medical and mental outcomes of PAE. For instance, a study compared recognizing and recording the features of PAE in 7- to 9-year-olds among a host of professionals (Andrews et al. 2018). Developmental pediatricians, geneticists, and neonatologists were the only group of professionals who correctly identified and reported the characteristic features of FAS.

In the future, specializing to correctly identify and intervene with those in the mental health system with PAE will require mental health professionals with global and public health perspectives. Programs of education and interventional application should be developed, implemented, and evaluated to examine the difference made in the clinical outcomes of those with PAE in the "new" mental health system (Clarke and Gibbard 2003). Knowledge of the features of the disorder directly affects recognition (Mukherjee et al. 2015). With high rates of underrecognition because of misdiagnosis, increasing identification of ND-PAE/FASD among mental health professionals in the future must be a prime goal to minimize the negative impacts of misdiagnosis and inappropriate interventions. Some initiatives are yielding results in making the mental health system more FASD informed (Brown et al. 2018). A recent study among mental health professionals confirmed that compared with a decade ago, clinicians were better in training, awareness, and recognition of the long-term consequences of PAE among their patients (Brown and Harr 2018). Awareness by these professionals should promote a health-related continuum beyond the individual patient's biomedical reality. Such a public health approach incorporates strategies in the health system and community. Professionals who value social justice and equity act as advocates for the vulnerable and disadvantaged, thereby emphasizing harm reduction and quality of life as important goals. The future of the patient and society depends on just such an appreciation of the wider health, social, and economic costs and benefits.

Future Considerations for Patients and Society

The future of effective care addressing all aspects of PAE and its mental disorder outcomes depends on advances in scientific evidence for recognizing its unifying patterns in patients. Effective care also involves adopting acceptable underlying mechanisms for the effects and complications of PAE vis-à-vis other mental disorders. Policies addressing PAE and service development are crucial for the future of patients with comorbidity. There is, however, a risk of overfocusing on the PAE to the exclusion of other closely related psychosocial disadvantages patients experience. This is because ND-PAE/FASD is readily recognized as a risk factor for adversity, given all the negative experiences (domestic violence, parental inadequacy or absence, poor support, poverty, malnutrition, lack of access to care, and ignorance) associated with it (Badry and Felske 2013). Remembering that paradigm is important, and future considerations within the field should focus also on the social determinants of health affecting individuals experiencing PAE. Rather than single out individuals and assign them total responsibility for their health, clinicians and the existing services should not ignore the economic and social inequalities and social marginalization common in this patient population.

Access to services depends significantly on the philosophy and policy of social and mental health service development. Diagnosis-dependent services insist on a diagnosis that excludes many and raises the impediment of having to obtain a clear diagnosis. Such a system risks excluding those with subthreshold and yet impaired disabilities and allows them to fall between the cracks. Other areas and clinical aspects of psychiatry have warmed up to the concept of subthreshold states. Subthreshold states of anxiety and depression coexist and have the capacity to produce significant impairment, especially in psychosocial functioning (Preisig et al. 2001). Because these states were often previously overlooked, clinicians are now, more than ever before, encouraged to understand epidemiology and service deficiencies and develop treatment strategies that reduce impairment. The future of the study of PAE and its mental disorder outcomes will benefit from an independent system of care. Such an impairment-dependent system has the advantage that it will reduce the emphasis on obtaining a diagnosis, but it also diminishes the chances of targeted approaches for known conditions rather than impairments.

An overarching treatment theme is how prevalent the services are that cater to those with the diagnosis and impairment. Countrywide differences exist in the organization of services, ranging from pedagogical foundations to systems of specialization and policy directed at the disability in question. In the United Kingdom, for instance, it is assumed that many with FASD and the mental disorder outcomes of PAE, even though not so diagnosed, are embraced by the learning disability system (at least 30%–40% of people with PAE have an IQ <70 and are included in learning disability services) (Mattson et al. 1997). Within such a service, health professionals, health and social establishments, and nongovernmental agencies exist to identify and intervene with those with FASD and other similar mental conditions such as autism, learning disorders, and intellectual disorders. A specific FASD service exists in different jurisdictions, for example, nongovernmental organizations (NOFAS in the United Kingdom and United States, Alcohol Healthwatch in New Zealand, FASD Network in Alberta, Canada). These focused services specialize in FASD and try to address the comorbid mental disorders by referral to mental health services or inclusion of mental health professionals in their multidisciplinary diagnostic and supportive teams.

Service development is not only dynamic; it is dependent on government policy. What is usually missing is inclusion of current best evidence to carve out policies that guide service development. It is recommended that establishment of services for the consequences of PAE—long-term disability and associated mental disorders—should be based on the best available and demonstrable evidence. At a minimum, services should be patient centered and cost-effective. An example of a specialized service for those with PAE and its consequences is a proposed level of service embedded within a six-tier model. This model is advocated because a similar one was used successfully for the delivery of mental and addiction services to the indigenous population of Canada (Anderson et al. 2017). Equally important is the amalgamation of mental health policy with existing health care policy but with the recognition of the added effect of the negative consequences of PAE. Heavy cost drivers for mental health care are linked to PAE, including the cost of disability, lack of productivity, and a shortened lifespan. Given the increased rates of mental disorders, adverse outcomes such as suicide, and a shortened life expectancy associated with high cost, benefits accrue when the mental health policies enacted and implemented adopt the lens of FASD (Anderson et al. 2017).

Future research requires an approach that is inclusive rather than divisive, based primarily on the best interest of patients. Data interpreted for scholarly and individualistic arguments do little to advance the health of the patient. Placing the patient first reduces the import of controversial arguments that focus on PAE as the sole agent of cognitive dysfunction without taking into account the wider psychosocial factors that play significant roles in the development of disorders. Certain critical reviews of the diagnostic guidelines assert that they emphasize precipitous yet unverifiable neurocognitive domain deficits. Verifiability has a place in ensuring that research is conducted in a highly rigorous manner; however, this should not be allowed to disenfranchise the vulnerable and "voiceless" patient. From the patient's perspective, the experience being misunderstood is perpetuated and prolonged by delays in obtaining a diagnosis. These diagnostic delays occur because recognizable patterns of neuropsychological deficits common in ND-PAE/FASD have yet to be developed.

Whereas strictly high-quality evidence informs treatment guidelines in medicine and psychiatry, this is yet to be the case in the study of PAE and its outcomes. The obstacles are real, and flexible approaches with scientific rigor are needed to confirm the value of the current level of evidence. Evidence informed by existing successful practice should be acceptable. It may not be at the level of double-blind, randomized controlled trials, but evidence of current practice can be studied to support aspects of care that lack guidelines. This is not an unusual approach; it is to be expected when there is no high-quality evidence available. In areas without double-blind, controlled findings, services depend on the next level of evidence to provide adequate care. Those services can then be subjected to clinical trials. In the area of medication treatment, for instance, the last double-blind clinical trial of medications completed for those with PAE was more than two decades ago. Problems associated with funding, stigma, research capacity, and insistence on monodiagnostic cases likely hinder progress in the field. Although this tide is turning, progress could be enhanced in the meantime through the adoption of practice-based evidence. Without compromising standards of care, outcomes are used to develop evidence (Millar et al. 2017). Current evidence for supplementation preventing or ameliorating the harmful effects of PAE, use of targeted approaches to correct specific neurocognitive deficits, and alternative treatments are transforming the field and should be encouraged with better funding.

Real-world practice equates to a real laboratory to examine the space of intervention for those with PAE. Findings about effective treatment can then be incorporated into existing practice. Obtaining information from multiple sources about groups of patients (e.g., those with specific mental disorder outcomes for PAE treated in different settings), scrutinizing the effectiveness of interventions, and applying regression analysis to the best outcomes through artificial intelligence will be relevant in the future. In the same manner, specific chemical indices, iron, choline, and zinc, analyzed in large samples of those affected by the consequences of PAE, with or without diagnosed mental disorders, could be a source of important information about identification and intervention. When indices are analyzed using machine learning, deductions could be used to formulate strategies, for example, recommending replacement therapy with megadoses of a given biochemical (e.g., amino acids, antioxidants) in those with a below-average level. The reasons for the deficiencies, genetic, developmental, or environmental, provide additional clinical research information. When levels are corrected, patient outcomes compared with those without deficiencies in their levels will be relevant in diagnosis and intervention.

Given the advances in neurophysiological detection of PAE-specific damage, the possibility of correcting damage through neurofeedback or transcranial magnetic stimulation is exciting. Considering its role in promoting myelin replacement, transcranial magnetic stimulation may have innovative therapeutic potential. Epigenetic findings are likely to give rise to DNA or gene therapies. With the information from practice-based evidence, a psychotropic medication algorithm will support efforts to identify effective medications that can then be subjected to high-quality clinical trials. Medications, psychotropic and nonpsychotropic, should be explored particularly, based on the oxidative stress hypothesis and the importance of limiting the role of a teratogen in organogenesis.

Future of Nonpharmacological Treatment

Success with psychological interventions in children and adolescents, such as addressing executive function and affect regulation, will revolutionize the care of adults with ND-PAE/FASD. Similarly, research-based development of social interventions, whether promoting sleep, financial independence, technology use, or the essential components of mentoring, is also a potential contributor to effective care.

Neuromodulation alters neuronal and synaptic properties through neurons or substances released by neurons. It changes how neurons act in the context of neuronal circuits and their interfaces to improve connection and function. The importance of neuromodulation in neurodevelopmental disorders such as epilepsy, ADHD, and depression implicates a similar role in ND-PAE/FASD in the future. Neurofeedback and external trigeminal nerve stimulation are common methods used to produce dynamic regulation of neuronal circuits. Changes in cortical excitability, neurotransmitter release, and signaling pathways result from nonpharmacological approaches. Noninvasive techniques such as transcranial magnetic stimulation and the stimulation of the supraorbital branch and the supratrochlear branch of the trigeminal nerve are said to modulate cortical and subcortical areas related to neuropsychiatric conditions. The increased activity in the areas that regulate attention, emotion, and behavior is said to be responsible for the estimated improvement in symptoms.

Conclusion

The increase in knowledge over the past half-century about the long-term effects of PAE on offspring is indicative of the kind of innovation anticipated in coming years. Animal studies and models will likely continue to inform the differential impact on the fetus of not just alcohol; this research will be crucial in making known the importance of other substances of abuse commonly used in pregnancy. The prevalence of substance use is increasing, and the effects in epigenetic terms of these substances will be pursued by scientists with interest. Systems of care should seriously consider whether the social return on investment in prevention, diagnosis, and intervention should be grouped together. Functional neuroimaging and advances in electrophysiology are at the cutting edge of diagnostic research and may assume clinical utility for individuals with ND-PAE/FASD. Systems of care should seriously adopt diagnosis and impairment-based models for supporting individuals. For any success in the recognition of ND-PAE/FASD, stigma should be actively addressed and combated at the policy level. For a time yet, practice and evidence will remain complementary to the success of interventions. With current double-blind trials in psychological interventions and anticipated trials of pharmacological therapies, it should become clear how interventions started early in life can change the trajectory of affected persons. Collaboration among specialists of the multidisciplinary team is key to knowledge translation and to the hope of promptly reducing the suffering of many and improving outcomes, no matter what system the affected person traverses.

CLINICAL PRACTICAL IMPLICATIONS

- Patients who report that their mothers exhibited clinical features of self-harm, depression, sexual victimization, or other risk factors associated with mental and substance use disorders should be screened for PAE.
- Clinical acumen will be needed to actively incorporate advances in genetics, imaging, and electrophysiology to improve the validity of ND-PAE/FASD diagnosis.

- "Screen and modify" should be the clinician's practice strategy that connects red flags with modification of approaches.

- Annual screening of children for consequences of PAE can be made simpler using deep machine learning focused on eye tracking and psychometric test results.

- PAE-related training and expertise and their application to patient evaluation form the cornerstones for the required change in the mental health and addiction systems.

- A history of PAE is a risk factor for adversity related to other social determinants of health.

- Mental health professionals should inquire about PAE in all clinical encounters.

- Systems that depend on diagnosis for services risk excluding those with ND-PAE/FASD who have subthreshold symptoms.

- Each successful treatment of ND-PAE/FASD should provide guideposts for the treatment of future patients.

References

Anderson T, Mela M, Stewart M: The implementation of the 2012 Mental Health Strategy for Canada through the lens of FASD. Canadian Journal of Community Mental Health 36(special issue):69–81, 2017

Andrews JG, Galindo MK, Meaney FJ, et al: Recognition of clinical characteristics for population-based surveillance of fetal alcohol syndrome. Birth Defects Res 110(10):851–862, 2018

Badry D, Felske AW: An examination of the social determinants of health as factors related to health, healing and prevention of foetal alcohol spectrum disorder in a northern context—the Brightening Our Home Fires Project, Northwest Territories, Canada. Int J Circumpolar Health 72(1):21140, 2013

Brown J, Harr D: Perceptions of fetal alcohol spectrum disorder (FASD) at a mental health outpatient treatment provider in Minnesota. Int J Environ Res Public Health 16(1): E16, 2018

Brown JM, Trnka A, Harr D, et al: Fetal alcohol spectrum disorder (FASD): a beginner's guide for mental health professionals. J Neurol Clin Neurosci 2(1):13–19, 2018

Brown JM, Bland R, Jonsson E, Greenshaw AJ: The standardization of diagnostic criteria for fetal alcohol spectrum disorder (FASD): implications for research, clinical practice and population health. Can J Psychiatry 64(3):169–176, 2019

Brown NN, Connor PD, Adler RS: Conduct-disordered adolescents with fetal alcohol spectrum disorder: intervention in secure treatment settings. Crim Just Behav 39(6):770–793, 2012

Chudley AE: Diagnosis of fetal alcohol spectrum disorder: current practices and future considerations. Biochem Cell Biol 96(2):231–236, 2018

Chudley AE, Conry J, Cook JL, et al: Fetal alcohol spectrum disorder: Canadian guidelines for diagnosis. CMAJ 172(5 suppl):S1–S21, 2005

Clarke ME, Gibbard WB: Overview of fetal alcohol spectrum disorders for mental health professionals. Can Child Adolesc Psychiatr Rev 12(3):57–63, 2003

Cook JL, Green CR, Lilley CM, et al: Fetal alcohol spectrum disorder: a guideline for diagnosis across the lifespan. CMAJ 188(3):191–197, 2016

Corrigan PW, Shah BB, Lara JL, et al: Addressing the public health concerns of fetal alcohol spectrum disorder: impact of stigma and health literacy. Drug Alcohol Depend 185:266–270, 2018

Corrigan PW, Shah BB, Lara JL, et al: Stakeholder perspectives on the stigma of fetal alcohol spectrum disorder. Addict Res Theory 27(2):170–177, 2019

de la Morena-Barrio ME, Ballesta-Martínez MJ, López-Gálvez R, et al: Genetic predisposition to fetal alcohol syndrome: association with congenital disorders of N-glycosylation. Pediatr Res 83(1-1):119–127, 2018

Fang S, McLaughlin J, Fang J, et al: Automated diagnosis of fetal alcohol syndrome using 3D facial image analysis. Orthod Craniofac Res 11(3):162–171, 2008

Grant TM, Brown NN, Graham JC, et al: Screening in treatment programs for fetal alcohol spectrum disorders that could affect therapeutic progress. Int J Alcohol Drug Res 2(3):37–49, 2013

Helgesson G, Bertilsson G, Domeij H, et al: Ethical aspects of diagnosis and interventions for children with fetal alcohol spectrum disorder (FASD) and their families. BMC Med Ethics 19(1):1, 2018

Longstaffe S, Chudley AE, Harvie MK, et al: The Manitoba Youth Justice Program: empowering and supporting youth with FASD in conflict with the law. Biochem Cell Biol 96(2):260–266, 2018

Lussier AA, Morin AM, MacIsaac JL, et al: DNA methylation as a predictor of fetal alcohol spectrum disorder. Clin Epigenetics 10:5, 2018

Manthey TJ, Knowles B, Asher D, Wahab S: Strengths-based practice and motivational interviewing. Adv Soc Work 12(2):126–151, 2011

Mattson SN, Riley EP, Gramling L, et al. Heavy prenatal alcohol exposure with or without physical features of fetal alcohol syndrome leads to IQ deficits. J Pediatr 131(5):718–721, 1997

Mattson SN, Foroud T, Sowell ER, et al: Collaborative initiative on fetal alcohol spectrum disorders: methodology of clinical projects. Alcohol 44(7-8):635–641, 2010

Millar JA, Thompson J, Schwab D, et al: Educating students with FASD: linking policy, research and practice. Journal of Research in Special Educational Needs 17(1):3–17, 2017

Miller WR, Tonigan JS: Assessing drinkers' motivation for change: the Stages of Change Readiness and Treatment Eagerness Scale (SOCRATES), in Addictive Behaviors: Readings on Etiology, Prevention, and Treatment. Edited by Marlatt GA, Vandenbos R. Washington, DC, American Psychological Association, 1997, pp 355–369

Moore ES, Ward RE, Wetherill LF, et al: Unique facial features distinguish fetal alcohol syndrome patients and controls in diverse ethnic populations. Alcohol Clin Exp Res 31(10):1707–1713, 2007

Mukherjee R, Wray E, Curfs L, Hollins S: Knowledge and opinions of professional groups concerning FASD in the UK. Adopt Foster 39(3):212–224, 2015

Preisig M, Merikangas KR, Angst J: Clinical significance and comorbidity of subthreshold depression and anxiety in the community. Acta Psychiatr Scand 104(2):96–103, 2001

Singal D, Brownell M, Hanlon-Dearman A, et al: Manitoba mothers and fetal alcohol spectrum disorders study (MBMomsFASD): protocol for a population-based cohort study using linked administrative data. BMJ Open 6(9):e013330, 2016

Soyka M, Kranzler HR, Hesselbrock V, et al: Guidelines for biological treatment of substance use and related disorders, part 1: alcoholism, first revision. World J Biol Psychiatry 18(2):86–119, 2017

Suttie M, Wozniak JR, Parnell SE, et al: Combined face-brain morphology and associated neurocognitive correlates in fetal alcohol spectrum disorders. Alcohol Clin Exp Res 42(9):1769–1782, 2018

Zhang C, Paolozza A, Tseng PH, et al: Detection of children/youth with fetal alcohol spectrum disorder through eye movement, psychometric and neuroimaging data. Front Neurol 10:80, 2019

Zuccolo L, Lewis SJ, Smith GD, et al: Prenatal alcohol exposure and offspring cognition and school performance: a 'Mendelian randomization' natural experiment. Int J Epidemiol 42(5):1358–1370, 2013

Appendix:
Abbreviations

ACE	adverse childhood experience
ADHD	attention-deficit/hyperactivity disorder
A&E/ER	accident and emergency/emergency room
ARBD	alcohol-related birth defects
ARND	alcohol-related neurodevelopmental disorder
ASD	autism spectrum disorder
BDNF	brain-derived neurotrophic factor
BRIEF	Behavior Rating Inventory of Executive Function
CanFASD	Canada Fetal Alcohol Spectrum Disorder Research Network
CBCL	Child Behavior Checklist
CD	conduct disorder
CDC	Centers for Disease Control and Prevention
CDG	Canadian diagnostic guidelines
CF	Coaching Families
CIFASD	Collaborative Initiative on Fetal Alcohol Spectrum Disorders
CJS	criminal justice system
CNS	central nervous system
D-KEFS	Delia-Kaplan Executive Function System
DSM	Diagnostic and Statistical Manual of Mental Disorders
DTI	diffusion tensor imaging
FA	fractional anisotropy
FABS	Fetal Alcohol Behavior Scale
FAE	fetal alcohol effects
FAEE	fatty acid ethyl esters
FAS	fetal alcohol syndrome

FASD	fetal alcohol spectrum disorder
FMF	Families Moving Forward
GoFAR	Go focus and plan, act, and reflect
HPA	hypothalamic-pituitary-adrenal axis
ICD	International Classification of Diseases
IDD	intellectual and developmental disorders
ILS	Independent Living Scale
IOM	Institute of Medicine
LHS	Life History Screen
MHS	mental health system
MILE	Math Interactive Learning Experience
MINI	Mini International Neuropsychiatric Interview
MRI	magnetic resonance imaging
MRS	magnetic resonance spectroscopy
ND-PAE	neurobehavioral disorder associated with prenatal alcohol exposure
NESARC	National Epidemiologic Survey on Alcohol and Related Conditions
NOFAS	National Organization on Fetal Alcohol Syndrome
NST	Neurobehavioral Screening Tool
ODD	oppositional defiant disorder
PAE	prenatal alcohol exposure
PCAP	Parent–Child Assistance Program
PCIT	Parent–Child Interaction Therapy
PET	positron emission tomography
pFAS	partial fetal alcohol syndrome
PFL	palpable fissure length
RAD	reactive attachment disorder
rTMS	repetitive transcranial magnetic stimulation
SAMHSA	Substance Abuse and Mental Health Services Administration
SPECT	single-photon emission computed tomography
TIP	Treatment Improvement Protocol
VABS	Vineland Adaptive Behavior Scales

Index

Page numbers printed in **boldface** type refer to tables or figures.